Common problems in primary care

Common problems in primary care

LYNNE LESAK GORLINE, R.N.C., M.S.
Family Nurse Clinician, Mid-South Family Practice
Foundation, Memphis, Tennessee

CHERYL CUMMINGS STEGBAUER, R.N.C., M.S.
Family Nurse Clinician and Assistant Professor,
Community Health Family Nursing Graduate Program,
University of Tennessee Center for the Health Sciences,
Memphis, Tennessee

With **53** illustrations

The C. V. Mosby Company
ST. LOUIS • TORONTO • LONDON   1982

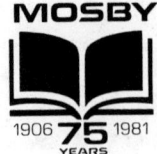

MOSBY

1906 **75** 1981
YEARS

A TRADITION OF PUBLISHING EXCELLENCE

Editor: Pamela L. Swearingen
Manuscript editor: Rebecca A. Reece
Design: Susan Trail
Production: Jeanne Gulledge

Copyright © 1982 by The C.V. Mosby Company

All rights reserved. No part of this book may be reproduced in any manner without written permission of the publisher.

Printed in the United States of America

The C.V. Mosby Company
11830 Westline Industrial Drive, St. Louis, Missouri 63141

Library of Congress Cataloging in Publication Data

Main entry under title:

Common problems in primary care.

    Includes bibliographies and index.
    1. Nursing.   2. Family medicine.   3. Ambulatory medical care.   4. Nurse practitioners.   I. Gorline, Lynne Lesak, 1950-   II. Stegbauer, Cheryl Cummings, 1947-   . [DNLM: 1. Nurse practitioners. 2. Primary health care. WY 128 G669c]
RT120.09C65   616   81-11143
ISBN 0-8016-1931-9   AACR2

GW/D/D 9 8 7 6 5 4 3 2 1   03/D/318

Contributors

CAROL M. ARMATIS, M.S., F.N.P.
Program Director, Family Nurse Practitioner Program, University of Vermont, Burlington, Vermont; formerly Assistant Professor, University of North Carolina at Chapel Hill, Chapel Hill, North Carolina

ANN M. BIDERMAN, R.N., M.S.
OB/GYN Nurse Practitioner, Ambulatory Reproductive Health Services, Women and Infants Hospital of Rhode Island, Providence, Rhode Island; formerly Department of Obstetrics, Gynecology and Reproductive Sciences, University of California, San Francisco, California

PATRICIA E. BRISLEY, R.N., M.P.H.
Family Nurse Clinician and Assistant Professor, Family Nursing Graduate Program, University of Alabama in Huntsville, Huntsville, Alabama; formerly Assistant Professor, Community Health Family Nursing Graduate Program, University of Tennessee Center for the Health Sciences, Memphis, Tennessee

MARY M. CRANE, R.N., M.S.
Family Nurse Practitioner and Assistant Professor, University of Evansville, Evansville, Indiana

LINDA LINDSEY DAVIS, R.N., M.S.N.
Adult Nurse Practitioner, Director, and Associate Professor, Adult Nurse Clinician/Practitioner Program, Old Dominion University, Norfolk, Virginia

SUZY H. FLETCHER, R.N., M.S.N.
Family Nurse Practitioner and Associate Professor, College of Nursing, University of South Florida, Tampa, Florida

WINIFRED STILL HAYES, R.N., M.S.
Adult Nurse Practitioner and Doctoral Candidate, School of Hygiene and Public Health, The Johns Hopkins University, Baltimore, Maryland; formerly Assistant Professor, Nell Hodgson Woodruff School of Nursing, Emory University, Atlanta, Georgia

SUE IHA, R.N., M.S.
Family Nurse Clinician, Joint Practice, Brookshire, Texas

MARGARET KRUCKEMEYER, R.N., M.S.N.
Family Nurse Practitioner, Veterans Administration Medical Center, Dayton, Ohio

STEPHANIE McGHEE, R.N., M.S.
Family Nurse Clinician, Exceptional Children's Clinic, University of Tennessee Center for the Health Sciences, Memphis, Tennessee

BARBARA CONWAY-RUTKOWSKI, R.N., M.N.
Coordinator, Nurse Consultation Services, Evansville, Indiana

CHERYL CUMMINGS STEGBAUER, R.N., M.S.
Family Nurse Clinician and Assistant Professor, Community Health Family Nursing Graduate Program, University of Tennessee Center for the Health Sciences, Memphis, Tennessee

RICHARD L. SWEET, M.D.
Associate Professor, Department of Obstetrics, Gynecology and Reproductive Sciences, University of California, San Francisco, California

BETTY L. WILSON, R.N., M.S.
Primary Care Nurse Practitioner and Assistant Professor, Department of Nursing Education, Meharry Medical College, Nashville, Tennessee

To my patient and loving husband,
Bill
and to my **family**
Lynne

To my loving and supportive husband,
Bill
and to my **mother** and **father**
Cheryl

Preface

The health care provider in a primary care setting faces a wide range of clinical problems. Current information on office management of these problems rarely is approached in a comprehensive manner. Often, out of necessity, nursing students in primary care are directed to medical literature that does not address nursing intervention—that which makes the extended role unique. In addition, nurse practitioners maintain their current knowledge by attending medical meetings or by reading medical journals. There is just evolving a cadre of nurses who can speak authoritatively on what nurses can and must do to provide nursing care to clients in ambulatory settings. It is our firm belief that nurses are an invaluable source of information about how to improve client outcomes in primary care. Often this involves synthesizing material found in traditional nursing literature and traditional medical texts to produce a totality of care that too few can boast they receive.

The purpose of this book is to bridge the gap between material found in written protocols or physical assessment manuals and the findings of current research literature. The book is designed to provide the practitioner with an update on management of common situations encountered in the ambulatory care setting. It is not a "how to" handbook for the beginning practitioner but a compilation of contributions from nurses with extensive clinical experience. The topics chosen represent those areas where the emphasis on nursing is less visible; hence many assume that the problem is purely "medical." Because nursing practice is based on nursing process, the book presents and develops problems in this format to include assessment, planning, implementation, and evaluation. By definition "implementation" means the actual giving of care, and "evaluation" means judging the effectiveness of the plan of care, based on the client's progress. Since the nursing process is a continuing cycle of evaluation based on the outcome of care actually given, the case studies presented herein illustrate these two parts of the nursing process. These clinical situations are written in a problem-oriented approach. To reduce confusion with nursing process terminology the term "problem" refers to the "assessment" portion of the SOAP format. Where no case study exists, implementation and evaluation are discussed in a separate section.

Nurse practitioners must deal with traditional nursing and traditional medical components of the client's health problems. The integration of these problems produces the totality of care. Therefore, we find it appropriate and essential that both nursing and medical diagnoses be addressed. One cannot care for the unified person without setting priorities, and one must never lose sight of the goal: to maintain health, to attain a higher level of wellness, or to achieve a dignified death.

A chapter on general physical assessment is not included in this book, because sufficient published material exists that covers this area well. Physical assessment in each chapter discusses specific assessment factors relevant to the client's initial problem. This will help the practitioner narrow the focus of interaction and thus produce more timely and appropriate goals for the client.

Finally, the recommendations for consultation and referral are general guidelines developed by the authors. Each individual practitioner must judge the need for referral on personal experience, availability of resources, and local customs and practices. The practitioner should always exercise great care in deciding the appropriate involvement of other health professionals. It is hoped that *Common Problems in Primary Care* will promote increasing excellence in practice as well as a higher level of wellness for those clients who are fortunate enough to receive the services of nurses in ambulatory care settings.

We wish to thank Jo Anne Chambers, Jean Swolensky, Jamie Boyd, Cindy Pommer, Nancy Erwin, and Shirley Pommer for typing the manuscript; Lee Donlevy for assistance with illustrations; and Dr. Beverly Bowns for her contribution to our professional growth.

Lynne Lesak Gorline
Cheryl Cummings Stegbauer

Contents

SECTION ONE		**Problems with alterations in comfort**
	1	Low back pain in the adult male, 3 Cheryl Cummings Stegbauer
	2	Knee pain and injuries in the adult runner, 26 Carol M. Armatis
	3	Assessing headaches in the adult client: focus on migraine, 68 Margaret Kruckemeyer
SECTION TWO		**Problems with body fluids**
	4	Anemia in the adult client, 87 Linda Lindsey Davis
SECTION THREE		**Problems with family coping**
	5	Sexuality during puberty, 101 Suzy H. Fletcher
	6	Divorce: potential for growth, 115 Barbara Conway-Rutkowski
	7	Caring for women during the climacteric, 125 Patricia E. Brisley
	8	Skin problems common to blacks: a nursing perspective, 147 Betty L. Wilson
SECTION FOUR		**Problems with nutritional alterations**
	9	Assessment and guidance of nutrition during the first year of life, 163 Stephanie McGhee
	10	Diverticular disease in the older adult, 192 Winifred Still Hayes

SECTION FIVE Problems with infectious diseases

11 Acute salpingitis, 213
Ann M. Biderman and Richard L. Sweet

12 Hepatitis type A: a community problem, 235
Sue Iha

13 Recurrent cystitis in the adult female, 252
Mary M. Crane

SECTION ONE

Problems with alterations in comfort

CHAPTER 1

Low back pain in the adult male

Cheryl Cummings Stegbauer

Estimates reveal that 75% of the U.S. population, at some point in their lives, experience low back pain (LBP) (Weis, 1975). This complaint, which equally affects men and women, frequently receives recognition as the most common problem seen by those specializing in musculoskeletal diseases. Even so, the cause of LBP is often obscure, and its incidence stands in contrast to the lack of scientific support for many commonly prescribed "conservative" treatments. In light of available research findings, one must question whether some therapies are effective or may even be harmful.

Many factors contribute to the lack of controlled research into LBP. First, LBP is not a single disease entity. Second, the anatomical structures involved are complex. Finally, before in vivo methods of measuring intradiscal pressure existed, hypothetical data provided the basis for conclusions about the load placed on the back by common activities.

The natural history of LBP contributes to the difficulties in evaluating and comparing different therapies. In summarizing the findings from several investigations, Nachemson (1969) reports that irrespective of the type of treatment, 70% to 80% of patients with LBP recovered within 2 months. Finneson (1977) surveyed a group of patients with verified lumbar disc protrusions who were treated without surgery. On initial questioning, about 50% were active and reasonably pain free. After 3 years, he again found that approximately 50% were satisfied with their status. However, a sizeable shift had occurred, with many who were formerly "incapacitated" becoming "pain free." Conversely, many pain-free individuals were incapacitated. Others report similar findings (Finneson).

The problem of LBP remains costly in economic and human terms. Nachemson (1976) reported 1,400 workdays lost annually per 1,000 workers in the United States. In the state of Washington, over 500,000 workdays were lost in 1 year because of compensable back injuries (Chaffin and Park, 1973). Rowe (1971) reported that LBP is second only to upper respiratory tract ailments in the average time lost for all employees at Eastman Kodak.

The impact of this disorder on the individual and family is evident because initial symptoms often occur in persons between 25 and 30 years old. This is a time when there are often young dependent children and when workers are establishing careers. In addition, the frequency of repeated episodes peaks at ages 40 to 45 (Nachemson, 1971). As Chaffin and Park concluded, LBP is a major source of cost and suffering to the world; it tends to strike younger workers and is recurrent.

This chapter discusses LBP as it occurs in the adult male. Back pain in children should always cause concern for the presence of a serious disease process. Pelvic conditions that may cause LBP in women are discussed in Chapter 13.

ANATOMY AND PHYSIOLOGY
Review of anatomy

An understanding of basic information related to the structure and function of the back greatly simplifies the discussion of LBP. The following anatomical facts figure heavily in the clinical picture. Anatomical relationships become clearer if one imagines the normal vertebral bodies and supporting structures as a single system (Fig. 1-1). The integrity of each part of the system is essential to effective and safe performance of the spine's function of locomotion, support, purposeful movement, and protection of the spine.

The lumbar spine consists of five superimposed vertebrae, massively designed to function as weight-bearing units. Between each vertebra is the intervertebral disc, a hydraulic cushion that facilitates motion, weight bearing, and shock absorption. The intervertebral disc is composed of a thick, tough outer layer, the annulus fibrosus, and a soft gelatinous core, the nucleus pulposus (Fig. 1-2). Because the nucleus is primarily fluid, it has hydraulic properties; that is, any external force exerted on a fluid in a confined space is transmitted equally throughout (Fig. 1-3). The upper and lower borders of the disc are formed by the cartilaginous end plates of the vertebral bodies. The peripheral fibers of the annulus are intertwining and insert directly into the rim of the vertebral body, and the central fibers insert into the end plates (Brashear and Raney, 1978). The intertwining fibers of the annulus provide protective elasticity and resistance to torsional stress (Fig. 1-4).

Several bony prominences compose the posterior portion of the vertebrae. The superior and inferior articular processes, or facets, guide the spine's movement (Fig. 1-5). The facets are actually arthrodial joints lined with synovial tissue and separated by synovial fluid. Variations in the planes of the facet joints, common in the lower lumbar area, may make the vertebral joints more vulnerable to torsional stress (Brashear and Raney). The transverse and spinous processes are points of muscle attachment. The more than 140 muscles in the back make it an area susceptible to strain from abuse and tension stress (Garrett and Ahmad, 1977). In addition to the support of strong muscles, ligaments hold the vertebrae together. The anterior longitudinal ligament begins at the second cervical vertebra and extends down the entire anterior surface of the vertebral bodies to the sacrum. The weaker, posterior longitudinal ligament extends downward from the first cervical vertebra, hugging the posterior surface of the vertebral bodies and intervertebral structures. Other posterior supporting structures are the ligamentum flavum, supraspinous ligament, and interspinal ligaments.

The sacrum articulates with the fifth lumbar vertebra, the ilium (upper portion of the hipbone), and the coccyx. The sacrum and the two hipbones form the bony pelvis.

There are three physiological curves in the spine: the lordotic curve of the cervical spine, the kyphotic curve of the thoracic spine, and the lordotic lumbar curve. Much is written about the possible role of lumbar lordosis in LBP. Fahrni (1975) proposed a cause-effect relationship between the position of the spine in "correct posture," and the presence of LBP. He, among others, observed the posture of people in Africa and India who sit cross-legged on the floor and work in positions that reduce the degree of lumbar lordosis. In contrast to westerners, they suffer little back strain and experience a much lower

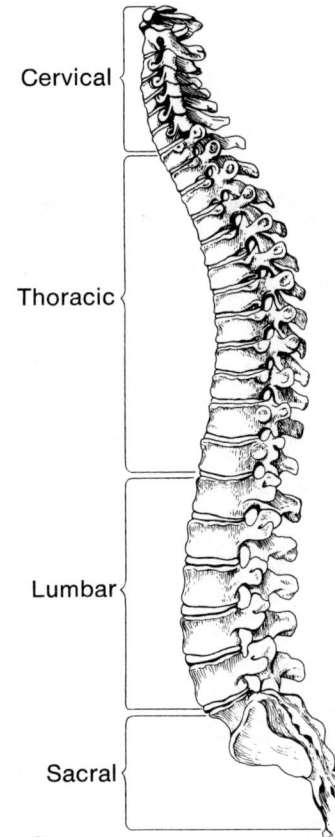

Fig. 1-1. Lateral view of the vertebral column.

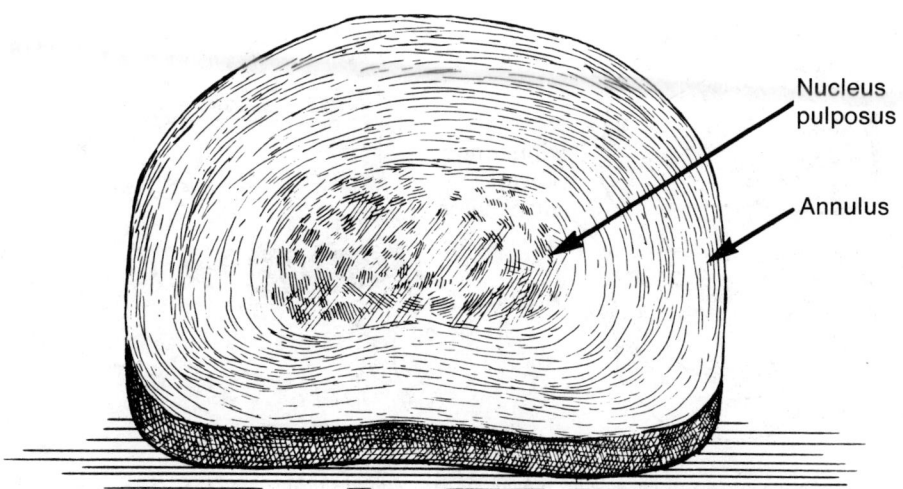

Fig. 1-2. Intervertebral disc formed by the annulus fibrosus and nucleus pulposus.

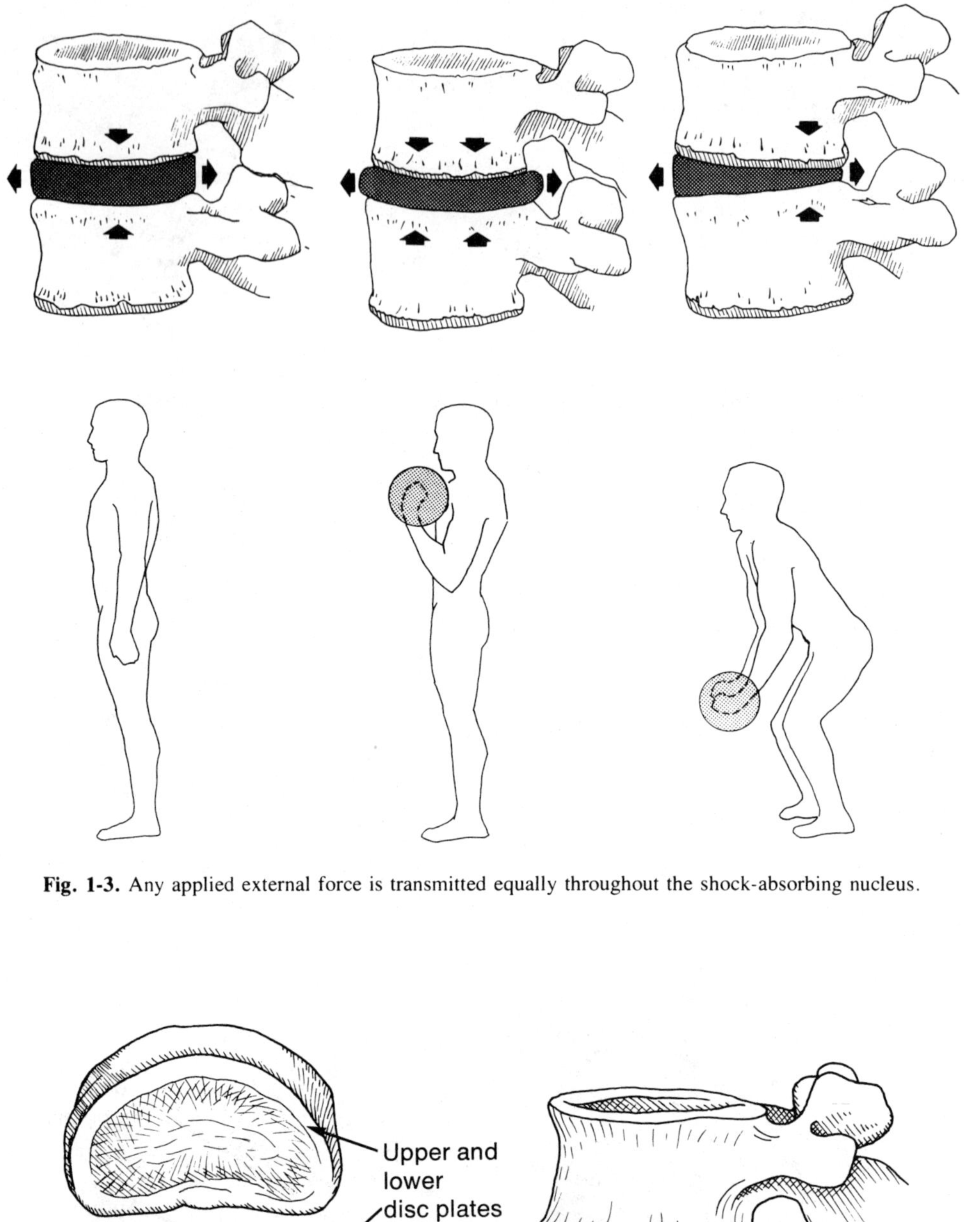

Fig. 1-3. Any applied external force is transmitted equally throughout the shock-absorbing nucleus.

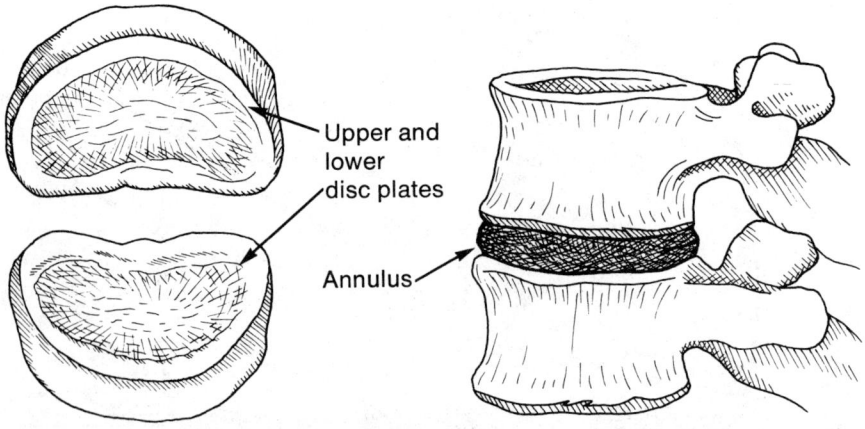

Fig. 1-4. Intertwining fibers of the annulus provide resistance to torsional stress. They insert into the edge of the vertebra and into the upper and lower disc plates.

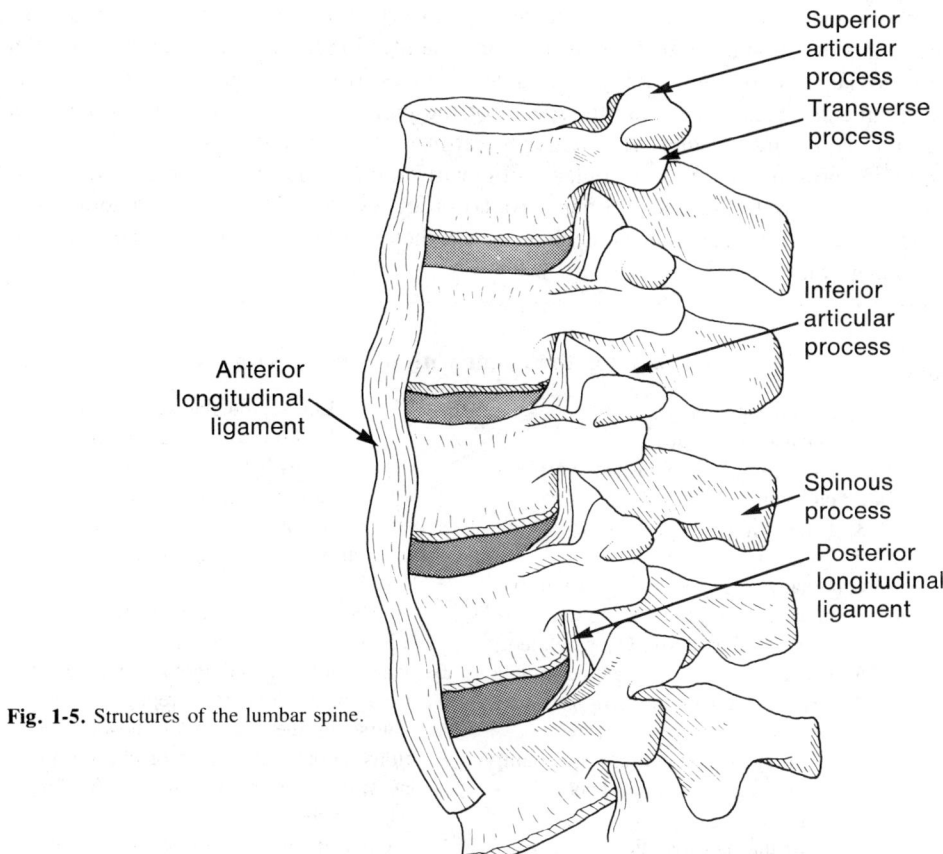

Fig. 1-5. Structures of the lumbar spine.

incidence of disc degeneration. Despite these observations, Nachemson (1969) reported no evidence to support the effectiveness of exercise programs in decreasing lumbar lordosis and pelvic tilt. Additionally, he cited Clemmesen and Simmelkiaer (1968), who show the difficulty in altering an adult's postural habit, even with intense exercise regimens.

Origin of pain

Although there is no complete agreement about the causes of LBP, Cailliet (1962) attempted to clarify its cause by describing the structures that are sensitive and insensitive to pain. The intervertebral disc and nucleus are free of any sensory nerve endings. Although the annulus has nerve endings, studies have not demonstrated sensory transmission from these nerves; therefore, the disc structures are considered pain insensitive. The ligamentum flavum, the interspinal ligaments, and the dura mater lie close to the disc but lack sensitivity to pain.

What, then, is the source of pain when degenerative changes in the nucleus and annulus decrease normal elasticity to allow encroachment of the disc on surrounding tissues? One sensitive structure is the posterior longitudinal ligament. Irritation of the ligament by an abnormal pressure produces pain (Cailliet). Another source of pain is the synovial tissue of the facet joints. This tissue has a rich sensory and vasomotor nerve supply. The facet joints are thought vulnerable to the same painful inflammatory reactions that affect the synovial tissue of other joints. Another source is irritation of the lumbosacral joints and ligaments. This causes painful spasm of the paravertebral muscles of the back and even the hamstring muscles. If disc degeneration is present, the muscle spasm can be a strong compressive force. Any contact with or irritation of the sciatic nerve (which arises from L-4, L-5, S-1, S-2 and S-3 nerve roots) produces pain along the dermatome of the involved root. However, other mechanical and chemical factors that may cause pain are also under study.

History for the client with low back pain

A. Present illness
1. What is your age?
2. How long have you had the present pain?
3. Did your pain begin suddenly or gradually?
4. What were you doing when the pain first began? Was injury involved? Was activity job related?
5. Have you recently engaged in any new or unconditioned physical activity?
6. When you first noticed the pain; where was it located? Has the location changed?
7. Does the pain radiate?
8. Have you had any symptoms (abdominal pain, fever, etc.) in addition to the back pain?
9. Have you noticed a "catch" in your back, or do you sometimes get "stuck" when you bend forward?
10. What makes your pain better?
11. What makes your pain worse?
12. How do you feel when you wake up in the morning?
13. Do you ever wake up during the night because of pain?
14. Is the pain better, worse, or unchanged when you:
    a. Bend forward to brush your teeth?
    b. Exercise?
    c. Cough or sneeze?
    d. Lie on your back?
    e. Lie on your side with your knees bent?
    f. Lie on your abdomen?
15. Have you noticed any unusual sensation in your extremities?
16. Have you experienced loss of bowel or bladder control?
17. Is an attorney helping you?

B. Past history, including past episodes of back pain, treatment regimens, and course of these episodes; hospitalizations; surgeries; serious or chronic illness; medications; immunizations, and TB skin testing

C. Family history, including back or joint problems, and malignancy

D. Life-style history
1. How long have you worked in your present job?
2. Are you able to carry out your usual daily activities?
3. How does your back pain affect your family life?
4. Are you experiencing stress or pressure at home or work? When did this pressure begin?
5. Are you experiencing pleasant or unpleasant changes in your life?
6. Do you exercise or play any sport? How often? How do you warm up and cool down?
7. Do you have any hobbies?
8. Is there any change in your sexual activity?

ASSESSMENT
Approach to the problem

The causes of LBP are numerous and terminology is confusing. A helpful approach to the clinical situation of back pain is to organize the assessment as a search for problems related to three things: the structural unit of the back; nerve root irritation; and local, systemic, or visceral disease processes (Table 1-1). The history is frequently the most valuable diagnostic tool (see p. 8). It should include risk factors related to age, sex, occupation, life-style, family history, and past events, such as previous malignancies. The presence or absence of findings during the physical examination provides supporting evidence to make the diagnosis (see below). The indications for laboratory tests are infrequent, since local or systemic disease process can often be excluded after the initial history and physical examination.

The appropriate use of lumbar x-ray films to assess LBP is a stimulus for discussion and investigation. The possible consequences of radiation exposure and cost are two areas of concern. Low back x-ray films are the largest single contributor to gonadal irradiation in the United States (Conners, 1973). The Advisory Committee on the Biological Effects of Ionizing Radiation (1972) suggests that low-level irradiation eventually could be responsible for a 2.5% to 25% increase in mutation-caused diseases. The potential radiation exposure to a client is substantial when one considers the recurrent nature of back pain and subsequent, repeated x-ray examinations. Also, reducing back x-ray use by 50% could result in estimated annual savings of $75 million (Rockey and others, 1978).

Essential physical examination for clients with low back pain

A. General observation
  1. Vital signs, height, weight
  2. Acute pain or distress
  3. Mobility and ease of movement
B. Musculoskeletal
  1. Back
    a. Birthmarks, skin tags, lipomata, hairy patches, discoloration
    b. Spinal curves
    c. Spinal deformity
    d. Iliac crest alignment
    e. Chest expansion
    f. Range of motion
    g. Spinal flexibility
    h. Tenderness of muscles, spinous processes, sacrum
  2. Extremities
    a. Leg lengths
    b. Peripheral pulses
C. Abdominal
  1. Masses
  2. Bruits
  3. Width of aorta
D. Rectal
  1. Guaiac
  2. Masses
  3. Prostate gland
E. Neurological
  1. Gait
  2. Reflexes
  3. Motor testing
  4. Sensory testing
  5. Valsalva's maneuver
  6. Straight-leg raising
  7. Femoral stretch test

Table 1-1. Approach to causes of low back pain in adult males

	Structural unit			Nerve root irritation
Characteristics	**Muscle strain**	**Spondylolisthesis**	**Degenerative disc**	**Herniated disc**
Onset	After unusual or unconditioned activity; with trauma; e.g., lifting	Sudden, with something "catching"; may occur with trauma	Insidious, mild to moderate pain; morning stiffness	Sudden, associated with lifting or other trauma
Age	NC*	NC	After 20; degeneration is progressive with age	20–40
Location of pain	Over muscles, no radiation	Pain over joint; lumbosacrum often involved; may mimic herniated disc	Radiates with nerve root involvement	Back and leg; rare presentation with leg pain only
Relieving factors	Heat	Rest, lying still; may ↓ with back flexion	Improves during day	Lying with knees flexed; side lying with back flexed
Effect of rest	Causes stiffness	Relieves	Causes stiffness in morning	Relieves
Aggravating factors	Motion, lifting, straining	Movement; may ↑ with back extension	Activity	Activity; Valsalva's maneuver, cough, sneeze
Physical findings	Paravertebral muscle tenderness; ↓ ROM 2° to muscle pain; no neurological signs; no systemic symptoms; muscles may be firm to rigid; spinal curves normal except with severe pain	Lipomata, hairy patch, and birthmarks suggest bony defect; tenderness over involved joint; deformity or abnormal spinal curve; no neurological signs unless mimics herniated disc	Negative	Positive neurological signs following involved nerve root; straight-leg raising and femoral stretch tests positive; percussion tenderness over involved area of spine; muscles tight and tender
X-ray findings	Negative	Normal or variable abnormal findings	Narrowing of disc	Negative, except with special tests, e.g., myelogram
Laboratory findings	Negative	Negative	Negative	Negative

*NC, noncontributory.

	Local disease		Systemic disease	Visceral disease	
	Pyogenic	**Tuberculosis**	**Ankylosing spondylitis**	**Abd. aortic aneurysm**	**Cancer of prostate gland**
	Insidious	Insidious; delay in seeking care as long as 6 mo	Insidious; may be precipitated by acute infection or trauma; morning stiffness	Asymptomatic stage; acutely abrupt onset; severe pain	Insidious; often asymptomatic until metastasis
	NC	NC	20-40	Most frequently over 40	Usually over 40
	Back; may involve severe spasm of back and hamstring muscles	Back, or radiates with nerve root involvement	Back pain usual presentation	Low back; may mimic herniated disc	Low back
	Eventually becomes severe and constant without relief	Eventually becomes constant	Stiffness relieved by exercise	NC	None
	Eventually interrupts sleep	Eventually interrupts sleep	May cause stiffness; pain often nocturnal	No effect	Does not relieve
	Movement	Motion; jarring motions	NC		NC
	Percussion tenderness over involved vertebrae; no neurological signs	Percussion tenderness over involved vertebrae; may present with neurological signs	Chest expansion < 3 cm at nipple line; ↓ forward bending; Schober's test ↑ <5 cm on forward bending; cervical limitation with back against wall; pressure over sacroiliac joints may reveal tenderness	Abdominal exam may reveal widened aorta, pulsating mass, and aortic bruit; commonly has other signs of vascular disease; may have neurological signs	Rectal exam significant; prostate gland reveals nodule or area of firmness; posterior lobe most often involved
	Normal or variable abnormal findings	May be abnormal; chest film may reveal primary site	Normal or variable abnormal findings	May outline mass; especially if aortic calcifications are present	Normal or variable abnormal findings
	ESR elevated; WBC normal or rarely >15,000	ESR elevated; WBC varies; urinalysis may help reveal primary; positive TB skin test	ESR elevated in 80%; HLA-B27 antigen in 96%; RA factor usually absent	Negative	Acid phosphatase elevated or normal; elevated alkaline phosphatase may occur with osteoblastic lesions

Continued.

Table 1-1. Approach to causes of low back pain in adult males—cont'd

	Structural unit			Nerve root irritation
Characteristics	Muscle strain	Spondylolisthesis	Degenerative disc	Herniated disc
Other	Tenderness always away from midline; LBP improves in 1 week and resolves by 2 weeks	NC		Often history of recurrent LBP; pain not relieved by rest or lasting all night suggests a tumor; café-au-lait spots, skin tags, or pedunculated tumors suggest neurofibromatosis and tumors, which may impinge on spinal cord and nerve roots

In looking at the questions surrounding the clinical usefulness of x-ray films to evaluate back pain in primary care, Rockey and associates studied 440 patients. These researchers concluded that back x-ray examinations have negligible diagnostic value in otherwise healthy patients under age 50 who have nontraumatic back pain. With few exceptions, I follow these guidelines. Radiography is essential when the client with back pain has a past history of malignancy. Additionally, a more conservative approach includes the client over 40, because of the increased incidence of metabolic and malignant disease during the fifth decade. Suspicion of a disease process such as ankylosing spondylitis, tuberculosis, or pyogenic infection of the spine should prompt radiological confirmation. In addition, spinal x-ray views are often necessary when the possibility of litigation or extensive financial compensation exists. Referral should be strongly considered for initial evaluation when medicolegal or Workmen's Compensation problems arise. When a condition requires more specialized evaluation, there are few indications for back x-ray examination before referral, in light of radiation exposure and duplication of tests. This is important because many agencies do not allow the release of films to the client, because of the possibility of loss.

Problems of the structural unit

Muscle strain. Investigation reveals that muscle strain is the most commonly seen cause of LBP. In a study group of 5,000 patients with LBP, 81% were classified as having muscle strain unrelated to skeletal disorders (Garrett and Ahmad).

Several important subjective and objective clues suggest muscle strain. The client usually reports some new, unusual, or unconditioned acitvity or recalls a specific injury, such

	Local disease		Systemic disease	Visceral disease	
Pyogenic	Tuberculosis	Ankylosing spondylitis	Abd. aortic aneurysm	Cancer of prostate gland
25% are diabetic; staphylococcus most common organism; fever rare unless abcess present	Rarely primary site; chest or genito-urinary tract usually primaty site	Familial clustering; low in blacks, high in some American Indian groups; may present as irridocyclitis and other systemic manifestations; may present with peripheral arthritis; associated with colitis, psoriasis, Reiter's syndrome	Immediate referral essential	Often no urinary symptoms; rectal exam necessary part of screening physical for males

as lifting. Rest stiffens the muscles, and movement aggravates the pain, which localizes to the muscles of the back. Muscles may be firm or rigid on palpation. Tenderness is always lateral to the midline, not over the vertebrae. Muscle pain causes a decreased range of motion. Except with severe muscle spasm, there are no deformities or abnormal curves of the spine. There are no positive neurological signs and no systemic symptoms. Except for some limited visceral conditions, such as prostatitis, all LBP unrelated to muscle strain should be referred for specialized evaluation.

Spondylolisthesis. Spondylolisthesis, a forward slipping of the vertebral body, occurs most often at the lumbosacral level because it is especially vulnerable to stress. This condition may relate to one of several underlying bony defects. It may be a painless condition, but trauma to the joint will cause a sudden onset of symptoms, with the complaint of something "catching" in the back. The pain is localized to the back or radiates down the leg and may increase with back extension and decrease with back flexion. An abnormal spinal curve is frequently present. Palpation over the spine may reveal abnormal alignment from one process to the other. Lipomata (fatty tumors), unusual hair patches (Faun's beard), birthmarks or excessive port wine marks on the back suggest bony defects and thus spondylolisthesis (Hoppenfeld, 1976). Except when spondylolisthesis mimics a herniated disc, there are no positive neurological signs and no evidence of systemic disease (Brashear and Raney).

Degenerative changes. Narrowing of the disc, decreased water content of the disc, fissures in the annulus, and lipping of the vertebral margins are all degenerative changes. There is no complete agreement on whether degenerative changes alone cause LBP. However, without question, degeneration begins at an early age, is progressive, and predisposes to bulging of the annulus or protrusion of disc material through the annulus or end plate. Two studies have addressed the relationship between degenerative changes and the existence of LBP. Magora and Schwartz (1976) considered the common x-ray findings of osteophytosis (spurring of vertebral margins) and degenerative osteoarthritis of the synovial joints of the back. They reported no relationship between these degenerative changes and the presence or absence of LBP. They concluded that the presence of these changes increases with obesity and age. Also, the changes may be predisposing factors but are not the direct cause of LBP. Therefore, immediately identifying these radiographic findings as the cause of LBP is unacceptable. Thorough assessment must continue until all other possible causes are excluded. The investigators also reported that activities such as prolonged sitting or standing and sudden maximal physical effort are important in triggering the onset of LBP.

Torgerson and Dotter (1976) compared the x-ray films of 387 subjects who had LBP with x-ray films from 217 asymptomatic controls, all of whom were 40 to 70 years old. They also concluded that osteophyte formation does not have a direct relationship to the presence or absence of LBP. However, degenerative disc disease (defined as narrowing greater than 2 mm at the center of the disc compared with the next normal lumbar space) appears to be a major cause of LBP.

Pain attributed to degenerative disc disease is described as mild to moderate, with morning stiffness (Brashear and Raney). Radiographic changes of the disc may be the only objective finding until rupture and nerve root involvement occur.

Nerve root irritation: disc herniation

A disc herniation refers to disruption of the annular fibers. With disruption of the annulus, three situations may occur. The nuclear material may prolapse, remaining confined by the outermost fibers of the annulus. The material may extrude or break through the annulus and lie beneath the posterior longitudinal ligament. Finally, the nucleus may sequestrate or break through the posterior longitudinal ligament and lie in the spinal canal (Macnab, 1977).

Disc herniation occurs most commonly in the 20- to 40-year age group, after degenerative changes begin (Brashear and Raney). A sudden onset of symptoms is associated with heavy lifting, trauma from severe torsion, or other stress to structures of the back. In some cases the pain progresses gradually, the major complaint being pain in the back and leg. Leg pain may occur at the onset of symptoms or can develop over a 2- to 3-day period. Usually there are previous episodes of back pain; leg pain may not be a feature of these episodes. Rarely, nerve root involvement may have only the symptom of leg pain rather than back pain that radiates to the leg. In this case, neurological signs, such as decreased deep tendon reflexes and motor weakness, provide clues to the problem. Activities that increase intraspinal pressure, such as coughing or sneezing, aggravate the pain. Rest, particularly with the knees flexed, decreases stretch of the nerve root, thus reducing discomfort. Any pain that increases with rest or persists all night suggests a tumor or other local disease process. This symptom is a significant historical finding, since several conditions, including benign and malignant tumors, can cause nerve root symptoms and mimic the clinical presentation of disc herniation. Differentiation of these conditions may be impossible without surgical exploration. However, the presence of café-au-lait spots, skin tags, or pedunculated tumors suggests neurofibromatosis tumors. These may involve the spinal cord or nerve root. Lipomata seen on the back may also extend to the cord, producing neurological symptoms (Hoppenfeld).

Positive neurological findings follow the pattern of the nerve root involved. They include decreased or absent deep tendon reflexes, muscle weakness, motor deficit, paresthesia, numbness, and loss of sphincter control.

Various examination techniques demonstrate nerve root irritation. Straight-leg raising—flexing the hip while extending the knee—stretches the sciatic nerve. During this test, the client is supine with the knees extended. The examiner slowly flexes the client's hip by raising a straight leg toward a 90-degree angle. The test result is positive if the client's leg pain is reproduced or increases. During straight-leg raising, pain that further increases with dorsiflexion of the foot and decreases when the knee is flexed strongly suggests nerve root irritation. Bilaterally positive results in straight leg–raising tests suggest a large disc herniation. When straight leg–raising tests are performed, it is important to distinguish between leg pain that is secondary to muscle stretch and pain radiating along the course of the nerve root.

The reverse leg–raising test, or femoral-stretch test, produces pain when a lesion involves the third or fourth lumbar roots. During this test the client is prone with the knee flexed at a 90-degree angle. The examiner then hyperextends the hip, stretching the femoral nerve and its root (Brashear and Raney). Radiating leg pain is a positive test result. Other objective findings include noncongenital deviations in the normal spinal curve, such as a lateral curvature or a flattened lumbar curve. Percussion over the area of the spine involving a herniation may produce tenderness. Tight, tender paravertebral muscles are also notable.

Local disease

Osteomyelitis. Although spinal infections are uncommon, they warrant discussion because of their potential severe consequences. Vertebral osteomyelitis is a disease of adults characterized by its insidious onset. Approximately 25% of affected individuals are diabetic. Staphylococcus is the most common offending organism (Macnab). The backache is often indistinguishable from that of mechanical strain. Its insidious onset and initial lack of x-ray findings frequently delay diagnosis for 8 to 10 weeks, or until the back pain becomes severe, constant, and interrupts sleep. Fever is uncommon unless there is abscess formation. As the infection advances, there are severe spasms of the paravertebral and hamstring muscles. Although nonspecific, an increased sedimentation rate is often found in this disease. The white blood cell count is normal or rarely greater than 15,000/mm^3 (Macnab).

Tuberculosis. Except in unusual cases, tuberculosis of the lumbar spine is not a primary lesion. It is commonly secondary to involvement of the lung or genitourinary tract. The insidious nature of this disease often leads to a delay in seeking care. Unlike pyogenic lesions, tuberculosis of the spine may initially have neurological signs. The sedimentation rate is increased, but the white blood cell count varies. Urinalysis and chest x-ray films help locate the primary site of infection. A positive TB skin test is suggestive but not diagnostic, since the positive test may represent a previous "conversion" and not active disease. The vague initial symptoms and nonspecific findings of early localized infections create confusion in diagnosis. However, with appropriate conservative therapy, the symptoms of acute muscle strain greatly decrease within 1 week and resolve within

2 weeks. The symptoms of localized infection and a poor response to symptomatic treatment should alert the practitioner to consider tuberculosis or osteomyelitis as a cause of low back pain.

Systemic disease: ankylosing spondylitis

The most commonly overlooked cause of back pain in young men is ankylosing spondylitis. This systemic rheumatic disorder is different from rheumatoid arthritis and classically associated with inflammation of the sacroiliac and spinal synovial joints. Back pain is the primary complaint, though the condition occasionally begins with an asymptomatic peripheral arthritis involving large joints—predominantly hips, knees, and shoulders. Acute iridocyclitis—inflammation of the iris and ciliary body—is a more unusual presentation and represents a systemic manifestation. Fever, anorexia, fatigue, weight loss, or anemia may also be present (Calabro, 1977).

Ankylosing spondylitis is a disease affecting men 10 times more often than women. In 80% of the cases the onset occurs when a man is 20 to 40 years old. As many as 3 million Americans may have the disease. The frequency is very low in American and African blacks and high in some North American Indian groups (Calabro).

Although the exact etiology is unknown, there is evidence of familial clustering, with a high incidence among monozygotic twins. There is a 90% frequency of the inherited antigen HLA-B27 in patients and their relatives (Calabro). The frequent association between ankylosing spondylitis and ulcerative colitis, regional enteritis, Reiter's syndrome, and psoriasis is due to the HLA-B27 antigen. The precise role the antigen plays is unknown; however, the risk of developing ankylosing spondylitis is 40 times greater in patients with ulcerative colitis who carry the B27 antigen (Calabro). Trauma or an acute infection may also precipitate spondylitis in predisposed individuals with the B27 antigen.

Recurrent nocturnal back pain and morning stiffness relieved by exercise are the symptoms usually present in the patient with ankylosing spondylitis. The course of the disease is progressive but rarely results in early severe disability. Other clues in the physical examination permit early diagnosis, which may prevent disability.

Costovertebral involvement occurs early and leads to decreased chest expansion. Costovertebral restriction should be considered when maximum chest expansion measured at the nipple line is less than 3 cm. A loss of spinal flexibility is evident when the patient cannot touch close to the floor on bending forward; distance on forward bending is measured from the fingertips to the floor. Schober's test also involves forward bending. While the patient stands erect, the examiner draws two marks: one on the spine at the level of the iliac crest, the other on the spine exactly 10 cm above the initial mark. The patient bends forward, and the examiner measures the new distance between the marks. If the new distance is less than 15 cm, early lumbar involvement is likely. Also, cervical flexibility should be assessed. The inability to touch the back of the head to the wall when the heels and back are against the wall and the chin is at carrying level suggests cervical limitation. Finally, pressure over the sacroiliac joints may reveal tenderness (Calabro).

Laboratory findings are helpful. The sedimentation rate is increased in 80% of the cases. Although an expensive test, the HLA-B27 antigen is present in up to 96% of patients with ankylosing spondylitis. Unlike rheumatoid arthritis, the rheumatoid factor is usually absent in spondylitis. Characteristic x-ray changes are diagnostic but may be absent in the early stages (Calabro).

Visceral disease

The back in many instances is the location of referred pain from thoracic, abdominal, and pelvic viscera. Generally, upper abdominal conditions refer pain to the lower thoracic and upper lumbar areas. Lower abdominal conditions refer pain to the lumbar area, and pelvic conditions to the sacral area. The absence of local signs of back disease indicate referred pain from other structures. Examples of localized signs are tenderness, limited range of back motion, and stiffness of the back. Referred back pain also occurs with relieving or aggravating factors related to the diseased organ; ulcer pain, for example, occurs when the stomach is empty (Isselbacher, 1980). Abdominal aortic aneurysm and prostatic diseases frequently involve pain referred to the back.

Abdominal aortic aneurysm. Recognition of an abdominal aortic aneurysm is essential because it is a potentially fatal condition. It is most often found in males over 40 years of age but may occur at any age (Schwartz, 1979). If the abdominal aneurysm is symptomatic, back pain is the most common symptom. This is because the aorta lies against the spine. Aneurysms may be symptomatic weeks or months before rupture. Abdominal examination, which is essential with the complaint of LBP, may reveal a pulsating epigastric or retroumbilical mass greater than 1 inch in diameter (Schwartz). An aortic bruit may be present. Other signs of vascular disease, such as cold feet and absent or weak peripheral pulses, may be found on assessment. Abdominal x-ray films may demonstrate an aneurysm, particularly in the presence of aortic calcifications. Immediate referral for surgical intervention may prevent a fatal rupture.

Cancer of the prostate gland. Cancer of the prostate gland is the most common cancer of men (Robbins and Angell, 1976). It usually occurs after 40, and the incidence increases rapidly with advancing age (Isselbacher). The sacral pain of chronic prostatitis occurs with dysuria and urinary frequency. However, carcinoma of the prostate gland with spinal involvement and lumbosacral pain is present frequently without urinary symptoms. A history of weight loss may accompany the back pain. Rectal examination is essential for screening because cancer of the prostate gland is often asymptomatic until metastasis occurs. An area of unusual firmness or a prostatic nodule, particularly in the posterior lobe close to the rectal wall, suggests cancer of the prostate gland and warrants referral (Robbins and Angell).

X-ray films of the back may not provide positive findings with metastasis, because radiographic evidence of bone destruction does not occur until it involves 50% of cancellous and 25% of cortical bone (Mennell, 1966). Therefore, normal x-ray findings do not exclude bone pathology.

In addition to bony metastasis, pelvic lymph node involvement also produces back pain. An elevated acid phosphatase level may indicate metastatic disease of the prostate gland; however, normal levels do not exclude it. Elevated levels of alkaline phosphatase may occur with metastatic bone lesions that are osteoblastic (Robbins and Angell).

PLAN FOR ACUTE MUSCLE STRAIN

Relief of back pain is one aspect in management of acute muscle strain. An additional consideration is to protect the spinal system. Each structure of the back is essential; when one part of the system, such as the muscle, is dysfunctional, it leaves other structures without support and more vulnerable to damage. The weakened structural system may expose the disc to excessive stress even during activities of daily living. Assuming that decreased intradiscal pressure is desirable, discouraging activities that increase disc pressures may prevent further injury. The following recommendations promote pain relief and protection of the spinal system.

Rest

Bed rest should be encouraged. With severe pain bed rest should continue until pain resolves. With mild pain even 1 day's rest may be sufficient because improvement is often rapid. In addition to the symptomatic relief provided by bed rest, there is evidence that the best position for relieving the load on the disc is the supine position (Nachemson, 1969). Sleeping in a prone position should be discouraged because it causes hyperextension of the spine. A firm mattress with a plywood board underneath provides support to the trunk to prevent undesirable motion of the spine. In a side-lying position, the top knee is flexed and a pillow placed beneath it to prevent rotation of the spine. Also, a pillow positioned behind the back may promote comfort and provide added support.

The back is further protected by individualized instructions to prevent activities that increase the load on the disc. The following findings from studies of disc pressures provide guidelines to teach habits that protect the back from increased disc pressure:
1. Sit with the back supported rather than unsupported. If possible, adjust a chair's backrest inclination between 100 and 110 degrees. For example, some typing or work chairs are adjustable and preferable to straight-back chairs (Anderson and others, II, 1974).
2. Stand at ease, with arms at the side, if unsupported sitting is the only other choice (Andersson and others, I, 1974).
3. When sitting, do not slump in the chair with knees extended. Sit with the hip and knee joints well flexed (Nachemson, 1969).
4. Avoid prolonged forward bending (Nachemson, 1969). Common activities that may demand this are vacuuming or gardening.
5. Lift objects keeping the back straight and using the leg muscles for strength (Nachemson, 1969).
6. Keep the object close to the body when lifting. This is as important as lifting with the back straight (Andersson and others, 1978).
7. Drive a car with an automatic transmission rather than a standard transmission, because depressing the clutch or shifting gears increases disc pressure (Andersson and others, IV, 1974).

Heat

The benefits of heat, cold applications, and various other methods of physiotherapy remain unproven in a controlled study (Nachemson, 1969). However, clients with muscle strain consistently report relaxation and relief of pain with heat application. This clinical observation suggests the need for controlled study.

Medication

Along with rest and heat application, medication may be necessary initially to relieve pain. Aspirin or acetaminophen (Tylenol), 650 mg every 4 hours as necessary, controls mild discomfort. Some clinicians prefer to give mild analgesics every 4 hours while the client is awake. In moderate to severe pain, aspirin combined with 30 mg of codeine given every 4 hours as needed may be necessary for the first few days. There are occasions when the pain is so severe that a more potent analgesic is necessary to achieve early pain relief and seems a necessity to allow rest. In this case physician consultation is necessary and hospitalization is a consideration. The client needs to know that any analgesic is temporary and not for long-term use.

The use of drugs to reduce muscle spasm is a common practice, and there are multiple drugs advertised for this purpose on the market. Diazepam (Valium) is used frequently for "muscle spasm." However, the usefulness of drugs to reduce spasm is poorly documented. Mooney and Cairnes (1978) noted that no description in the literature relates myoelectric activity to chronic back pain in an individual "at rest in a supported position." They failed to demonstrate myoelectrical activity of the back in individuals in bed traction complaining of severe back pain and spasm. The recurrent nature of LBP creates the potential for chronic drug use. Mooney and Cairnes reported that diazepam is the most common drug causing habituation in clients referred to their Spinal Pain Center. I find muscle relaxants of little clinical use in the management of LBP. The effects of multiple medications "are not well substantiated, they are too costly, and drug dependence is to be avoided whenever possible" (Mooney and Cairnes, p. 55). The use of medications other than analgesics should be avoided in the treatment of LBP for these reasons.

Stress management

Although many studies attempt to address the psychological aspect of back pain, the problem remains a complex one. With muscle strain, psychological stress at least aggravates an existing condition and interferes with rest. Often the client is "too busy" to rest. Many clients are unaware of the degree of stress in their lives and only view "negative" events as stress producing or requiring coping mechanisms. The Social Readjustment Rating Scale (SRRS) by Holmes and Rahe (1967) helps evaluate stressful events in everyday life (Table 1-2). Various life events are given values called life change units. These quantify the degree of stress for events experienced by the client and are added to total the number of life change units for 1 year.

The following suggestions utilize the SRRS as a preventive measure and were designed by Holmes to be given to patients:

1. Become familiar with the life events and the amount of change they require.
2. Put the scale where you and the family can see it easily several times a day.
3. With practice you can recognize when a life event happens.
4. Think about the meaning of the event for you and try to identify some of the feelings you experience.
5. Think about the different ways you might best adjust to the event.
6. Take your time in arriving at decisions.
7. If possible, anticipate life changes and plan for them well in advance.
8. Pace yourself. It can be done even if you are in a hurry.
9. Look at the accomplishment of a task as a part of daily living, and avoid looking at such an achievement as a "stopping point" or a "time for letting down."

10. Remember, the more change you have, the more likely you are to get sick. Of those people with over 300 Life Change Units, for the past year, almost 80 percent get sick in the near future; with 150 to 299 Life Change Units, about 50 percent get sick in the near future; and with less than 150 Life Change Units, only 30 percent get sick in the near future. So the higher your Life Change Score, the harder you should work to stay well.*

Exercise

Abdominal muscles relieve the load on the back during lifting (Frost, 1973). They also minimize torque, bending, and shear stress in the lumbar spine (Farfan, 1975). Health care providers often prescribe exercises to strengthen the back and abdominal muscles and to increase mobility of the spine. However, there are few controlled studies on the clinical effects of these exercises. Additionally, the available studies raise the question of potential harm from increased disc load during commonly prescribed isotonic exercises, such as sit-ups. Measurements of the disc pressure during performance of frequently prescribed exercises revealed that "all the common isotonic exercises resulted in intradiscal pressures that were higher than those measured in standing and even in straining and jumping" (Nachemson and Elfström, 1970, p. 31). For example, sit-up exercises, with knees both bent and extended, increase the load on the lumbar spine to equal that when leaning forward with 10-kg weights in each hand (Nachemson and Elfström). A contradiction is that authors who promote these exercises often attempt a decrease in the load on the back by discouraging other activities, such as bending forward and lifting. There are alternatives to isotonic exercises. Isometric exercises show the least increase in intradiscal pressure (Nachemson, 1969). Studies by Kendall and Jenkins (1968, 1978) and by Lidstrom and Zachrisson (1970) demonstrate favorable clinical response with the isometric exercises (which they describe) rather than isotonic exercises.

For practitioners determining who needs "low back exercises," there is no evidence that clients with LBP have weak back and abdominal muscles unless they are incapacitated for more than 1 month (Nachemson and Lindh, 1969). Clients with chronic back pain and incapacitation for periods of 1 month or more need rehabilitation including isometric abdominal exercises and exercises for quadriceps strengthening to ease lifting using knee extensors. The management of chronic LBP is complex and beyond the scope of this chapter. Mooney and Cairns describe a team approach that seems essential to management of this multifaceted problem. A physical therapist is valuable for teaching the exercises, monitoring the client's progress, and progressing exercises as needed.

Several adjunctive treatment measures may be beneficial, including low-heeled shoes and correction of obesity to prevent exaggerated lumbar lordosis. The contribution of obesity to degenerative changes is also a consideration in encouraging weight loss. With severe back strain back braces prescribed by an orthopedic surgeon may aid in controlling the acute problem.

After recovery from an acute episode of LBP not involving prolonged incapacitation, it is important that the client begin an exercise, such as swimming or walking, which promotes general fitness. When an individual trains and becomes accustomed to activities,

---

*From Holmes, T.H. Cited in Smith, C.K., and others: Life change and illness onset: importance of concepts for family physicians, J. Fam. Pract. **7:**975, 1978.

Table 1-2. The Social Readjustment Rating Scale*

Life event	Mean value
1. Death of spouse	100
2. Divorce	73
3. Marital separation from mate	65
4. Detention in jail or other institution	63
5. Death of a close family member	63
6. Major personal injury or illness	53
7. Marriage	50
8. Being fired at work	47
9. Marital reconciliation with mate	45
10. Retirement from work	45
11. Major change in the health or behavior of a family member	44
12. Pregnancy	40
13. Sexual difficulties	39
14. Gaining a new family member (e.g., through birth, adoption, oldster moving in, etc.)	39
15. Major business readjustment (e.g., merger, reorganization, bankruptcy, etc.)	39
16. Major change in financial state (e.g., a lot worse off or a lot better off than usual)	38
17. Death of a close friend	37
18. Changing to a different line of work	36
19. Major change in the number of arguments with spouse (e.g., either a lot more or a lot less than usual regarding childrearing, personal habits, etc.)	35
20. Taking on a mortgage greater than $10,000 (e.g., purchasing a home, business, etc.)	31
21. Foreclosure on a mortgage or loan	30
22. Major change in responsibilities at work (e.g., promotion, demotion, lateral transfer)	29
23. Son or daughter leaving home (e.g., marriage, attending college, etc.)	29
24. In-law troubles	29
25. Outstanding personal achievement	28
26. Wife beginning or ceasing work outside the home	26
27. Beginning or ceasing formal schooling	26
28. Major change in living conditions (e.g., building a new home, remodeling, deterioration of home or neighborhood)	25
29. Revision of personal habits (dress, manners, associations, etc.)	24
30. Troubles with the boss	23
31. Major change in working hours or conditions	20
32. Change in residence	20
33. Changing to a new school	20
34. Major change in usual type and/or amount of recreation	19
35. Major change in church activities (e.g., a lot more or a lot less than usual)	19
36. Major change in social activities (e.g., clubs, dancing, movies, visiting, etc.)	18
37. Taking on a mortgage or loan less than $10,000 (e.g., purchasing a car, TV, freezer, etc.)	17
38. Major change in sleeping habits (a lot more or a lot less sleep, or change in part of day when asleep)	16
39. Major change in number of family get-togethers (e.g., a lot more or a lot less than usual)	15
40. Major change in eating habits (a lot more or a lot less food intake, or very different meal hours or surroundings)	15
41. Vacation	13
42. Christmas	12
43. Minor violations of the law (e.g., traffic tickets, jaywalking, disturbing the peace, etc.)	11

*Reprinted with permission from: *Journal of Psychosomatic Research,* Vol. 11, Holmes, T.H., and Rahe, R.H., "The Social Readjustment Rating Scale," copyright 1967, Pergamon Press, Ltd.

a pattern of regular movements develops, which is less likely to cause LBP. Regular exercise three to four times a week rather than infrequent exercise or weekend sports activities should be encouraged.

CASE STUDY
Subjective

Dan Taylor is a 33-year-old clothing store manager seeking treatment for his first episode of LBP. He has a 3-day history of mild to moderate pain limited to the lower back. He first noticed the pain while bending forward to brush his teeth. Although he is uncomfortable, he continues to work. Mr. Taylor considers himself healthy and is concerned about the significance of this new problem. Almost any movement aggravates the pain, and a hot shower or lying on the floor provides temporary relief. The condition improves after a night's rest, although his muscles seem "stiff" in the morning. He takes no medication for the pain, but did try to "work out the soreness" by exercising, without achieving relief of symptoms. On initial questioning he says that he is unaware of any unusual activity, but later he recalls helping a friend chop wood for an hour the day before the pain began. No other back symptoms exist, such as "catching" in the back or being "stuck" in one position. There is no history of fever, abdominal pain, urinary symptoms, muscle weakness, paresthesia, or loss of sphincter control. He reports no history of hospitalizations, surgeries, or serious or chronic illnesses. He recalls a broken right arm at age 15. He does not take any medications presently; he is allergic to codeine. His immunizations are current.

The review of systems is noncontributory.

Family history is noncontributory, except that his grandfather died at 75 with cancer of the prostate gland.

Life-style. Mr. Taylor has been married for 5 years and describes his relationship with his wife as very good. His wife is pregnant with their first child, due in 2 months. They bought a house and plan to move within the next 2 weeks. Although he is excited about the changes in his life, he is aware of pressure to "get things done" before the baby's birth. The client was recently and unexpectedly offered a job promising financial advancement above his presently secure position. He is indecisive about the job change. After the baby is born, his wife plans to leave her work as a teacher for about 1 year.

Mr. Taylor stopped smoking 4 years ago after using tobacco for 6 years. He does not drink alcohol. His only exercise is tennis once or twice a month. He has never had a weight problem and prefers fruits and vegetables to higher-calorie foods.

Objective

General. Ht, 6 ft; wt, 185 lb; BP, 118/76; T, 98.4; P, 74; R, 18. He is in no acute distress, although he guards his back when changing position from sitting to lying or sitting to standing.

Musculoskeletal. Inspection of the spine reveals no skin lesions, masses, or discoloration. There are no abnormal spinal curves or deformity, and iliac crests are level. There is mild palpatory tenderness over the paravertebral muscles in the lumbar area; the muscles are firmer on the right side of the spine. The spine is nontender to palpation and percussion. Schober's test reveals a 16.5-cm measurement with forward bending. Chest measurement reveals 40 cm on expiration and 48 cm on inspiration.

Lower extremities. Bilateral leg lengths measure 95 cm from the anterior superior iliac spine to the medial malleolus. There is no deformity or malalignment noted. Peripheral pulses are strong and equal bilaterally.

Abdomen. There is no tenderness; bowel sounds are active. No abdominal bruit, masses, or organomegaly is present, and the aorta is not widened.

Neurological. Straight-leg raising is negative. Sensory and motor testing is intact in lower extremities, without evidence of muscle atrophy. Deep tendon reflexes are 2+ in all extremities.

Rectal. There are no masses. The prostate gland is nontender, without nodules or unusual firmness. The stool guaiac test is negative.

Problems

1. Low back pain secondary to acute muscle strain
2. Alteration in comfort
3. Lack of knowledge related to prevention of back injury
4. Role change

Plan

Rest. Mr. Taylor was instructed to lie down as often as possible until his 1-week return visit. He was to follow the guidelines for positions of rest for the back and to avoid any lifting. Teaching included the importance of rest in providing pain relief and allowing recovery without additional injury. The nurse was aware that curtailing activity is often the most difficult part of treatment for those not in severe pain. Therefore, instructions stressed the short duration of this limitation. An additional focus was on restructuring his schedules and activities to allow initial bed rest. Other teaching points included expected outcomes. Mr. Taylor understood that his pain should resolve within 1 week if he followed treatment guidelines. After the pain resolved, he was to return gradually to his normal activities. (This encouragement may improve compliance. Also, it prevents unnecessary restriction of future activities because of fear of recurrent injury.)

Heat. Mr. Taylor was encouraged to continue the warm showers, which were providing pain relief. The use of a heating pad was suggested, with caution given against falling asleep while using the pad.

Medication. Because of the mild nature of Mr. Taylor's pain, his history of relief with heat and rest, and his allergy to codeine, aspirin was the drug of choice. He was instructed to take 10 grains of aspirin every 4 hours, as needed for pain. If he experienced symptoms of gastric irritation, he was to substitute acetaminophen for pain relief.

Stress management. Mr. Taylor spoke of feeling much "pressure" in his life. For this reason, the SRRS was provided, along with discussion of the tool and the guidelines for its use. He agreed to consider this scale at a convenient time.

Evaluation

At his 1-week return Mr. Taylor was symptom free. He continued to follow the guidelines for activity and safe positioning presented at the first visit. He returned to a light work schedule after 2 days' rest. By the end of a week he resumed his usual work. During the week he and his wife discussed the new job offer. They reviewed the SRRS and totaled 272 units for the year. They decided that with major life changes, a new baby, purchase of a new home, and loss of his wife's income, they would both be happier and feel less stressed if he remained in his present job for the time being. With resolution of his acute problem, Mr. Taylor agreed to schedule time for a complete health assessment, including planning an exercise program for general fitness.

REFERENCES

Advisory Committee on the Biological Effects of Ionizing Radiation: The effects on population of exposure to low levels of ionizing radiation, Washington, D.C., 1972, National Academy of Sciences–National Research Council.

Andersson, B.J., and others: Lumbar disc pressure and myoelectric back muscle activity during sitting. I. Studies on an experimental chair, Scand. J. Rehabil. Med. **6:**104, 1974.

Andersson, B.J., and others: Lumbar disc pressure and myoelectric back muscle activity during sitting. II. Studies on an office chair, Scand. J. Rehabil. Med. **6:**115, 1974.

Andersson, B.J., and others: Lumbar disc pressure and myoelectric back muscle activity during sitting. IV. Studies on a car driver's seat, Scand. J. Rehabil. Med. **6:**128, 1974.

Andersson, B.J., and others: Quantitative studies of the load on the back in different working postures. In Grimby, G., editor: Physical demands and the disabled: a methodological survey, Stockholm, 1978, Almquist och Wiksell.

Brashear, H.R., and Raney, R.B.: Shand's handbook of orthopedic surgery, St. Louis, 1978, The C.V. Mosby Co.

Brown, M.: Muscular mechanism of the lumbar spine and the position of power and efficiency, Orthop. Clin. North Am. **6**:233, 1975.

Calabro, J.J.: Early diagnosis and management of ankylosing spondylitis, Med. Times **105**:80, 1977.

Cailliet, R.: Low back pain syndrome, Philadelphia, 1962, F.A. Davis Co.

Chaffin, D.B., and Park, K.S.: A longitudinal study of low back pain associated with occupational weight lifting factors, Am. Ind. Hyg. Assoc. J. **34**:513, 1973.

Clemmesen, S.M., and Simmelkiaer, A.S.: Investigation on the inclination of the surface of the sacral vertebra to the horizontal plane and its relationship to pelvic tilt and to posture. In Program of Fifth International Congress of Physical Medicine, Montreal, 1968, p. 62.

Conners, J.P.: Summary: remarks by Gatlin, J. Cited in summary report and proceedings of the Conference on Low Back X-rays in Pre-employment Physical Examination, Chicago, 1973, American College of Radiology.

Dehlin, O., and Berg, S.: Back symptoms and psychological perception of work, Scand. J. Rehabil. Med. **9**:61, 1977.

Fahrni, W.H.: Conservative treatment of lumbar disc degeneration: our primary responsibility, Orthop. Clin. North Am. **6**:93, 1975.

Farfan, H.F.: Muscular mechanism of the lumbar spine and the position of power and efficiency, Orthop. Clin. North Am. **6**:135, 1975.

Finneson, B.E.: Nonsurgical treatment of low back pain, J. Neurosurg. Nurs. **9**:54, 1977.

Frost, H.M.: Orthopaedic biomechanics, Springfield, Ill., 1973, Charles C Thomas, Publisher.

Garrett, J.T., and Ahmad, M.D.: The industrial back problem: role of the industrial hygienist and ergonomics, Am. Ind. Hyg. Assoc. J. **38**:560, 1977.

Gracovetsky, S., and others: A mathematical model of the lumbar spine using an optimized system to control muscles and ligaments, Orthop. Clin. North Am. **8**:135, 1977.

Hanson, P.G., and others: Clinical guidelines for exercise training, Postgrad. Med. **67**:120, 1980.

Hardy, J., editor: Rhoads' textbook of surgery principles and practice, ed. 5, Philadelphia, 1977, J.B. Lippincott Co.

Holmes, T.H., and Rahe, R.H.: The social readjustment rating scale, J. Psychosom. Res. **11**:213, 1967.

Hoppenfeld, S.: Physical examination of the spine and extremities, New York, 1976, Appleton-Century-Crofts.

Hult, L.: Cervical, dorsal and lumbar spinal syndromes, Acta Orthop. Scand. Suppl. **17**:1, 1954.

Isselbacher, K.J., and others, editors: Harrison's principles of internal medicine, ed. 9, New York, 1980, McGraw-Hill Book Co.

Kendall, P.H., and Jenkins, J.M.: Lumbar isometric flexion exercises, Physiotherapy **54**:158, 1968.

Kendall, P.H., and Jenkins, J.M.: Exercises for backache: a double-blind controlled trial, Physiotherapy **54**:154, 1978.

Lidstrom, A., and Zachrisson, M.: Physical therapy on low back pain and sciatica, Scand. J. Rehabil. Med. **2**:37, 1970.

Macnab, I.: Backache, Baltimore, 1977, The Williams & Wilkins Co.

Magora, A.: Investigation of the relation between low back pain and occupation, Scand. J. Rehabil. Med. **5**:181, 1973.

Magora, A., and Schwartz, A.: Relation between the low back pain syndrome and x-ray findings, Scand. J. Rehabil. Med. **8**:115, 1976.

Mennell, J.M.: Differential diagnosis of visceral from somatic back pain, J. Occupat. Med. **8**:477, 1966.

Mooney, V., and Cairns, D.: Management in the patient with chronic low back pain, Orthop. Clin. North Am. **9**:543, 1978.

Nachemson, A.: Physiotherapy for low back pain patients, Scand. J. Rehabil. Med. **1**:85, 1969.

Nachemson, A.: Low back pain—its etiology and treatment, Clin. Med. **78**:18, 1971.

Nachemson, A.: The lumbar spine: an orthopedic challenge, Spine **1**:59, 1976.

Nachemson, A., and Elfström, G.: Intravertebral dynamic pressure measurements in lumbar discs, Scand. J. Rehabil. Med. **2**(suppl. 1):1, 1970.

Nachemson, A., and Lindh, M.: Measurement of abdominal and back muscle strength with and without low back pain, Scand. J. Rehabil. Med. **1:**60, 1969.
Pederson, O.F., and others: Back pain and isometric back muscle strength of workers in a Danish factory, Scand. J. Rehabil. Med. **7:**125, 1975.
Robbins, S.L., and Angell, M.: Basic pathology, ed. 2, Philadelphia, 1976, W.B. Saunders Co.
Rockey, P.H., and others: The usefulness of x-ray examination in the evaluation of patients with back pain, J. Fam. Pract. **7:**455, 1978.
Rowe, L.M.: Low back disabilities in industry: an updated position, J. Occupat. Med. **13:**476, 1971.
Schwartz, S.I., editor: Principles of surgery, ed. 2, New York, 1979, McGraw-Hill Book Co.
Smith, C.K., and others: Life change and illness onset: importance of concepts for family physicians, J. Fam. Pract. **7:**975, 1978.
Torgerson, W.R., and Dotter, W.E.: Comparative roentgenographic study of the asymptomatic and symptomatic lumbar spine, J. Bone Joint Surg. [Am.] **58:**850, 1976.
Weis, E.B.: Stresses at the lumbosacral junction, Orthop. Clin. North Am. **6:**83, 1975.
Wiltse, L.L., and Rocchio, P.D.: Preoperative psychological tests as predictors of success of chemonucleolysis in the treatment of the low-back syndrome, J. Bone Joint Surg. [Am.] **57:**478, 1975.

CHAPTER 2

Knee pain and injuries in the adult runner

Carol M. Armatis

Throughout history humans have used running for various purposes. In earliest times running was essential to existence; later the Greeks viewed running as a sport. Over time, technology lessened the need for running as an element of survival. Similarly, as sports became more numerous, diverse, and specialized, running was less popular as a source of entertainment. By the middle of the twentieth century, running was not an amusement or recreational habit of the general populace.

In 1968 Kenneth H. Cooper wrote *Aerobics*. His book linked running to a healthier life (Cooper, 1968). Some medical sources further supported running by connecting it to a reduced rate of coronary disease. Also, innumerable lay articles published in *The Jogger* and *Runner's World* reported remarkable physical and physiological changes linked to running (Blazina and others, 1973). These were increased muscle strength, decreased respiratory and heart rates, increased energy, more efficient use of glucose, hypotension, increased high-density lipoproteins, and decreased hematocrit (Mangi and others, 1979).

In addition, James F. Fixx (1977) proposed psychological reasons for running, which he termed the "brain-body phenomena." These included the need to master one's existence, live at one's pace, submerge the self in a greater cause, assert without hurting others, and balance stress and relaxation.

Many seek the physiological and psychological rewards of running. A Gallup poll estimated that there are 23 million Americans who run or jog (Carpenter, 1978). Like any other physical activity, running can stress body structures. It places an increased load or stress on the lower extremities, particularly on the knee joint. The concern of this chapter is the vulnerability of the knee, a critical structure in running. The conditions presented in this chapter are those common running injuries related to chronic stress and overuse. Most of these conditions begin as simple soft tissue injuries, such as strains, sprains, and bursitis. Over time, as running continues and mileage increases, additional overloading occurs. This overload may lead to more chronic or even acute articular, cartilaginous, and ligamentous injuries. Thus preventive measures are a vital part of the treatment plan. The discussion includes the etiology, assessment, plan for treatment, prevention, and rehabilitation, and evaluation of these common problems.

REVIEW OF ANATOMY

The knee is a complex joint. The running motions of flexion and extension demonstrate that the knee is not merely a hinge formed by the femur and the tibia. During flexion, the tibia actually glides posteriorly over the femoral condyles (Fig. 2-1). When the foot is planted, the final few degrees of full knee extension are accompanied by 10 degrees of internal rotation of the femoral condyles on the tibial fossae (Hoppenfeld, 1976). When the foot is free, there is the same degree of external tibial rotation about the femoral condyle. With the foot planted or free, this rotation allows the femoral condyle to lock the knee joint in full extension. This "lock home" or "screw home" mechanism provides stability to the fully extended knee.

The cruciate ligaments are passive stabilizers of the knee joint (Fig. 2-1). These ligaments are the main stabilizers during flexion and gliding movements (Hertel and Schweiberer, 1978). They also play an important role in supporting the knee during the 10-degree rotary movement.

The menisci are two C-shaped cartilages. Each meniscus attaches to the intercondylar notch of the tibia, and fills the space between the femoral condyle and tibial fossa (Fig. 2-2). They form concave depressions into which the femoral condyles fit. The menisci have four functions: to bear weight, to absorb shocks, to stabilize the joint, and to facilitate rotational movement. Because of their attachment to the cruciate ligaments, they assist in stabilizing the knee during rotary movement.

The synovial membrane surrounds the articular components of the joint. It is vascular and contains sensory nerve fibers for pain. Effusion in this compartment or capsule can be due to numerous clinical situations. Examples are infection, any of the systemic collagen diseases, or metabolic diseases. Additionally, it may be the by-product of articular car-

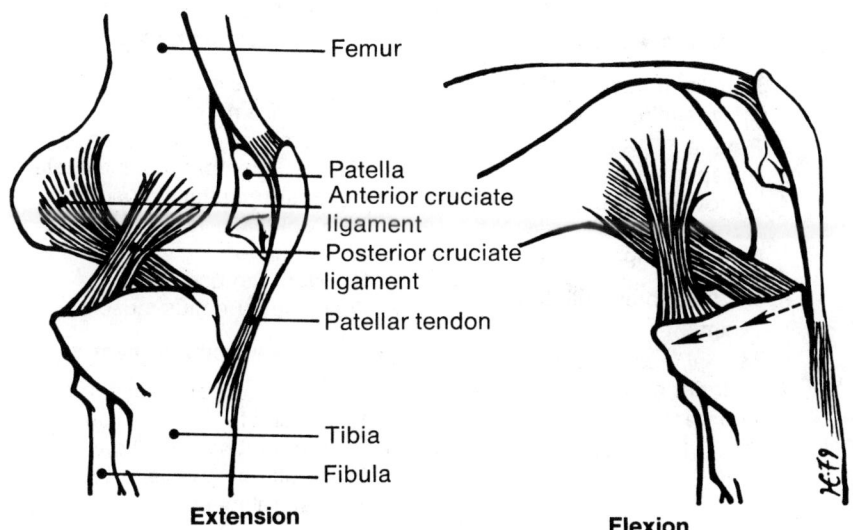

Fig. 2-1. Gliding motion of the left tibiofemoral joint (medial femoral condyle is removed).

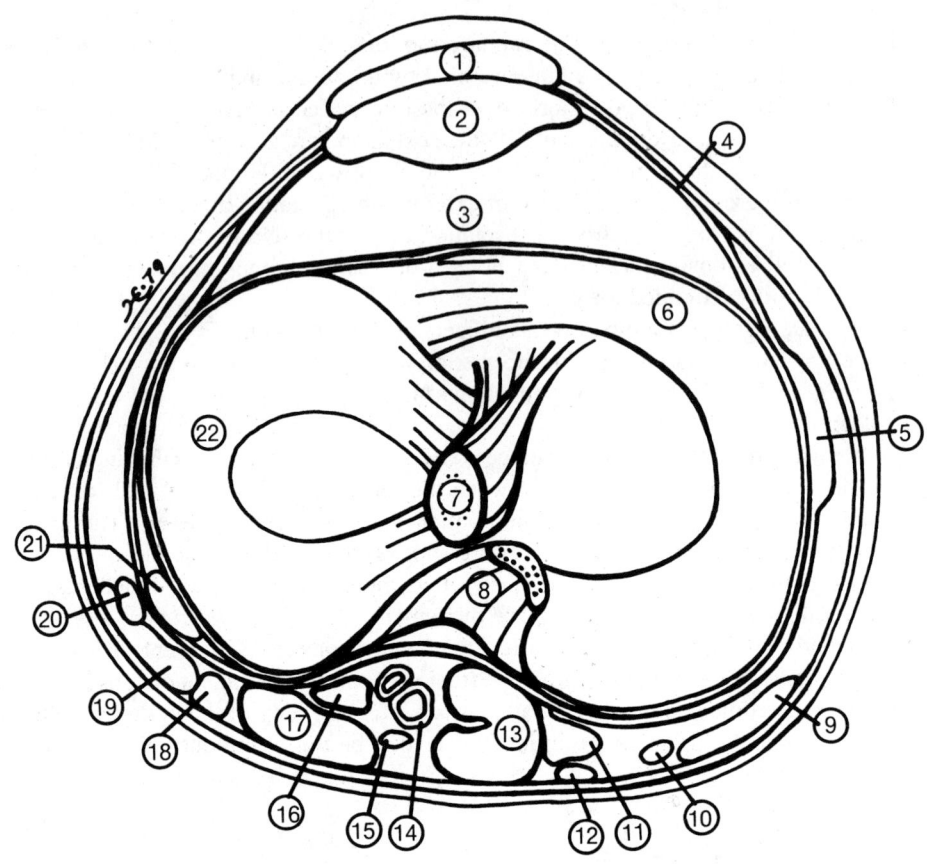

Anterior compartment

1. Patellar tendon and infrapatellar bursa
2. Patella
3. Infrapatellar fat pad
4. Synovial membrane

Medial compartment

5. Medial (tibial) collateral ligament
6. Medial meniscus
7. Anterior cruciate ligament
8. Posterior cruciate ligament

Posterior compartment

9. Sartorius muscle
10. Gracilis muscle
11. Semitendinosus muscle
12. Semimembranosus muscle
13. Gastrocnemius muscle
14. Popliteal artery
15. Tibial nerve
16. Plantar muscle
17. Gastrocnemius muscle

Lateral compartment

18. Common peroneal nerve
19. Biceps femoris tendon
20. Fibular collateral ligament
21. Popliteal muscle
22. Lateral meniscus

Fig. 2-2. Cross section through the left knee joint.

Knee pain and injuries in the adult runner 29

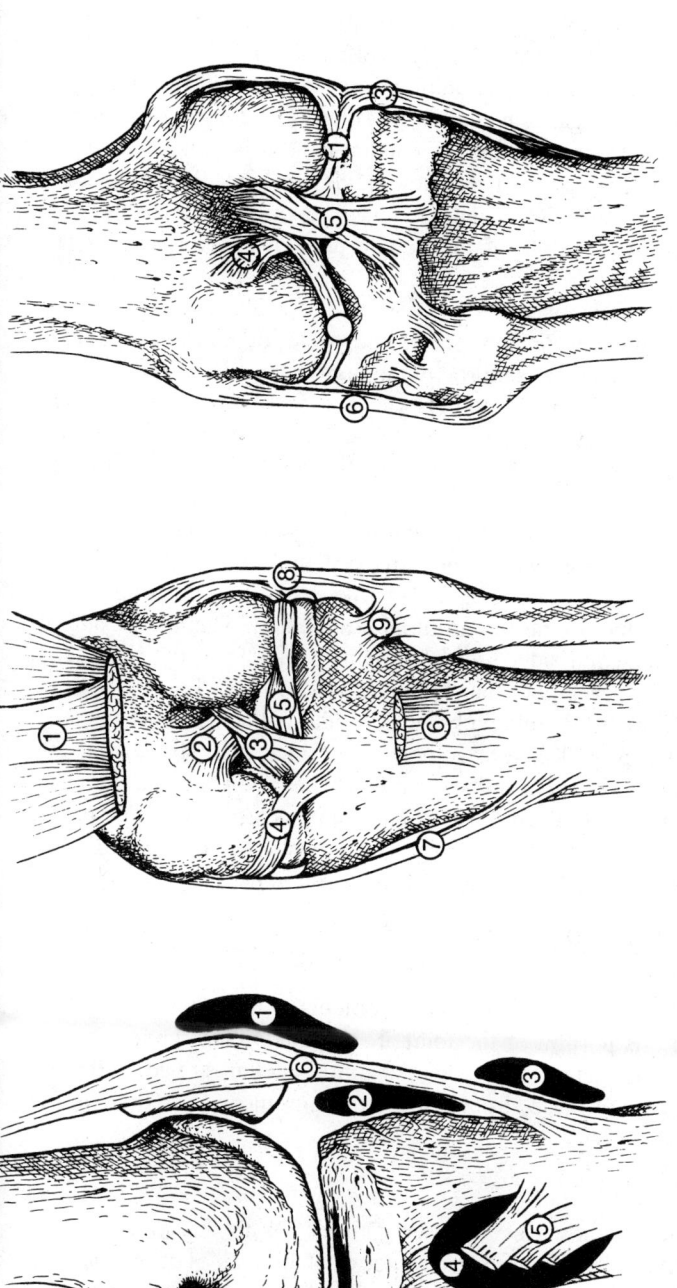

Medial view of left knee showing significant bursae

1. Prepatellar bursa
2. Deep infrapatellar bursa
3. Superficial infrapatellar bursa
4. Pes anserine bursa
5. Pes anserine tendon unit
6. Patellar tendon

Anterior view of left knee (patella removed)

1. Quadriceps muscle tendon unit
2. Posterior cruciate ligament
3. Anterior cruciate ligament
4. Medial meniscus
5. Lateral meniscus
6. Patellar tendon
7. Medial collateral ligament
8. Fibular collateral ligament
9. Tibiofibular ligament

Posterior view of left knee

1. Medial meniscus
2. Lateral meniscus
3. Tibial collateral ligament (medial)
4. Anterior cruciate ligament
5. Posterior cruciate ligament
6. Fibular collateral ligament (lateral)

Fig. 2-3. Medial, anterior, and posterior views of the left knee.

tilage or bone damage. Injury to the membrane itself or neighboring structures (ligaments, meniscus, tendons, or infrapatellar fat pad) may produce effusion.

The patella is another important structure in running movements. It lies on the anterior aspect of the knee beyond the joint capsule and bursae (Figs. 2-1 and 2-2). The quadriceps tendon suspends the patella proximally, and the patellar tendon suspends it distally. The patellar-femoral joint is a gliding joint. The patella slides up and down the intercondylar groove of the femur as the knee flexes and extends. The vastus medialis muscle-tendon attachment to the superomedial pole of the patella prevents lateral shift of the patella from the intercondylar groove.

The structures that prevent hyperextension are the posterior capsule and the hamstring muscle-tendon unit. The posterior capsule consists of the posterior oblique ligament, oblique popliteal ligament, and part of the semimembranous tendon. The capsule is an important stabilizer during external tibial rotation (Hertel and Schweiberer; Mains and others, 1977). The hamstrings are powerful flexor muscles. By attaching to either side of the anterior aspect of the tibia, they produce lateral and rotary stability and prevent anterior displacement of the tibia (Fig. 2-3).

The powerful quadriceps muscle provides the main dynamic stabilization of the knee joint. Stability is due primarily to a massive ligamentous system on the lateral, medial, and part of the posterior surface of the knee (Fig. 2-3). This system, comprising strong fibrous bands, provides a brace effect to the femorotibial articulation. The lateral side of the knee is more stable than the medial side. Lateral support comes from the two distal condyles of the femur, which form a bipod (James and others, 1978). The very dense fibrous band called the iliotibial tract, the relatively weak fibular collateral ligament, and the posterior lateral capsule also provide lateral support. The increased strength in the lateral ligamentous system allows less opportunity for injury when the knee is in motion.

The medial aspect of the knee is less protected by ligamentous structures. The prime stabilizing structure is the medial collateral ligament. The posterior oblique ligament increases medial stability, particularly during external tibial rotation.

ASSESSMENT AND PLAN FOR PROBLEMS IN THE ANTERIOR COMPARTMENT

The anterior compartment is the site of most knee problems in the adult runner. The predominant structures within this portion of the joint are the quadriceps tendon, suprapatellar bursa, synovial membrane, patella and its tendon, infrapatellar fat pad, and anterior portions of both menisci. Any of these structures can sustain injury from the chronic stress of running.

Peripatellar pain

Peripatellar pain is commonly known as "runner's knee." With this problem, the runner complains of discomfort either medial to, lateral to, or on both sides of one patella. Historically, the clinical picture is benign. The client's pain relates only to running. Any other weight-bearing movement, such as ascending or descending stairs, is usually painless. Other signs or symptoms, such as effusion, "giving way," "popping," or "clicking" of the knee, are absent.

Peripatellar pain may involve structural instability of the foot. The instability allows excessive foot pronation during the stance phase of running, thus transmitting increased stress to the knee (American Academy of Orthopaedic Surgeons, 1975; Cailliet, 1973; Sheehan, 1972). Additional stresses may exist. These environmental stresses include inappropriate shoes and running surfaces (Mangi and others; Sheehan, 1972). The practitioner must question the particulars of the running routine: Have the running shoes been changed? Has the running course been changed to hills or uneven surfaces?

The physical assessment must include a thorough examination of the runner's lower extremities (see p. 32). This determines the presence of anatomical variations leading to excess pronation of the foot and resultant peripatellar pain. Such variations are Mortions' foot, flatfeet, and unequal leg lengths ($>\frac{3}{8}$ inch) (James and others). Examination of the runner's shoes is important with any complaint of knee pain (Table 2-1).

Morton's foot is the most frequent anatomical variation associated with excess pronation of the foot (Sheehan, 1978) (Fig. 2-4). When Morton's foot is present, providing good support to the first metatarsal heads is imperative. Various methods may accomplish this. First, foot supports can offer stability to the first toe and decrease the stress on the second metatarsal (Fixx; James and others). Such supports are Dr. Scholl's Flexors or Spenco Insoles shaped to provide Morton's foot extension (Fig. 2-5). If these are unavail-

Table 2-1. Guidelines for running shoes for feet without anatomical variations or previous injuries

Shoe part	Design characteristics
Toe box (tip of shoe to metatarsal joint)	Rounded tip
	Allowance of no more than 1 index finger width (up to ½ inch) from end of toe to end of shoe when standing
	All 5 toes should dorsiflex easily
	Sole—1 to 2 layers thick and flexible
Forefoot (from metatarsal joint to talar joint)	Tongue—padded and seamless
	Last—straight or U-box lacing
Heel	Sole—flexible to 70°-90° easily
	Height—½-⅝ inch greater than shoe body
	Width—beveled to a slight flare at outsole
	Counter—stiff, providing stability
	Achilles' pad—molded well and producing no friction
	Ankle collar—molded well and producing no friction
Sole	Basic construction—3 layers of shock-absorbing material beginning at heel, tapering to 2 layers at metatarsal joint and then 1 layer at shoe toe
	Insole—in contact with total foot, comfortable, and without friction
	Midsole—cushioning material; no foot movement present between insole and midsole
	Outsole bottom layer—waffle design

Physical examination of the knee in the adult runner

A. Anatomical variations
1. Leg
   a. Length
      (1) True length
      (2) Apparent length
      (3) Length of femur
      (4) Length of tibia
      (5) Length of foot
   b. Shape
      (1) Tibial torsion (15° to 20° normal)
      (2) Genu
         (a) Recurvatum
         (b) Valgum (3 inches between malleoli)
         (c) Varum (2 inches between condyles)
2. Knee
   a. Patella
      (1) Position (normal, high, low)
      (2) Pain/no pain to 45° luxation
      (3) Peripatellar, retropatellar facet
      (4) Patellar tendon
3. Foot
   a. Longitudinal arch
      (1) Pes planus (rigid or supple arch)
      (2) Morton's foot

B. Range of motion
1. Leg
   a. Flexion
   b. Extension
   c. Abduction and adduction (of hip)
2. Foot
   a. Flexion
      (1) Dorsal
      (2) Plantar

C. Muscles
1. Size
   a. Thigh girth
   b. Calf girth
2. Strength (0 to 5)
   a. Quadriceps
   b. Hamstring
   c. Hip flexors

D. Gait
1. Stance phase
2. Swing phase

E. Maneuvers
1. Joint line tenderness
   a. Anteromedial
   b. Midmedial
   c. Posteromedial
   d. Anterolateral
   e. Midlateral
   f. Posterolateral
2. Ligamentous tenderness
   a. Medial compartment (or capsule)
   b. Medial collateral ligament
   c. Fibular collateral ligament
3. Pes anserinus tenderness
4. Ligamentous laxity with:
   a. Forced valgus at 0° flexion
   b. Forced valgus at 30° flexion
   c. Forced varus at 0° flexion
   d. Forced varus at 30° flexion
5. Rotary stability tests
   a. Anterior drawer with neutral foot
   b. Anterior drawer with 15° external rotation
   c. Posterior drawer with neutral foot
   d. Posterior drawer with 15° external rotation
6. McMurray's test
   a. Internal rotation (click, pop, grating pain)
   b. External rotation (click, pop, grating pain)

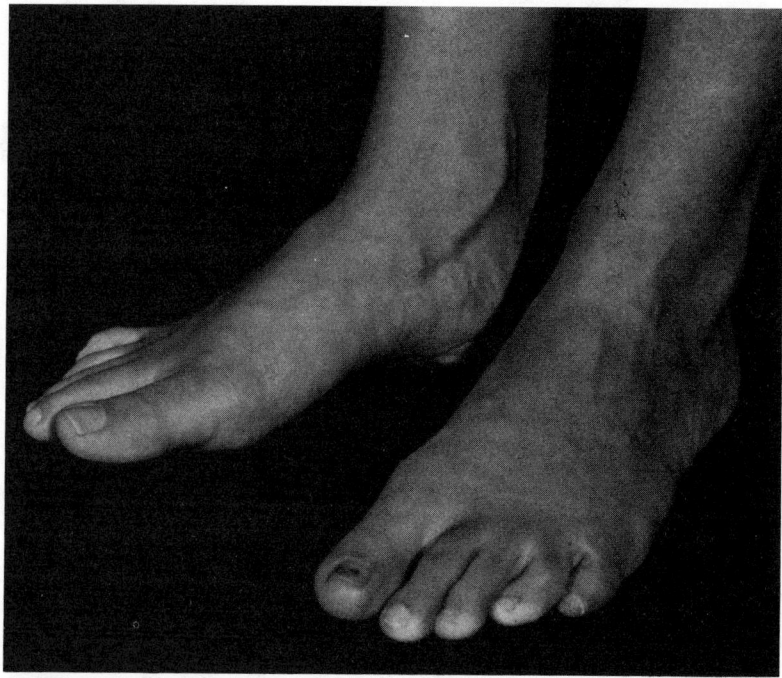

Fig. 2-4. Three characteristics of Morton's foot are (1) short, hypermobility of first (great) toe metatarsal; (2) displacement of sesamoid bones (plantar surface); and (3) long second metatarsal bone with a thickened shaft.

able, ¼-inch moleskin, cork, or orthopedic felt is usable, if it follows the configuration suggested in Fig. 2-5. The second support is a well-cushioned shoe with a rigid heel counter and solid shank. These features decrease the possibility of excessive pronation. Also, one should suggest that the runner maintain the present running frequency, distance, time, and surface for a period of 7 to 10 days. This allows the foot and knee to adjust to the flexible orthotics or the change in shoes, and usually prevents aches or blisters that can accompany the inserts or new shoes. Also, introducing only one of these therapeutic alternatives at a time is advisable.

Pes planus, also known as flatfoot, is another common anatomical variation leading to excessive foot pronation. In pes planus, the medial longitudinal arch is lost. If the arch is absent only when one stands (and not when one sits), the flatfoot is supple and is correctable with arch supports. The use of a Dr. Scholl's 611 or Procomfort arch support often provides sufficient correction to prevent excessive stress to the knee. Another device that may be successful is a flexible longitudinal lift, or wedge. It is contoured to the concavity of the arch when it is not bearing weight (Sheehan, 1978). The wedge is made from dense foam, felt padding, or moleskin.

At times arch supports may not correct pes planus, or they may overcorrect the condition. Overcorrection leads to additional knee and foot problems. Either circumstance can be avoided by keeping the runner's routine static for approximately 1 to 2 weeks. During this time, proper positioning of the support should be checked.

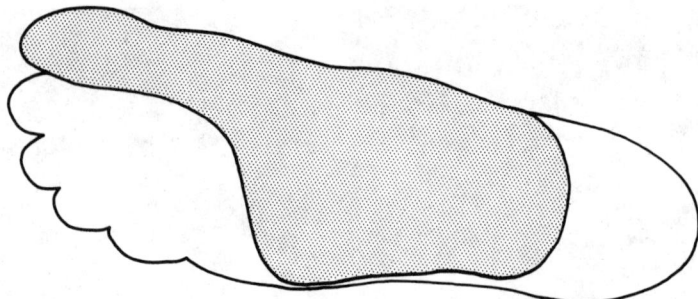

Fig. 2-5. Morton's foot extension. The insole ends at the junction of the metatarsotarsal joint of the second, third, fourth, and fifth toes but extends beyond the distal phalanx of the first toe.

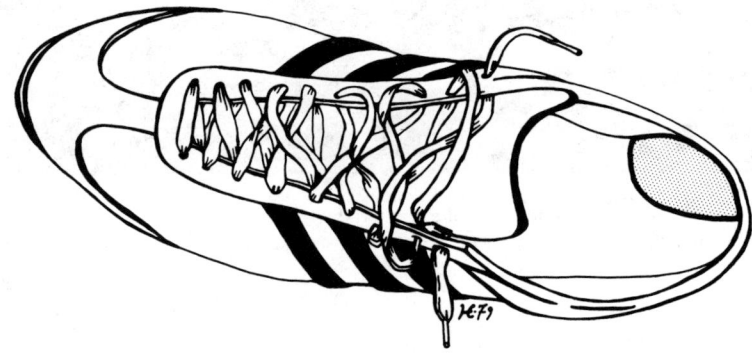

Fig. 2-6. The medial heel lift extends no farther than 1 inch in length and no wider than halfway across the width of the calcaneus bone.

The runner may have a rigid flatfoot (arch absent when sitting and standing) or unresponsive, supple flatfoot. If so, referral to a sports podiatrist or orthopedist for possible permanent orthotics or correction is appropriate.

Another common cause of excessive foot pronation is leg length discrepancy. Discrepancies in leg length can be "true" or "apparent," depending on the cause. True discrepancies are actual differences in the leg length as measured bilaterally from the anterior superior iliac spine to the medial malleolus. Apparent discrepancies give the appearance of unequal leg lengths because of other problems such as scoliosis. Bilateral measurement from the umbilicus to the medial malleolus reveals an apparent discrepancy.

Discrepancies of 1 cm or less can be corrected with medial heel lifts beveled to fit the contour of the calcaneus (Fig. 2-6) (American Academy of Orthopaedic Surgeons). Any discrepancy greater than 1 cm occurring with a history of low back pain complaints needs review by an orthopedist. This professional may provide orthotic equipment and may prevent debilitating problems. Also, the underlying cause of an apparent discrepancy may need orthopedic attention.

The vastus medialis muscle-tendon unit is another structure subject to stress when there is excessive pronation of the foot or of the leg (Fig. 2-3). Strain of this unit is usually due to imbalance between the vastus medialis muscle and the stronger hamstring muscles, or to changes in the running routine. The latter should be suspected if the runner reports adding extra miles or hills or a change from flat to uneven surfaces. Even running against traffic instead of with traffic or running inside on a banked track creates an uneven surface.

The physical examination demonstrates concentrated soreness of the medial border of the patella. Also, there is a dull aching sensation spreading upward into the muscle belly during quadriceps muscle contraction. Usually there is minimal swelling, a stable joint with a full range of motion, and no retropatellar pain. A progressive stretching and strengthening exercise program for the quadriceps muscle is the treatment (see stretching and strengthening exercises provided at end of chapter).

Infrapatellar bursitis

The infrapatellar bursa lies behind the patellar tendon and in front of the fat pad. In most people there is no communication between the bursa and the knee joint. The infrapatellar fat pad separates the two. The cause of the bursitis is repeated overactivity, which causes friction between the patellar tendon and the upper tibia and fat pad. The runner complains of pain over the bursa on complete passive flexion and complete active extension of the knee. Tenderness circumscribes the patellar tendon but is more notable under its edges. Gently picking up the tendon with two fingers elicits pain when the fingers move behind the tendon. If the inflammation progresses, including increased fluid formation, a bulge may be evident on either side of the tendon. Pressure on one side of the fluid bulge causes a bulge on the other side (O'Donoghue, 1976).

Differentiating infrapatellar bursitis from inflammation and swelling of the fat pad is not always possible. The latter may exhibit swelling and tenderness that is deeper and more posterior to the tendon. Complete extension of the knee may also be painful or impossible. With this clinical sign, lesions of the medial meniscus are essential considerations (see Meniscial Injuries). Overlooking a meniscial injury can have serious consequences in terms of the future welfare of the joint. A displaced, complete, or buckethandle tear of the medial meniscus may be present (Smillie, 1978). Bursitis, fat pad inflammation, or medial meniscus tear may prohibit complete extension of the knee and produce effusion. Thus it is usually difficult to distinguish the simple traumatic bursitis from a more serious meniscus tear. Because of the diagnostic difficulty, orthopedic consultation is necessary. Also, it should be remembered that runners may come for treatment with knee effusions unrelated to running and secondary to other serious conditions. Orthopedic referral allows examination of knee aspirates and facilitates accurate diagnosis and appropriate treatment.

Patellar tendinitis

The four motor components of the quadriceps muscle are the medialis, intermedius, lateralis, and rectus. They originate from the femur, and their tendon muscle fibers converge over the patella and join with the patellar tendon. The patellar tendon proceeds downward to the tubercle of the tibia, where it inserts. Stress can occur at any point along this continuum. Pain, tenderness, and mild swelling are present at the weakest link in the chain.

The majority of runners experience discomfort or pain at the patellar region as a result of excessive strain to the quadriceps muscle and to the patellar tendon. These runners mention increasing their distances and adding hills to their routine. The onset of pain is insidious. Pain is usually present at the inferior pole of the patella or over the tibial tubercle. There is local swelling and tenderness. The client commonly complains of pain over the patella when moving, particularly on descending hills or stairs. Climbing and descending stairs create in the patellar tendon a force of 3.3 times the body weight (Reilly and Martens, 1972). Another complaint is knee stiffness after sitting for any length of time. Gentle palpation over the tendon reveals a creaking sensation.

Other conditions may appear initially with the signs and symptoms of patellar tendinitis. The clinical confusion arises when the biomechanical stabilizing structures of the knee obscure a severe injury. Thus the mild signs and symptoms do not reflect the extent of damage. The lack of effusion or swelling is particularly misleading. In gross ligamentous injuries, for example, the joint decompresses, and synovial fluid and blood flow into the soft tissue of the lower leg. Slight effusion results, allowing continuation of the client's normal activities. In the case of patellar tendon swelling, the provider must evaluate the cruciate, lateral, and medial ligaments and the medial meniscus to exclude quadriceps compensation in the presence of a severe ligamentous injury.

The location of pain at the inferior pole of the patella helps distinguish patellar tendinitis from chondromalacia patellae (see Recurrent Dislocated Patella). In both conditions the client complains of pain on descending stairs or hills. However, patellar tendinitis causes knee stiffness after sitting, and chondromalacia does not.

Management of patellar tendinitis is contingent on determining the degree of strain and the involvement of other structures. Blazina and others suggest three levels of injury to determine therapy: (1) pain only after running, without functional impairment; (2) pain both during and after running, but still without functional impairment; and (3) pain during and after running, prolonged duration of pain, and functional impairment. For levels 1 and 2, therapy consists of decreasing running distances and reducing or modifying running routines for hills. This should be coupled with the application of local heat immediately after the run or the use of a warm-water Whirlpool. Another salient feature of the therapy is adequate stretching of the quadriceps muscle before and after the run (see Plan for Prevention and Rehabilitation of Knee Injuries). For level 3 strains, referral to an orthopedist is appropriate for consideration of surgical intervention or more radical nonsurgical procedures, such as splints, casts, and daily physical therapy (O'Donoghue; Smillie).

Recurrent dislocated patella

All disclocations of the knee involve disruption of certain groups of ligaments. The more common dislocation of the adult runner is the chronic patellofemoral dislocation. In this case, the client may report previous episodes of acute subluxation. Previous episodes predispose the client to recurrent dislocations from the stress of running.

The basic mechanism for patellar dislocation occurs when the quadriceps muscle relaxes. With dislocation, the patella passes laterally over the femoral condyle as the knee extends. Although dislocation usually results from a blow to the medial aspect of the normal knee, anatomical variations can promote subluxation without the exogenous force. For example, subluxation is common among females because of their wide pelvis and internally angulated femurs (Glinz, 1978). People with genu valgum, or knock knees, demonstrate a similar condition. Although a clinical entity in its own right, patella alta (high-riding patella) is the most common single cause of subluxation (Smillie). Dislocation is rare with genu varum, or bowlegs (Hughes and Hogue, 1977).

Other factors that predispose a runner to patellar dislocation from minor stress on the knee can exist. These include: (1) a deficient vastus medialis muscle, (2) a shallow patellar groove or a relatively flat lateral femoral condyle, and (3) a convex lateral facet of the patella.

Historically, when dislocation is complete, the diagnosis is obvious. In mild cases, in which the patella slips momentarily over the edge of the condyle, the complaint usually is insecurity or incidents of giving way. These may be followed by small recurrent synovial effusions (Smillie). The client notes vague anteromedial knee pain and some difficulty descending inclines. Tenderness of the patella with pressure may suggest subluxation. These symptoms are similar to those of a torn meniscus and can mislead the examiner. Sometimes the mechanism of injury helps differentiate recurrent subluxations and torn menisci. In meniscial tears, giving-way incidents occur from stepping on a stone or encountering an uneven surface; either of these mechanisms produces a forceful rotational motion. In recurrent subluxations, the giving way occurs when the patient simply turns or, in most cases, recalls, no particular movement. Regardless of the manner of injury, the possibility of meniscial damage should be considered until it is excluded by definitive evidence.

On examination the alignment of the patella in standing and sitting positions should be studied. With the client sitting, the direction that each patella faces should be noted. Lateral displacement of one patella may indicate instability. Additional data can be obtained by observing the patella in the femoral groove as the knee extends. Whether the patella moves into a lateral position as the knee comes toward complete extension should be noted. With the client standing, the presence of genu valgum or varum, the patella's position, and whether the patella is normal or high riding are also determined (Hoppenfeld). The difference in the circumference of the right and left quadriceps muscles 4 to 6 inches above the midpoint of the patella is also measured to provide information about the volume of the vastus medialis muscle.

The single most important clinical sign of patellar instability is a positive response during the apprehension test. During this test the client displays apprehension or fear of patellar dislocation. The test is administered with the client supine. The client's knee is flexed at 45 degrees, and the patella is forced laterally; the patella may partially slip or sublux. A "zero" response is one in which the client shows no apprehension, indicating a stable patella. With a grade 1 response, the client shows mild anxiety; with a grade 2 or higher, the client has a marked reaction with concomitant muscle tensing. With grade 3 or 4 responses, the client invariably shows extreme anxiety, indicating patellar instability. If the runner displays a grade 2 response or above on the apprehension test, referral to an orthopedist is in order.

Many therapies exist for recurrent dislocated patella. There is no proof of one completely effective therapy (Cailliet). For the primary care provider it is imperative to exclude meniscus involvement before using conservative treatment. For mild degrees of dislocation the runner's routine and shoes should be investigated to eliminate uneven surfaces, worn-out shoes, and muscle imbalance. The client should begin quadriceps-stretching exercises and then graduated weight-resistive exercises (see Plan for Prevention and Rehabilitation of Knee Injuries). These maintain and ultimately improve the strength and stabilizing effects of the vastus medialis.

Chondromalacia patellae denotes a condition of pain arising from a cartilaginous abnormality on the posterior surface of the patella. Theoretically, the lesion undergoes three phases: (1) localized cartilage softening, swelling, and fibrillation, with yellowing and loss of brightness; (2) the appearance of an area of fragmentation and fissuring; and (3) erosion of the cartilaginous pieces (Bandi, 1977). Studies show that 40% to 50% of the runners who seek treatment for knee problems have this condition (Baumann, 1978; Cailliet). Some authors attest to the young (under age 25) athlete's propensity to develop chondromalacia. However, data from autopsy investigations indicate that abnormal asymptomatic chondromalacia appears with increasing frequency as age increases and that by age 35 everyone has abnormal cartilage (Baumann).

The etiology of chondromalacia patellae is complex. Most practitioners agree that an external cause is usually necessary to transform a latent asymptomatic condition into a symptomatic, painful one. However, histological examinations reveal that endogenous mechanical factors of the knee joint can precipitate the pain. In addition, the cartilage is avascular and relatively free of sensory nerves. Therefore, a secondary synovitis is the primary cause of pain (Bandi).

Similar clinical presentations may confuse chondromalacia patellae with peripatellar pain (runner's knee). Both conditions have a history of anterior knee pain that worsens during and after a period of increased running. What distinguishes chondromalacia patellae are four additional clinical features: (1) the occasional history of a direct blow to the knee in months or years in the past, (2) a retropatellar pain elicited during flexion and extension of the knee by the gentle pressing of the patella against the femoral condyle, (3) a retropatellar pain accompanied by a sensation of grating or crepitation when gentle pressure is exerted over the patella, and (4) a history of momentary knee locking (James and others).

Physical examination must include the entire range of leg and knee maneuvers. The alignment of the client's legs should be viewed anteriorly and laterally to determine whether the anatomical variations mentioned above are present. Particular attention should be paid to the patella's position throughout flexion, neutral position, and extension maneuvers. The practitioner should look for patellar instability and patella alta and, additionally, for excessive pronation of the foot and its causes. With the client's knee in full extension, valgus and varus stress is placed over the tibial condyles. Abnormal lateral movement indicates tibiofemoral instability. Joint stability is determined by performing this same maneuver with the knee in 30 to 40 degrees of flexion. Finally, meniscial involvement is determined by performing McMurray's test. It is unusual for the menisci to cause retropatellar pain. However, because of the anatomical proximity and similar clinical presentation of meniscial injuries, it is not unusual for both to occur simultaneously (Smillie). In pure chondromalacia patellae McMurray's test and maneuvers for stability are rarely positive. X-ray results in the early stages of chondromalacia patellae are normal. Even in advanced stages the only abnormal finding may be an irregular posterior surface on the lateral x-ray view.

The number and frequency of locking episodes usually determine the treatment for chondromalacia patellae. When there are no episodes, therapy initially consists of correcting structural instabilities of the foot with orthotics and a good running shoe. Depending on the degree of pain, reducing mileage and restricting running are important. In addition to restriction of running, isometric quadriceps exercises are done until pain decreases to occasional episodes upon stress. Then weight-resistive exercises are introduced. The other treatment of choice is operative. Data substantiate that surgical correction of the underlying cause, such as patella alta or traumatic damage, greatly improves the prognosis (Bandi). Thus orthopedic referral for consideration of surgery is necessary if the pain interferes with activities of daily living or if the symptoms are severe or unresponsive to treatment and exercise (Smillie).

ASSESSMENT AND PLAN FOR PROBLEMS IN THE MEDIAL AND LATERAL COMPARTMENTS

The medial and lateral compartments house the most important biomechanical structures of the knee. The soft tissues (ligaments, muscle-tendon units, capsule, and menisci) produce an engineering phenomenon yet to be duplicated in machines. The interrelationships of ligaments and muscle-tendon units maintain the integrity and stability of the joint to such a fine balance that ascribing specific functions to any ligament is difficult. However, from a clinical viewpoint, importance of the ligaments becomes clearer. The medial collateral ligament is a frequent site of minor injuries. The anterior and posterior cruciate ligaments, although not directly involved in most running injuries, may stabilize the joint with meniscus injury. Likewise, the muscle-tendon units of the quadriceps and hamstrings depend on all of the ligaments for stability during movement.

Excessive stretching produces injuries to the muscle-tendon units and ligaments of the knee. Each structure within the medial and lateral compartments has a specific functional range of stretch. Exceeding this range produces varying degrees of injuries. In 1966 the Subcommittee on Classification of Sports Injuries of the American Medical Association classified *strains* as muscle-tendon unit injuries and *sprains* as ligamentous injuries (Craig, 1973). As noted in Tables 2-2 and 2-3, there are similarities between a strain and a sprain. However, the classification system cited above is helpful in determining the severity of an acute injury.

A detailed account of the circumstances of an injury helps to differentiate whether it is a strain or a sprain and to determine its severity. Because the majority of runners have an overuse syndrome, the most important assessment data are running history, training routines, training equipment, and complete bilateral leg examination. In most cases this evaluation establishes a definite diagnosis.

Tendinitis

To most beginning runners and even some "ultramarathoners," tendinitis is a nemesis. It occurs before the tendon thickens and strengthens enough to tolerate the stress

Table 2-2. Strains

Diagnosis	Cause	Symptoms	Signs	Pathological changes	Sequelae
First degree	Trauma to a portion of the musculotendinous unit from excessive, forcible stretch (e.g., increased running distance from 5 to 12 miles)	Sharp, localized pain aggravated by movement or tension of the particular unit; interference with endurance	Local tenderness and swelling; mild muscle spasm; ecchymosis probably within fibers and not seen for days, if at all; no loss of joint function or muscle strength	Local mild inflammation; disruption of a few fibers	Chronic tendinitis, periostitis; recurrent strains
Second degree	Trauma from violent contraction or excessive, forcible stretch (e.g., abrupt stop while running full speed)	Localized pain aggravated by movement or tension of the unit	Moderate to diffuse swelling and muscle spasm; localized tenderness; impaired muscle function and strength; ecchymosis	Torn fibers without disruption	Calcification at muscle origin or tendon insertion; permanent disability
Third degree	Exogenous force in addition to violent contraction or excessive, forcible stretch (e.g., abrupt stop while running)	Immediate severe pain and disability	Usually immediate severe spasm, swelling, ecchymosis, hematoma; loss of muscle function; usually a palpable gap or bulge	Complete rupture of muscle or tendon; may have an avulsed fracture at tendinous attachment	Permanent disability

Table 2-3. Sprains (acute ligamentous injuries)

Diagnosis	Cause	Symptoms	Signs	Pathological changes	Sequelae
First degree	Abnormal motion of joint (e.g., tripping over curbstone while walking)	Initial pain with injury; then relatively pain-free thereafter	Mild point tenderness over ligament; little or no localized swelling; joint stable; no functional loss or abnormal motions	A few fibers torn; small hemorrhage	Recurrence
Second degree	Abnormal excessive motion of joint; may be combined with exogenous trauma (e.g., fall while running)	Initial pain with injury and pain with movement (mild to severe)	Point tenderness over ligament; pain elicited with joint stress evaluations; more diffuse swelling; ecchymosis; no abnormal motion in any direction	Partial tear, at least ½ of fibers intact; hemorrhage localized or more diffuse	Recurrence; persistent instability; possible progressive degenerative changes of joint
Third degree	Abnormal, excessive motion of joint; violent exogenous trauma (e.g., side block to flexed knee)	Pain; immediate and continued loss of function	Marked tenderness, swelling, and hemorrhage; possible deformity of joint; marked abnormal motion with minimal stress maneuvers	Complete tear of the ligament, with or without bony fragment	Persistent instability and disability

and the repetitious motions of running. Inflammation may occur in any of the tendons surrounding the knee joint. More commonly involved are the quadriceps tendon, patellar tendon, hamstring tendons, pes anserinus tendons, and gastrocnemius muscle (Fig. 2-3).

The running history of a client with tendinitis usually indicates either a change of running surface (such as hills or hard concrete or pavement) or a 20% to 50% increase in the daily or weekly running distance. If the runner is a relative beginner, increased stress occurs before the tendons and muscles have time to accommodate. The more advanced runner often adds or increases the frequency of speed work involving sprints. In either case, the stress exceeds the stretching potential of the muscle-tendon unit. A description of the runner's warm-up and cool-down regimens may reveal inadequate stretching or overstrengthening of the unit involved. The hamstrings as well as the gastrocnemius and soleus muscles are much stronger than their antagonists, the quadriceps muscles. This muscle imbalance establishes a risk for more severe injury. The runner diagnoses and manages most first-degree strains. It is the injury's recurrence and increasing interference with running that finally prompt the runner to seek treatment.

Initially, if the signs and symptoms of the tendinitis are similar to those of first-degree strains, symptomatic treatment should be offered. This includes applying ice within the first 24 to 48 hours and reducing swelling with a compression bandage. Ten grains of aspirin 4 times a day for 3 days may reduce inflammation. Thereafter, the client applies moist heat to the knee, especially during the warm-up. In addition, the client institutes stretching and strengthening exercises for the injured unit and its antagonists for correction of muscle imbalance. The running routine and regimen should be restructured to remove the stress-producing portion. This allows continuation of running without further injury. This regimen is individualized according to the runner's goals and present running distances, speed, and ability. Generally, a gradual progression of distance is emphasized. For example, I recommend no more than a 10% to 15% increase in distance each week. Alternating hard and easy days is encouraged, and "grinning and bearing the pain" is discouraged.

When the tendinitis is more severe and parallels a second-degree strain, the aim of treatment is protection of the injured knee and prevention of further damage. A second-degree strain and more severe tendinitis represent a problem with compliance because most runners want to continue running. However, only complete rest allows approximation of fibers for normal healing and prevents scarring and calcification or ossification. Depending on the individual and unit involved, an orthopedist may splint, apply a compression bandage, or apply a cylinder cast until the acute symptoms subside (3 to 4 weeks). If the onset of the swelling occurred immediately with the pain, a hematoma is probable and the orthopedist may aspirate for pain relief and fluid examination.

If the runner's history includes frequent episodes of tendinitis and a clinical picture similar to a second-degree strain, early rupture of the unit should be considered. Another consideration is an avulsed fracture of the tibia, which may be difficult to identify by x-ray examination. It is best to promptly refer the client for further evaluation and possible surgery.

Ligamentous injuries

The classification, assessment, and management of ligamentous problems compose the most complex, enigmatic aspect of sports injuries. In order to overcome the confusion regarding these injuries, the Committee on Research and Education of the American Orthopaedic Society for Sports Medicine, in July 1977, formulated a classification of knee joint instabilities. This model attempts to describe the instability in terms of the direction of tibial displacement and the ligamentous deficits elicited with various stress maneuvers. When using this classification, one must remember that the degree of trauma as well as the degree of instability determines the degree of injury. In chronic injuries the degree of instability is more important because little acute trauma occurs. The overall categories of the classification include: (1) one-plane instabilities—medial, lateral, anterior, and posterior; (2) rotary instabilities—anteromedial, anterolateral, posterolateral, and posteromedial; and (3) combined rotary instabilities—anterolateral-postereolateral, anterolateral-anteromedial, and posteromedial.

One-plane instabilities are evaluated by two classic stress maneuvers: the abduction/adduction stress tests and the drawer sign. The first maneuver, abduction/adduction stress tests, measures lateral and medial instabilities, respectively. To perform the abduction stress test, varus stress is placed on the tibia with the knee in nearly complete extension and the ankle stabilized. A noticeable gap palpable in the lateral joint line represents a major instability. The structures involved are the fibular collateral ligament, lateral capsular ligament, anterior cruciate ligament, arcuate popliteus complex, and biceps tendon. With the knee in 30 degrees of flexion the same maneuver is performed. Positive results indicate laxity, with or without a complete tear of the fibular collateral ligament (Muller, 1977). The adduction stress test is performed with the client's knee in the same position, but valgus stress is placed on the tibia. The tibia moving away from the femur in extension represents another major instability. Involved are the medial (or tibial) collateral ligament, medial capsular ligament, anterior cruciate ligament, posterior oblique ligament, and medial portion of the posterior capsule. All varus and valgus instabilities with a gap of 25 mm or more indicate a cruciate ligament tear (Hertel and Schweiberer). With the knee in 30 degrees of flexion, only the medial capsular ligament and medial (or tibial) collateral ligaments are involved. Lack of appreciable rotary instability verifies involvement of the medial capsular ligament and medial collateral ligament.

To evaluate posterior and anterior instabilities the drawer sign maneuver is performed. With the client supine, the knee flexed at a 90-degree angle, and the foot flat on the table, the tibia is pushed backward (posterior sign) and then is pulled forward (anterior sign). A positive anterior or posterior drawer sign demonstrates a lesion of the corresponding cruciate ligaments and lesion of at least one lateral ligament (Hertel and Schweiberer). A positive anterior sign is more common because the incidence of damage to the anterior cruciate ligament is higher than that to the posterior cruciate ligament. A positive anterior or posterior sign is tibial movement greater than 1 cm in the corresponding direction (DeGowin and DeGowin, 1969). A few degrees of tibial movement are normal as long as there is equal movement on the opposite knee. Rotary maneuvers provide additional information concerning the involvement of specific structures.

Rotary and combined rotary instabilities are evaluated with a variation of the drawer sign, the rotary drawer sign. During this test the client's knee is kept in a semiflexed position and the foot in 15 degrees of external rotation. Then posterior or anterior force is smoothly applied to the tibia. Anteromedial rotary instability exists when the medial tibia plateau rotates anteriorly, with a medial opening of the joint line. The structures involved are the medial capsular ligament, medial (or tibial) collateral ligament, posterior oblique ligament, and anterior cruciate ligament. This is the most sensitive test for revealing an isolated tear of the medial capsular ligament when there is one-plane instability in knee extension and the anterior cruciate ligament is intact (Hertel and Schweiberer). With anterolateral instability, the lateral tibia plateau rotates forward with excessive lateral opening of the joint line. Involved are the lateral capsular ligament, arcuate ligament complex, and anterior cruciate ligament. Posterolateral instability is similar to anteromedial instability, but there is posterior rotation of the tibia with a lateral opening. This instability involves the lateral capsular ligament, biceps tendon, anterior cruciate ligament, and arcuate ligament complex.

Description of the remaining combined rotary instabilities is simple. Violent trauma inflicted to the knee results in multiple tears in the medial, lateral, and posterior compartments. This renders the knee functionless for most sporting events (Muckle, 1978).

Acute ligamentous injuries. Most runners develop these injuries from falling while running over uneven surfaces or by catching their foot in a hole. Determining the ligaments involved and the extent of their injury requires careful reconstruction of the circumstances: Was the runner immediately disabled or able to continue? What was the quality of the initial pain? When did the swelling occur? What therapies were tried? Did the knee lock?

Different degrees of damage to the knee ligaments depend on the degree of stress and the position of the knee at the time of injury. The medial ligaments are the most commonly injured. The stability of these ligaments is evaluated by the adductor test, the anterior drawer sign, and the rotary drawer sign. However, determining which ligaments are involved is difficult. For the purpose of management, sprains are divided into first degree, second degree (partial tear), and third degree (complete tear, with or without bone fracture).

First-degree sprains are mild ligamentous injuries occurring at either the attachment to the bone or to its midsection. The joint is stable, and there is no blood in the joint or the soft tissue. Additionally, there is no effusion, locking, or pain on normal (gentle) range of motion.

Management is symptomatic and directed toward the prevention of sequelae. Immediate application of a compression bandage and ice may reduce any swelling. This is continued for 24 to 48 hours until acute symptoms abate and is followed with the application of moist heat, especially before running. The client may wear a compression bandage for 2 weeks or less. Immobilization is unnecessary, since it leads to decreased quadriceps strength and subsequent reinjury. The amount, time, and running distance depend on the individual runner. Initially, a 24-hour rest from running assists the healing process. Swimming is a substitute exercise, if the client tolerates only short running distances. The client begins active leg exercises for the hamstrings and quadriceps within 24 hours, followed by weight-resistive exercises. The progress of rehabilitation is rapid, with ligament healing anticipated within 14 days. More severe sprains necessitate orthopedic referral.

A second-degree sprain is a ligamentous injury that interferes with the strength of the ligament. This injury may involve only a few fibers to half of the ligamentous fibers. The signs and symptoms follow a pattern similar to that of a first-degree sprain but are more severe. There is joint swelling and possible ecchymosis in the soft tissues. The other positive findings include pain with duplication of the direction of force and position of the knee during injury, pain during any of the instability maneuvers, and muscle spasms. However, with gentle extension the flexion spasms will subside. The prominent finding is joint stability in any direction, including rotary. X-ray examination with multiple views rules out any possible fracture. Excluding concurrent meniscial injury is imperative especially if there is a history of locking and incomplete extension of the knee during examination. The goals of management are to safeguard the weakened joint structure and to prevent future injuries or disabilities. The duration of treatment varies. Some individuals would benefit by hospitalization, others by home therapy, and the majority by a combination of physical therapy and home care.

A client infrequently experiences a complete tear (third-degree sprain) from running. Although rare, this should always be a consideration when a ligamentous injury is being evaluated. The signs and symptoms of this type of injury are even more severe than those of first- and second-degree sprains. There is immediate disability and a sensation that the knee gave way or subluxed. Usually the runner needs assistance into the primary care site and is unable to bear weight on the injured knee. Hemarthrosis, swelling, and perhaps a deformity of the knee are evident. If present, instability is a confirmatory finding. However, a torn ligament, particularly the anterior cruciate, may not show any major instability. The treatment of choice is prompt surgical repair. A small percentage of othopedists use conservative treatment, but only rarely.

Chronic ligamentous injuries. Seasoned runners frequently present vague complaints of "loose knees" or "water on the knee." These symptoms occur when they begin new routines such as high-mileage training or anaerobic sprints. Occasionally, the beginning runner also develops these symptoms. The client's history usually reveals an old knee injury during adolescence or young adulthood. In most men the old injury occurred during a contact sport, such as football, basketball, or rugby. In women it more likely occurred during a fall or a car crash. In addition, treatment was inadequate or the rehabilitation program excluded a knee-strengthening regimen. The common terms for these problems are instability and chronic or idiopathic synovitis. These are not diagnoses but merely symptoms of an underlying problem.

Commonly reported ligaments of the chronic unstable knee are the medial (or tibial) collateral, the anterior cruciate, the posterior cruciate, and very rarely the lateral collateral ligament (Muckle; O'Donoghue). The principal complaint is a feeling that the knee may give way. As the laxity of the ligaments progresses, distance running becomes increasingly difficult. As ligament strength continues to deteriorate, the intervals of trouble-free running become shorter with possible difficulty in descending stairs or jumping down from heights. If a meniscus injury is also present, there may be a history of knee-locking episodes.

The physical examination reveals varying degrees of quadriceps wasting. Previously mentioned tests for joint stability show laxity of the involved ligament. Comparison with the normal knee verifies a small amount of instability. The practitioner should also search for signs of a meniscus tear. In most cases management of chronic instability involves referral to an orthopedist for reconstruction of the ligament. Most surgeons agree that reconstruction cannot make an unstable knee a normal one; at best it reduces the symptoms to a tolerable level.

The onset of the effusion in chronic, idiopathic synovitis occurs in association with unaccustomed activity, such as extra miles and the addition of sprints. The effusion develops over a matter of hours, but it may go unnoticed until the next morning. There is very little local heat, and pain varies according to the amount of distention of the synovial membrane. Paradoxically, as the frequency of these episodes increases, the pain decreases although the injury may be worsening.

In the physical examination the practitioner should compare the swollen knee with the normal one. There may be complete absence of the contours in the medial and lateral side or only slight irregularity. On palpation, recent serum effusion feels "boggy." Ballottement of the patella is possible in large effusions, but "milking" the suprapatellar pouch distally can reveal minor effusions. With hemarthrosis, palpation is usually more "doughy." Careful manipulation freely moves the leg through the complete range of motion. If there is a meniscial injury, a fixed flexion contracture of 10 to 40 degrees may be present. Pain accompanying the stress maneuvers may indicate the old injury.

The effusion of idiopathic synovitis is secondary to trauma. However, determining the etiology of any effusion is essential for treatment of the underlying cause. Evaluation of all historical data and clinical measurements are necessary before establishing the diagnosis of idiopathic synovitis secondary to trauma. Also, the epidemiological pattern for systemic diseases places the adult runner at risk. Although the effusion itself is not usually considered an emergency, prompt examination of synovial fluid is important. Examination of joint aspirates is an important factor in identifying systemic problems.

Despite the effusion, most runners will want to continue their running routines. It is imperative that they understand the importance of complying with referral for expert evaluation. Exclusion of a systemic or infectious condition is essential. Additionally, allowing the knee to remain distended can lead to enzymatic destruction of the articular cartilage (Puhl and Cotta, 1978). Also, studies show that adding strain to the joint before resolution of a simple effusion may result in a torn meniscus (Muckle, Smillie).

Meniscial injuries

Meniscial injuries are common to anyone participating in sports. Even everyday activities expose the menisci to vertical compression, horizontal deviation, and rotary forces sufficient to cause injury. Although these structures are relatively passive in their function, speculation is that injury to a meniscus may cause subsequent degenerative joint changes (Muckle).

Certain predisposing factors enchange the mechanism of injury. After age 30 the risk of injury increases. Necessary nutritional substances in the joint are thought to break down at this time. Because the blood vessels are only in the periphery and nutritional metabolism depends on the interfacing synovial fluid, interference with this pathway can cause degenerative or trauma-induced changes (Smillie).

In most healthy adults anatomical variations can produce increased risk of injury when running. This is particularly true of runners with genu valgum, varum, and recurvatum outside the normal range (Smillie). This risk further increases with laxity of the ligaments and poor muscle tone of extensor and flexor muscles. Therefore, the likelihood of meniscus injury increases for beginning runners and for those without a balanced program of stretching and strengthening exercises.

Even in the acute meniscial injury signs and symptoms are quite vague. Pain, a prominent feature, localizes to the medial or lateral joint line of the affected meniscus. The aching discomfort may be deep or localized to the contralateral side of the injury (Smillie). Typically when a meniscus tears extensively, it may displace and cause locking. A locked knee usually flexes but will not fully extend; occasionally a muscle spasm interferes with both. If there is a history of locking but none is evident on examination, this sign should heighten concern of both a torn meniscus and a torn cruciate ligament.

Frequently there is a history of the knee giving way. Although there are multiple causes for this symptom, by far the most common is a torn meniscus. If the cause is insufficiency of the quadriceps or cruciate ligament, the symptom occurs on descending stairs or jumping down from a height. When the cause is a torn meniscus, the symptom is the result of a simple sudden turn or walking on an uneven surface.

In a meniscial injury the vastus medialis muscle is smaller in the injured knee. This results in a 1- to 2-mm difference in the girth of the quadriceps muscle, usually because of the loss of full extension. Also, results of McMurray's test and Apley's test are positive.

McMurray's test is performed with the client supine. The practitioner stands next to the affected knee and flexes it until the knee touches the buttock. The foot is rotated laterally; then the knee is extended to a 90-degree angle. The click of a torn meniscus can be felt and heard.

The client lies prone for Apley's test. The practitioner stands next to the affected knee, flexes the knee to 90 degrees, and rotates the foot laterally. While holding this position, the practitioner presses downward on the sole of the foot. This causes compression of the tibial condyles on the femoral condyles. Pain indicates a medial meniscus tear. Physical findings are not the only indicators for referral. The prime reason for referral is the history of locking or repeated episodes of giving way, or both.

PLAN FOR PREVENTION AND REHABILITATION OF KNEE INJURIES

All but a few injuries are preventable. The most convincing evidence of that comes from veteran runners, who sustain far fewer injuries than the beginning runner. It is critical for all runners to understand that running does not provide flexibility. Running chiefly strengthens the posterior leg muscles and leaves their antagonists relatively weak. To prevent these imbalances, which can produce or exacerbate injuries, a primary care provider should encourage a routine program of stretching and strengthening exercises.

Stretching exercises

Figs. 2-7 through 2-13 provide a sample program of stretching exercises. Most of the stretching exercises illustrated here pattern hatha yoga asanas (Iyengar, 1977). This program does not follow the traditional asanas order and is not a full catalogue of possible positions. The practitioner can incorporate the following principles into any stretching program to prevent overstretching and possible subsequent injuries:

1. Demonstrate these exercises for the runner who has never done stretching exercises before.
2. Each exercise is divided into phase 1 (prestretch) and phase 2 (stretch).
3. Do each exercise *slowly* and at the runner's own pace.

48 *Problems with alterations in comfort*

4. Never hold the breath. Breathe slowly and deeply through the nostrils. Time inspiration during phase 1, before the stretch, and expiration as the runner moves into the stretch, or phase 2.
5. Hold the stretch position from 5 to 30 seconds. Continue to breathe while holding the position. Repeat the stretch 3 to 5 times.
6. Remind the runner that not everyone initially achieves all the stretches.
7. Do not force the stretch positions either by jerking or by bouncing.
8. Do all stretches daily before running.

Suggested stretching exercises
QUADRICEPS

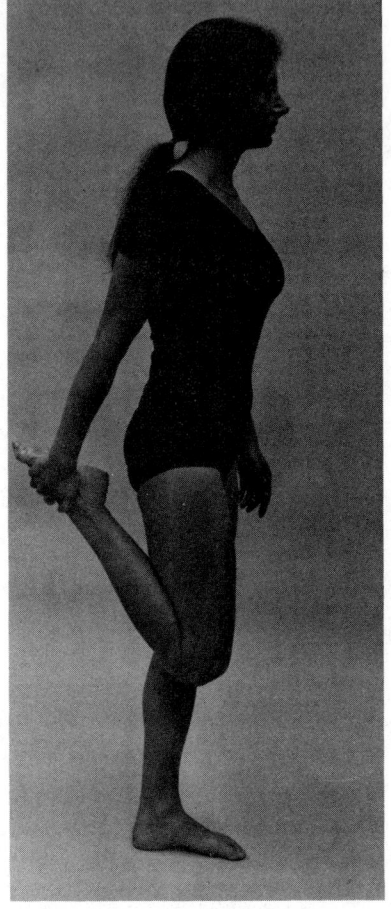

Fig. 2-7

Phase 1 (Fig. 2-7)
1. Stand erect or lie in the prone position; use a wall for balance if necessary.
2. Flex the knee and hold this position by grasping the ankle.
3. Bring the heel toward the buttocks slowly.

Phase 2
4. Extend the knee slowly toward the back, keeping the back straight and the opposite foot planted.
5. Hold the stretch 5 to 30 seconds. Repeat 3 to 5 times.
6. Repeat this sequence with the opposite leg.

HAMSTRINGS

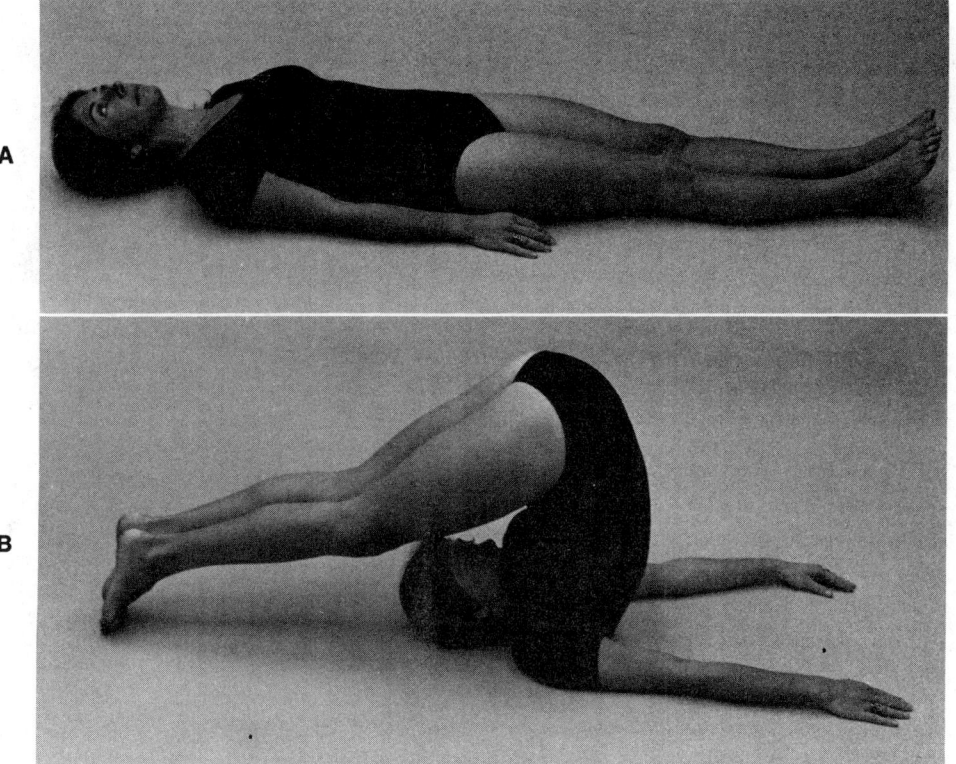

Fig. 2-8

Phase 1 (Fig. 2-8, *A*)
1. Lie supine.
2. Flex the hips with the knees extended, bringing both legs above the hips.
3. Continue slowly moving the legs in an arc over the head.

Phase 2 (Fig. 2-8, *B*)
4. With legs parallel, lower the toes to the ground.
5. If back, neck, or leg discomfort occurs, do not continue. Also, separate the knees and legs in a split position to ease discomfort.
6. Hold the position for 5 to 30 seconds. Do not tense in the hold position; relax all muscles. Repeat 3 to 5 times.
7. Reverse the movement to return to the supine position. Flexed knees ease the return.

50 *Problems with alterations in comfort*

HAMSTRINGS—cont'd

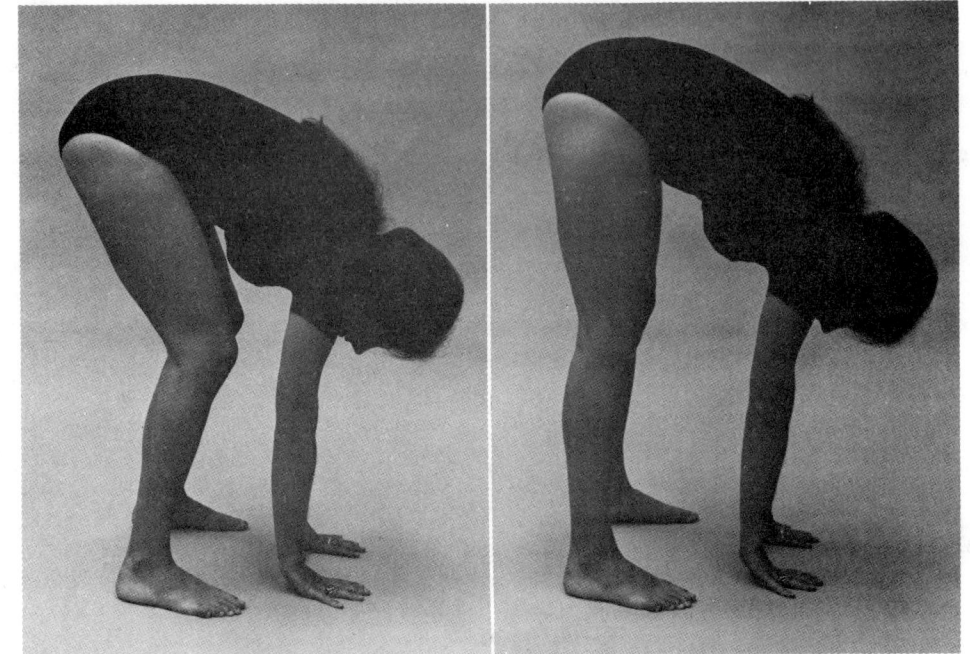

Fig. 2-9

Phase 1 (Fig. 2-9, *A*)
  1. Stand erect and flex at the waist.
  2. Flex the knees.
  3. Place the palms (or fingers) flat on the ground.
Phase 2 (Fig. 2-9, *B*)
  4. Slowly straighten the knees.
  5. Hold the position 5 to 30 seconds. Repeat 3 to 5 times.

HAMSTRINGS

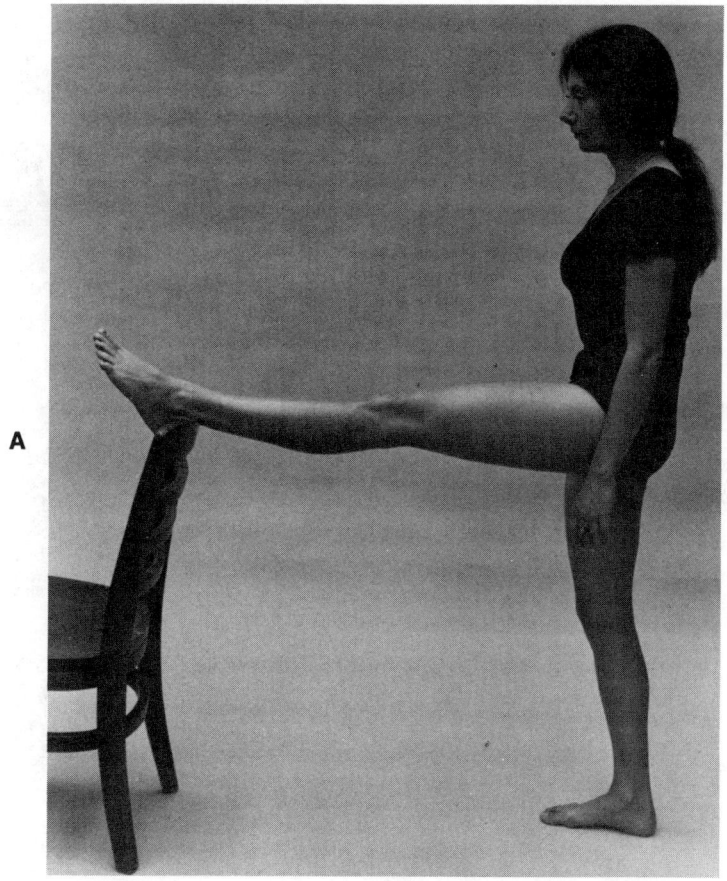

Fig. 2-10 *Continued.*

Phase 1 (Fig. 2-10, *A*)
1. Stand erect; place the heel on a waist-high table or chair.
2. The elevated leg is at a right angle to the opposite leg.

HAMSTRINGS—cont'd

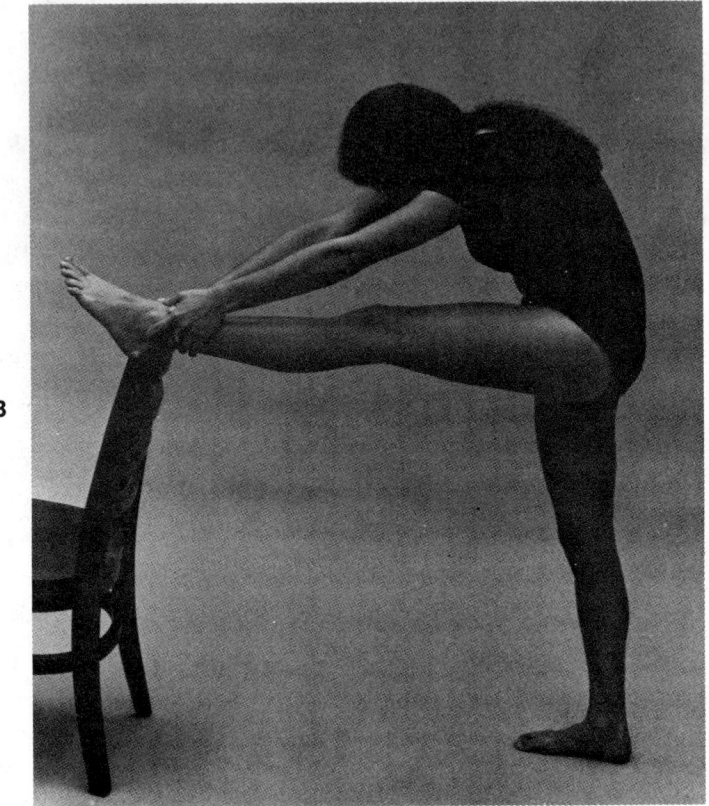

Fig. 2-10, cont'd

Phase 2 (Fig. 2-10, *B*)
   3. Flex at the waist and grasp the elevated ankle with both hands.
   4. Bring the nose toward the elevated knee.
   5. Hold the position 5 to 30 seconds. Repeat 3 to 5 times.

GASTROCNEMIUS AND ACHILLES TENDON

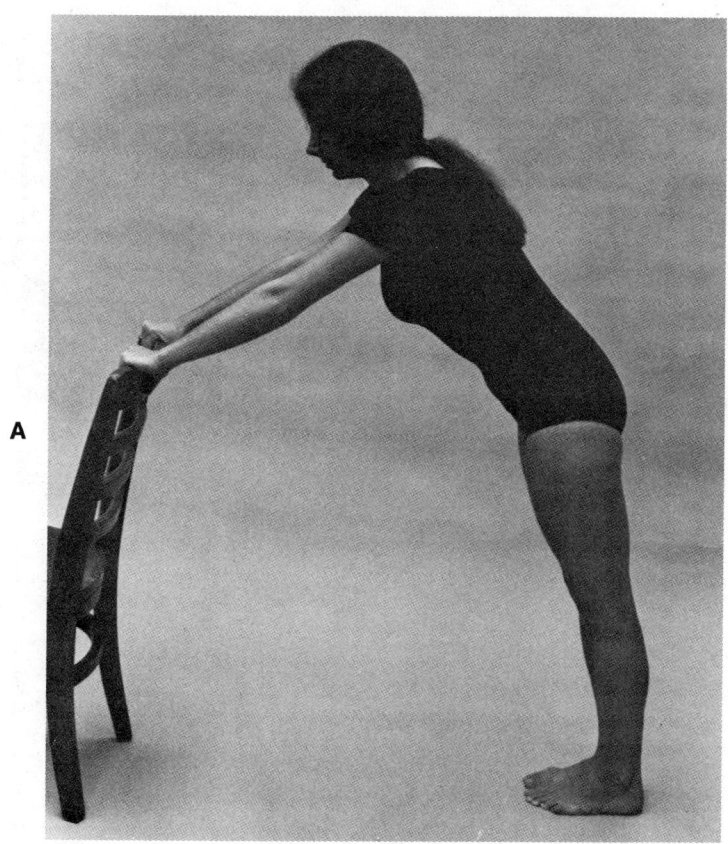

Fig. 2-11

Continued.

Phase 1 (Fig. 2-11, *A*)
1. Place the palms flat on the wall at shoulder height or grasp a chairback.
2. Move away from the wall or chair until the heels begin to lift.

54 *Problems with alterations in comfort*

GASTROCNEMIUS AND ACHILLES TENDON—cont'd

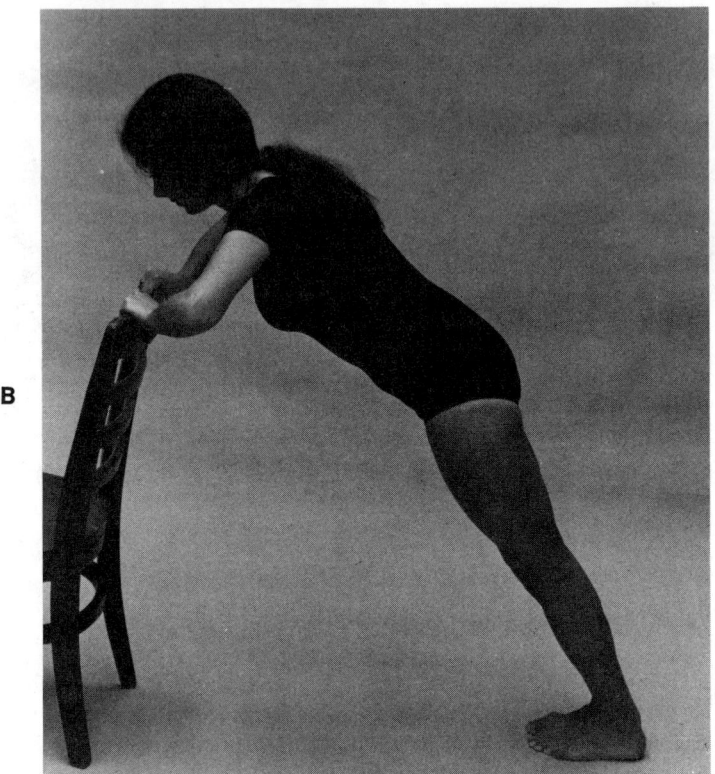

Fig. 2-11, cont'd

Phase 2 (Fig. 2-11, *B*)
   3. Flex at the elbows; keep them down.
   4. Bring the nose to the wall (or as close as comfortable) slowly.
   5. Hold the position 5 to 30 seconds. Repeat 3 to 5 times.

ABDUCTOR MUSCLES

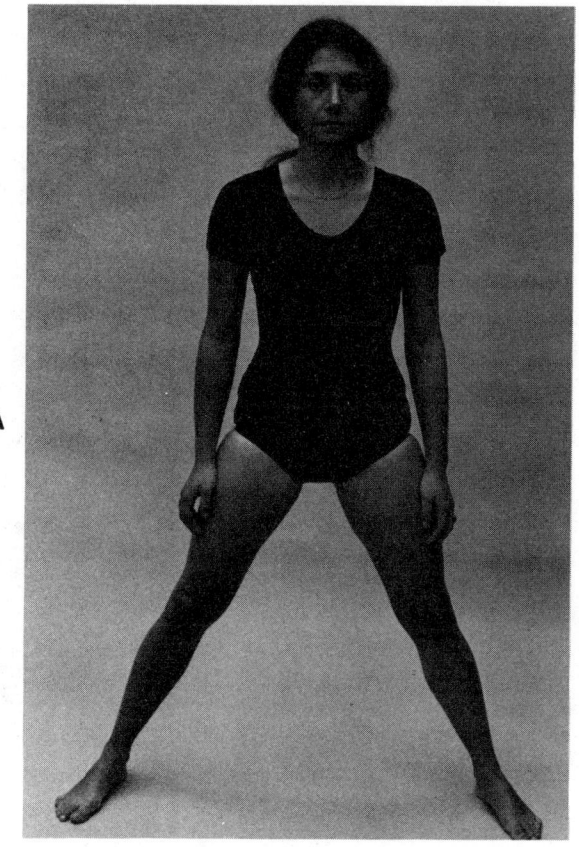

Fig. 2-12

Continued.

Phase 1 (Fig. 2-12, *A*)
1. Stand erect and spread the legs apart to a comfortable split.
2. Keep the knees extended with the toes pointing forward.

56 *Problems with alterations in comfort*

ABDUCTOR MUSCLES—cont'd

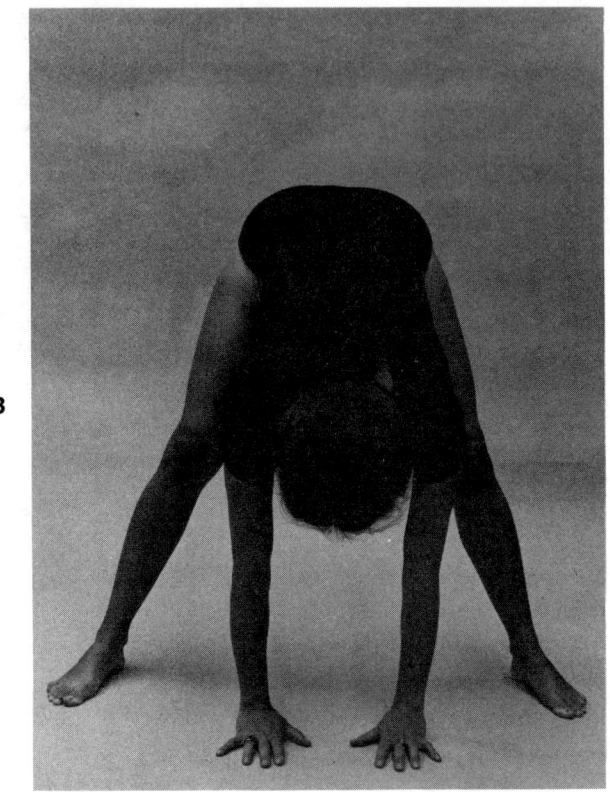

Fig. 2-12, cont'd

Phase 2 (Fig. 2-12, *B*)
   3. Flex at the waist.
   4. Place the hands on the floor; keep the knees extended.
   5. Slowly spread the feet farther apart to a comfortable position.
   6. Hold the position 5 to 30 seconds. Repeat 3 to 5 times.

ABDUCTOR MUSCLES

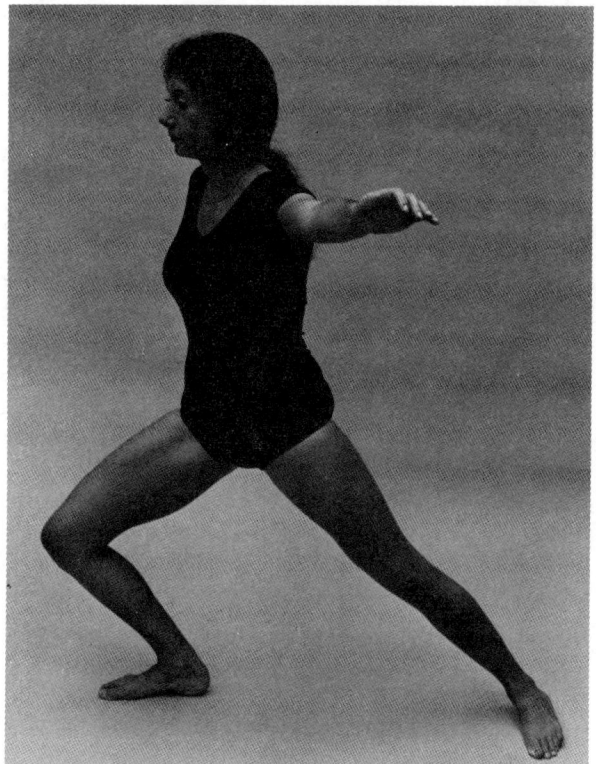

Fig. 2-13

Phase 1 (Fig. 2-13)
1. Stand erect, the forward foot pointing ahead.
2. Keep the rear foot at a right angle, with the entire sole flat on the floor.
3. Move the feet apart to a comfortable stretch.

Phase 2
4. Slowly flex the knee of the front foot to a 90-degree angle.
5. Look forward, using the arms as balance.
6. Hold the position for 5 to 30 seconds. Repeat 3 to 5 times.

See also isometric quadriceps exercises.

Strengthening exercises

Isometric and resistive exercises strengthen the quadriceps and abductor muscles of the legs. The use of weights is optional. The individual should gradually progress from isometric exercises to weight-resistive exercises.

Some seasoned runners with healthy knees can begin with weight-resistive exercises to strengthen the quadriceps muscles. Initially the runner does these exercises daily for both legs. The client sits on the edge of a table that is taller than waist high. The client performs each weight-resistive exercise slowly and for 3 sets of 10 to 15 repetitions. A high number of repetitions with low weight resistance increases the endurance but not the strength of the muscles. Muscles only strengthen when brought to the point of fatigue; in the vernacular, they "burn."

The initial amount of weight to use is usually determined through trial and error. The guiding principle is use of sufficient resistance to obtain the maximum effort of the muscle. For most sedentary people, 5 to 10 pounds is a safe beginning range, with a maximum weight of 45 pounds. Only one leg is weighted and exercised at a time. When the runner performs repetitions easily, an additional 1-pound weight can be added each day until the maximum is reached. Between each set of exercises the runner should rest the leg for 1 minute by laying it on a nearby chair. This removes the added traction on the quadriceps muscle when the knee is flexed. Once a program is begun, weight-resistive exercises can be done every day for a week, then every other day thereafter. If a swimming pool is available, walking in waist-high water in all directions simulates weight-resistive exercises. A 50-yard walk in the pool or a walk until the muscle group begins to quiver or burn is a good start.

Orthopedic consultation should be sought when exercises are used to rehabilitate an injured knee. Early consultation is necessary because exercises for rehabilitation should begin early to prevent further muscle atrophy. The exercises are modified according to the muscles involved, the extent of the injury, and the goal of the program.

Isometric strengthening exercise

QUADRICEPS

Phase 1 (Fig. 2-14, *A*)
1. Stand erect with the back flush to the wall.
2. Keep the feet parallel and away from the wall at a distance the length of the femur.

Phase 2 (Fig. 2-14, *B*)
3. Slowly slide down the wall.
4. Stop when the knees are at a right angle.
5. Hold the position 10 to 90 seconds or until a slight burning occurs in the muscle.
6. Keep a chair or table nearby to assist in returning to the starting position.
7. Repeat 3 to 4 times after a 1- to 2-minute rest.

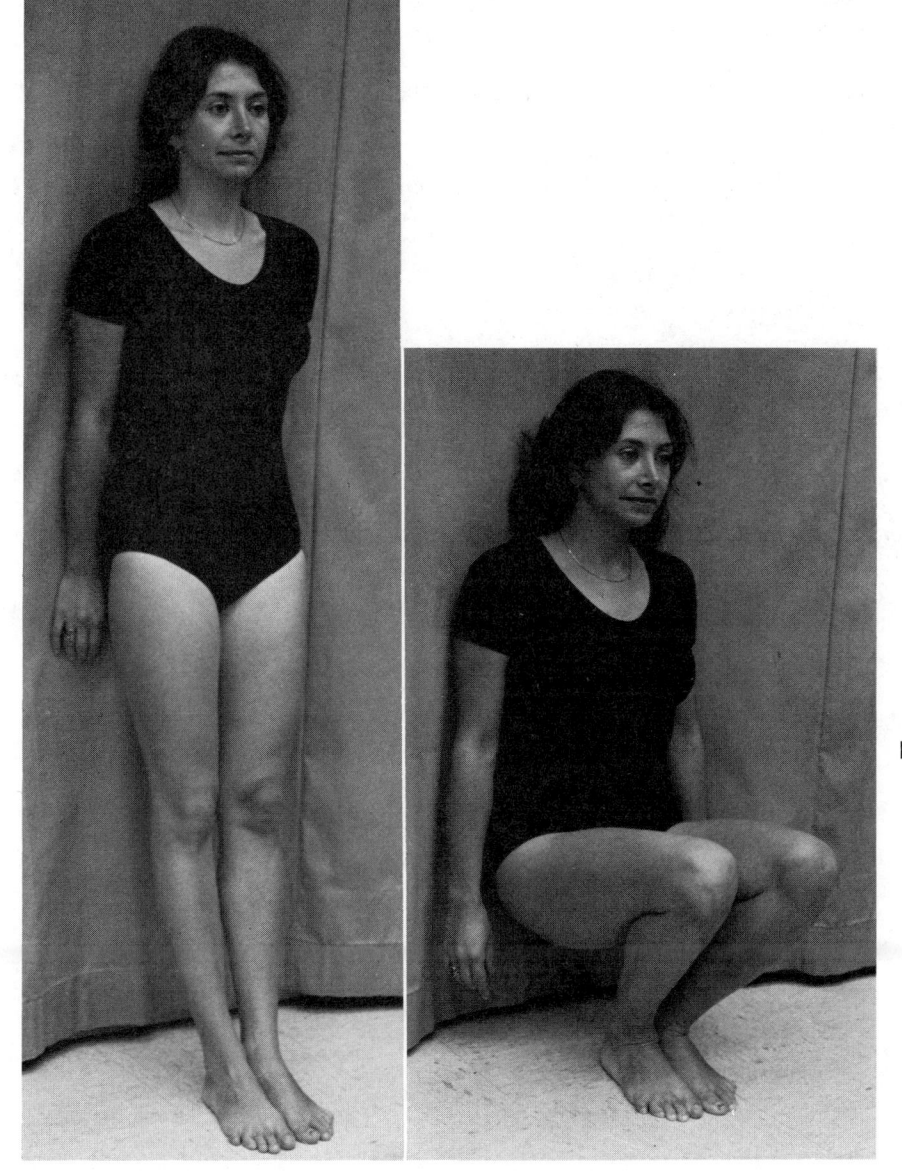

Fig. 2-14

60 *Problems with alterations in comfort*

Weight-resistive strengthening exercises
QUADRICEPS (EXTENSOR ACTION)
Phase 1 (Fig. 2-15, *A*)
 1. Lean backward at the waist, supporting the weight with the hands.
 2. Place a folded towel (3 to 4 inches thick) under the distal femur.

Phase 2 (Fig. 2-15, *B*)
 3. Fully extend the weighted leg and lock the knee.
 4. Hold for a count of 3 to 10 seconds.
 5. Slowly lower to the same count or longer.
 6. Repeat 30 times, resting 1 minute between each set of 10. Rest the weighted foot on a chair between each set of 10.
 7. Exercise the opposite leg.

Knee pain and injuries in the adult runner 61

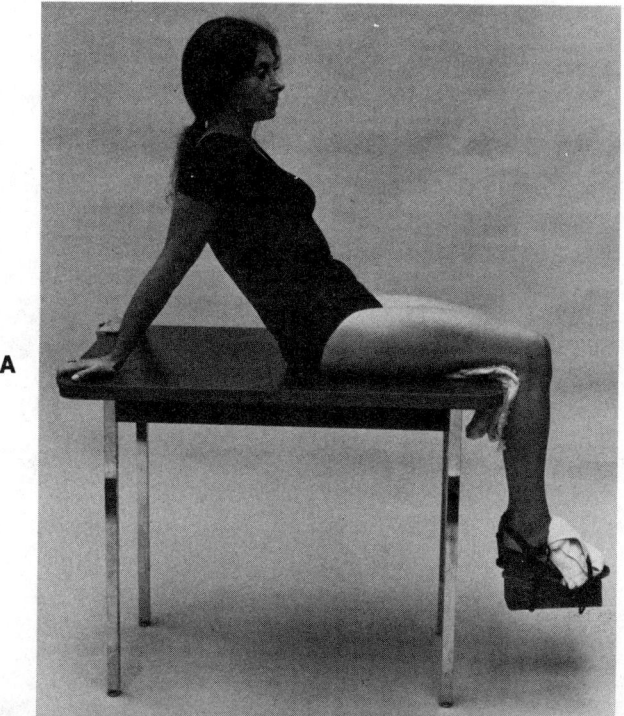

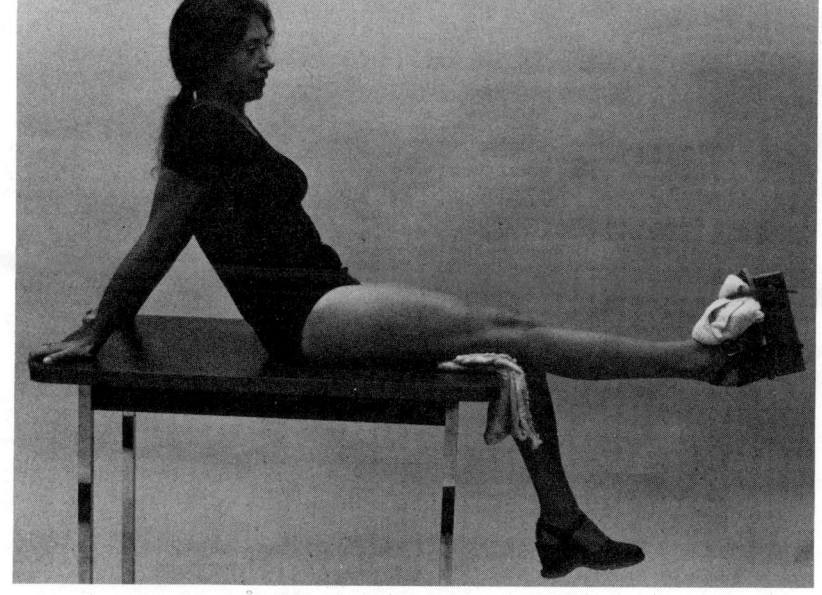

Fig. 2-15

QUADRICEPS (FLEXOR ACTION)

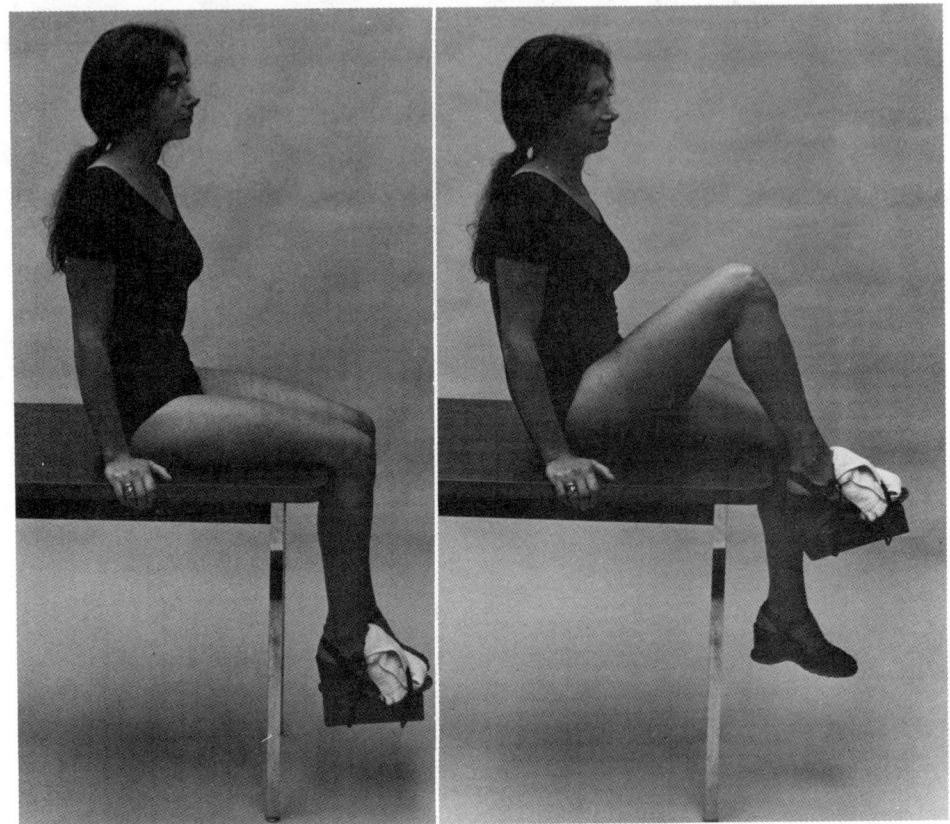

Fig. 2-16

Phase 1 (Fig. 2-16, *A*)
1. Sit, keeping the back straight.
2. Position the knees 1 inch from the table edge.

Phase 2 (Fig. 2-16, *B*)
3. Bring one knee toward the chest as high as possible.
4. Hold for a count of 3 to 10 seconds.
5. Slowly lower the knee to the same count.
6. Rest the weighted foot on a chair to release pulling action.
7. Repeat 30 times, resting 1 minute between each set of 10.

HAMSTRINGS

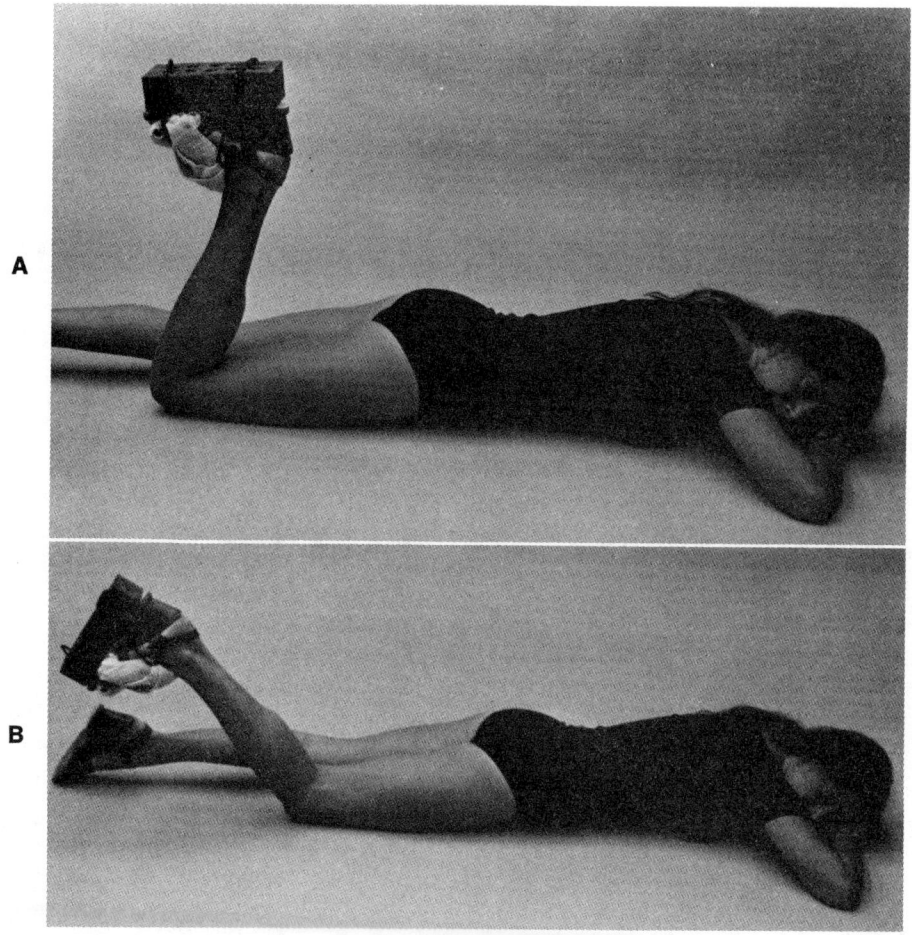

Fig. 2-17

Phase 1 (Fig. 2-17, *A*)
 1. Lie prone.
 2. Flex the knee, bringing the heel to the buttocks.
 3. Hold for a count of 3 to 10 seconds.
Phase 2 (Fig. 2-17, *B*)
 4. Slowly lower the knee to the same count.
 5. Repeat 30 times, resting 1 minute between each set of 10.

64 *Problems with alterations in comfort*

ABDUCTORS/ADDUCTORS

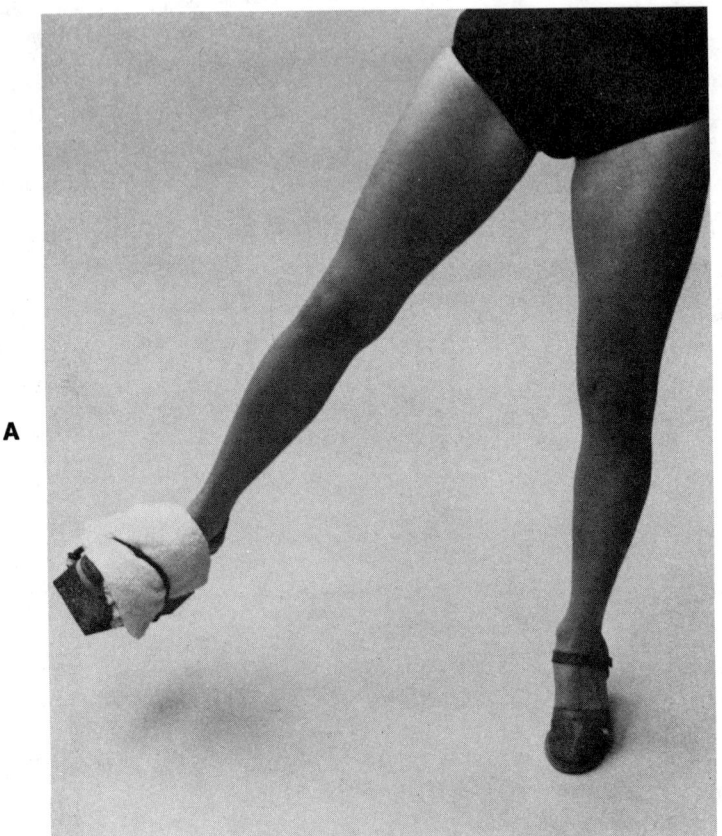

Fig. 2-18

Phase 1 (Fig. 2-18, *A*)
1. Either stand or lie supine.
2. Position the weighted foot 12 inches in front of the body.
3. Swing the foot out, abducting the leg as far as comfortable.

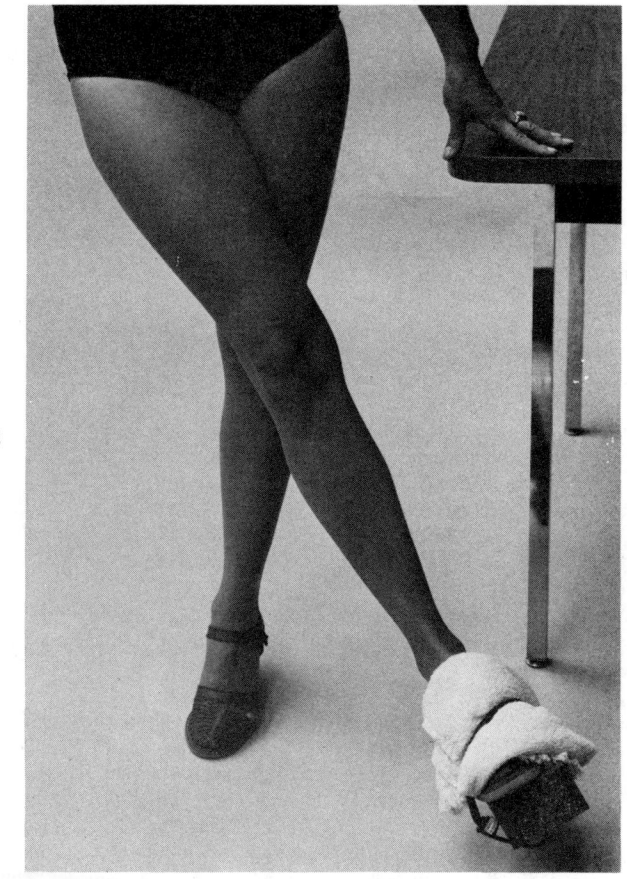

Fig. 2-18, cont'd

Phase 2 (Fig. 2-18, *B*)
    4. Hold for a count of 3 to 10 seconds.
    5. Slowly return the foot to the same count.
    6. Continue the return past the other foot.
    7. Repeat 30 times, resting 1 minute between each set of 10.

SUMMARY

Besides encouraging running to enhance physical and mental health, providers have a responsibility to caution the potential, beginning, and experienced runner. First, running has its risks; among them is temporary to permanent injury to the knee. Second, signs or symptoms of old or new knee injuries need immediate attention for diagnosis and treatment. Finally, stretching and strengthening exercise programs can prevent imbalances of the leg muscles that produce new injuries or exacerbate old ones.

REFERENCES

American Academy of Orthopaedic Surgeons: Atlas of orthotics: biomechanical principles and application, St. Louis, 1975, The C.V. Mosby Co.
American Orthopaedic Association: Manual of orthopaedic surgery, Chicago, 1972, The Association.
Bandi, W.: Trauma-induced chondromalacia patellae. In Hungerford, D.S., editor: The injured knee, New York, 1977, Springer-Verlag New York Inc.
Baumann, L.L.: Retinacular release: indication, technique, results. In Hastings, D.E., editor: The knee: ligament and articular cartilage injuries, New York, 1978, Springer-Verlag New York Inc.
Blazina, M.E., and others: Jumper's knee, Orthop. Clin. North Am. **4:**655, 1973.
Cailliet, R.: Knee pain and disability, Philadelphia, 1973, F.A. Davis Co.
Carpenter, M.: See Dick run! See Jane run! Sci. Digest **84:**8, Aug. 1978.
Colson, J.H., and Armour, W.J.: Sports injuries and their treatment, London, 1975, Stanley Paul & Co. Ltd.
Committee on Research and Education: Report, presented at the Third Annual Meeting of the American Orthopaedic Society for Sports Medicine, California, July, 1977.
Cooper, K.H.: Aerobics, New York, 1968, Bantam Books Inc.
Craig, T.T.: Comments in sports medicine, Chicago, 1973, American Medical Association.
DeGowin, E.L., and DeGowin, R.L.: Beside diagnostic examination, ed. 2, London, 1969, The Macmillan Press Ltd.
Editors of Runner's World: The complete runner, Mountain View, Calif., 1974, World Publications.
Fetto, J.F., and Marshall, D.V.M.: Medial collateral ligament injuries of the knee: a rational for treatment, Clin. Orthop. **132:**206, 1978.
Fixx, J.F.: The complete book of running, New York, 1977, Random House Inc.
Glinz, W.: Arthroscopy in articular cartilage injury. In Hastings, D.E., editor: The knee: ligament and articular cartilage injuries, New York, 1978, Springer-Verlag New York Inc.
Hertel, P., and Schweiberer, L.: The biomechanics and pathophysiology of knee ligaments. In Hastings, D.E., editor: The knee: ligament and articular cartilage injuries, New York, 1978, Springer-Verlag New York Inc.
Hoppenfeld, S.: Physical examination of the spine and extremities, New York, 1976, Appleton-Century-Crofts.
Hughes, J.L., and Hogue, R.E.: Basic rehabilitation principles of persons with leg length discrepancy: an overview. In Hungerford, D.S., editor: Leg length discrepancy, New York, 1977, Springer-Verlag New York Inc.
Huizinga, J.: Homo ludens: a study of the play element in culture, translated by R.F.C. Hill, London, 1949, Routledge & Kegan Paul.
Iverson, L.D., and Clawson, D.K.: Manual of acute orthopaedic therapeutics, Boston, 1977, Little, Brown & Co.
Iyengar, B.K.: Light on yoga, New York, 1977, Schocken Books Inc.
James, S.L., and others: Injuries to runners, Am. J. Sports Med. **6:**40, 1978.
Khasigian, H.A., and others: Body type and rotational laxity of knee, Clin. Orthop. **130:**228, 1978.
MacBryole, C.M., editor: Signs and symptoms: applied pathologic physiology and clinical interpretation, ed. 4, Philadelphia, 1964, J.B. Lippincott Co.
Mains, D.B., and others: Medial and anterior-posterior ligament stability of the human knee measured with a stress apparatus, Am. J. Sports Med. **5:**144, 1977.
Mangi, R., and others: The runner's complete medical guide, New York, 1979, Summit Books.
Mirkin, G., and Hoffman, M.: The sports medicine book, Boston, 1978, Little, Brown & Co.

Morscher, E.: Etiology and pathophysiology of leg length discrepancies. In Hungerford, D.S., editor: Leg length discrepancy, New York, 1977, Springer-Verlag New York Inc.
Muckle, D.S.: Injuries in sports, Bristol, 1978, John Wright & Sons Ltd.
Muller, W.: The knee joint of the soccer player. In Hungerford, D.S., editor: The injured knee, New York, 1977, Springer-Verlag New York Inc.
O'Donoghue, D.H.: Treatment of injuries to athletics, ed. 3, Philadelphia, 1976, W.B. Saunders Co.
Puhl, W., and Cotta, H.: The pathophysiology of damage to articular cartilage. In Hastings, D.E., editor: The knee: ligament and articular cartilage injuries, New York, 1978, Springer-Verlag New York Inc.
Ramamurti, C.P.: Musculoskeletal disorders. In Leitch, C.J., and Tinker, R.V., editors: Primary care, Philadelphia, 1978, F.A. Davis Co.
Reilly, D.T., and Martens, M.: Experimental analysis of the quadriceps muscle force and patello-femoral joint reaction force for various activities, Acta Orthop. Scand. **43:**126, 1972.
Ruttman, A., and Kieser, C.: The importance of arthrography following trauma to the knee joint. In Hungerford, D.S., editor: The injured knee, New York, 1977, Springer-Verlag New York Inc.
Sheehan, G.A., editor: Encyclopedia of athletic medicine, Mountain View, Calif., 1972, World Publications.
Sheehan, G.A.; Medical advice for runners, Mountain View, Calif., 1978, World Publications.
Smillie, I.S.: Injuries of the knee joint, ed. 5, Edinburgh, 1978, Churchill Livingstone.
Strauss, R.H.: Sports medicine and physiology, Philadelphia, 1979, W.B. Saunders Co.
Yocum, L.A.: The deranged knee: restoration of function, a protocol for rehabilitation of the injured knee, Am. J. Sports Med. **6:**51, 1978.

CHAPTER 3

Assessing headaches in the adult client: focus on migraine

Margaret Kruckemeyer

"Headache" commonly describes all pains of the head, face, and related structures. It is estimated that 42 million Americans seek care yearly to obtain relief from headaches (Diamond, 1979a). In addition, the United States has 20 million migraine and 100 million tension headache sufferers (Basmajian, 1979). However, the problems of headaches is not a new one. With the advent of written language were descriptions of the eye symptoms of migraine victims.

Headache is a symptom that demands identification of an underlying cause. This chapter presents the assessment of the client with headache. Emphasis is on the historical factors that differentiate the multiple causes of this complaint. Physiology, the plan of care, and the case study focus on migraine headaches, since this type of headache exemplifies a chronic problem requiring client teaching and knowledgeable self-care.

PHYSIOLOGY
Origin of head pain

Since the adult skull is a rigid structure, the space within it is strictly defined. Any change occurring within this space produces pain. Knowledge of the pain-sensitive structures within the cranium is essential to determine the factors producing and influencing headache. Pain-sensitive structures of the cranium fall into three categories: intracranial structures, extracranial structures, and nerves (Table 3-1). Direct stimulation of these pain structures by traction, distention, or dilation results in pain. The pain is transmitted mainly by the trigeminal nerve, the sensory pathway of the anterior two thirds of the posterior one third of the head. The most common cause of headache is alterations in the size of blood vessels within the skull. This particularly involves the extracranial arteries (Hannington, 1977).

Physiological factors in migraine

Etiology. Vascular headaches of the migraine variety result from dilation of the intracranial and extracranial arteries (Edmeads, 1979). This arterial dilation causes an excruciating, throbbing, pulsating head pain worsened by exertive efforts. Two factors pri-

Table 3-1. Causes of headache classified by areas of cranium and their pain-sensitive structures

Area	Pain-sensitive structure	Causes of headaches

Intracranial	Cranial sinuses and their tributaries
	Dural and cerebral arteries
	Parts of dura mater (in vicinity of large vessels)
		Traction
		   Space-occupying lesions (tumors, hematomas, abscesses, aneurysms)
		Dilation
		   Migraine, vasodilating agents (monosodium glutamate, nitrites, histamine, alcohol)
		   Metabolic factors (hypoxia, hypercapnia, hypoglycemia)
		   Drug reactions (foreign protein, caffeine withdrawal, carbon monoxide poisoning)
		   Hypertension, pyrexia
		Distention
		   Meningeal processes (meningitis, hemorrhage, encephalitis, post-lumbar puncture, post-pneumoencephalogram, head injury)

Extracranial	Skin, scalp, fascia, eye, nasal sinuses, teeth	Inflammation of cranial arteries (temporal arteritis) Diseases of eye (glaucoma, eyestrain, iritis) Diseases of ear, nose, throat (sinusitis, allergic rhinitis) Diseases of teeth (root abscess, temporomandibular joint dysfunctions) Diseases of neck (arthritis, cervical fibrositis, spondylitis) Trauma
Nerves	Trigeminal Facial Glossopharyngeal Vagus Second and third cervical	Excessive stimulation of trigeminal or glossopharyngeal nerves ("ice cream headache") Neuralgias (trigeminal—tic douloureux) Inflammation of nerves (tumor, aneurysm, central lesions—multiple sclerosis)
Other		Psychogenic (hypochondriasis, severe anxiety, severe depression, conversion reactions)

marily control vascular changes: the sympathetic nervous system and humoral substances such as the vasoconstrictors (serotonin, noradrenaline, adrenaline) and the vasodilators (neurokinin, bradykinin, histamine, and prostaglandin E_1) (Lance, 1978). Much research focuses on the interplay between these controlling factors and stress as the cause of vascular responses. Studies on migraine-prone individuals refer to triggering, or precipitating, factors and list sympathetic nervous system stimulants. These stimuli, whether external or internal, demand physiological adaptation. This usually occurs as a sympathetic nervous system response releasing catecholamines (Hannington, 1973). Any stimuli or substances that cause or mimic a change in catecholamine metabolism may trigger a migraine attack (see p. 70).

Trigger factors such as a change in eating patterns, fasting, excessive carbohydrate ingestion at one meal, or eating foods containing vasoactive amines may precipitate a migraine attack in a susceptible individual. There is controversy about the importance of tyramine, a vasoactive amine, in producing headaches. Some studies confirm, while others deny, that ingestion of tyramine (without monamine oxidase inhibitors) provokes

Trigger factors in migraine headaches

A. Physical/systemic
 1. Hypertension
 2. Local head and neck pains: muscle spasms, toothaches
 3. Sleep disturbances: overuse of sleeping pills, nightmares, insomnia
 4. Hormonal changes: menstruation, premenstrual period, menopause
 5. Fatigue: both mental and physical
 6. Overexertion: lifting heavy weights, straining with bowel movements, prolonged bending and stooping

B. Environmental
 1. Inclement weather: sudden changes in barometric pressure, e.g., thunderstorm
 2. Change of climate: hot and humid or hot, dry, windy conditions
 3. Loud noise: especially high-pitched constant sounds
 4. Bright lights: glare from sun or from artificial lighting, prolonged focusing on television or cinema screen, flickering disco lights

C. Foods
 1. Chicken livers, pickled herring, canned figs, nuts, pods of broad beans, cheese, chocolate, citrus fruits, fried foods, and pastries
 2. Additives: monosodium glutamate (MSG), nitrites (hotdogs, cured meats)
 3. Irregular eating habits: irregular mealtimes, irregular meals, dieting and fasting

D. Drugs
 1. Alcohol: especially wine
 2. Medications: oral contraceptive pills, vasodilating agents (histamine, marijuana)
 3. Overuse: vasoconstrictors, caffeine (coffee, tea, Coca-Cola), nicotine (tobacco), ergotamines (methysergide maleate [Sansert])

E. Psychosocial
 1. Stress or tension
 2. Psychosocial imbalance: anxiety, worry, depression, excitement, shock, anger, frustration, any other strong emotion

migraine headaches (Dalton, 1977). In the absence of conclusive data, clinicians have adopted a conservative approach recommending that foods and beverages containing vasoactive amines be eliminated from the diet of clients with migraine (Dalessio, 1979). A nationwide survey in England of food intake 24 hours before spontaneous migraine attack revealed ingestion of cheese by 40%, chocolate by 33%, alcohol by 23%, and citrus fruits by 23% (Dalton, 1977).

Stimulation of catecholamine release occurs during hypoglycemia. It also exerts a profound effect on the tone of the cranial blood vessels (Dalessio). Reactive hypoglycemia may occur after an excessive carbohydrate load and precipitate headaches in susceptible persons. Hypoglycemia also may occur during fasting or skipped meals. Dalton noticed that some migraine subjects experienced an attack after a 5-hour gap between daytime meals or an overnight gap exceeding 13 hours. Headaches resulting from fasting gaps seem dependent on the energy expenditure of the client. For example, a meal at 6:00 PM may be adequate unless the migraine sufferer follows it by strenuous exercise without additional food. Hannington (1973) believes that the unifying factor in the cause of migraine lies in a disturbance of amine metabolism. More research is necessary to explain such unanswered questions as:

Why does migraine tend to run in families?

Why do blood vessels in migraine sufferers appear to react to certain stimuli in a way that results in headache?

Why do women suffer from migraine attacks related to the timing of menses or ovulation?

What triggers the drop in blood levels of serotonin, a powerful vasoconstrictor, at the onset of a migraine attack?

Why do migraine attacks usually subside as one grows older?

Course of events during migraine. Many investigators consider the blood vessel changes in the cerebral and meningeal circulation to be the basis for the prodroma, course, symptoms, signs, and sequelae of the migraine attack (Lance). Backers of the vascular theory believe that the migraine attack has three phases: vasoconstriction, vasodilation, and edema. Some victims report that, before the onset of an attack, they experience symptoms which suggest a hypothalamic disturbance. These symptoms are euphoria or other mood changes, increased appetite and thirst, craving sweet things, or feeling drowsy.

In the first phase, vasconstriction of certain cranial arteries produces preheadache phenomena such as central visual disturbances, weakness, dizziness, or speech difficulties. After the vasoconstrictive phase, vasodilation and subsequent headache begin. There is documentation of a drop in serotonin levels during the vasodilation phase (Lance).

As vasodilation persists, the walls of the cranial arteries thicken and edema occurs in the surrounding tissues. Wolff (1972) isolated neurokinin from the edematous areas. This enzymelike bradykinin causes further vasodilation and enhances the permeability of the capillaries, which increases the edema. As the attack enters the edematous stage, the head pain becomes dull and steady. Some victims experience nausea, vomiting, dryness of the mouth, diaphoresis, or chilling. Following prolonged distention of the cranial arteries and prolonged pain, contraction of the skeletal muscles of the head and neck may occur. This causes further discomfort. The attack may continue for a few hours or for days.

In addition, the mechanism of migraines involves many factors that are not fully understood. It is clear, for example, that vasomotor disorders are not necessarily painful or demonstrated by the painless preheadache phenomena of migraine. Inflammatory reactions seem to contribute to the development of the associated pain. Researchers are becoming more aware of the relationship between pain and events related to inflammation, such as blood clotting and immune mechanisms.

ASSESSMENT

Perhaps one half of those seeking treatment for headaches are treated symptomatically without regard to diagnosis. Many do not recieve a careful history or neurological examination, which are the keys in determining the underlying cause of head pain (Diamond, 1979a).

History

The characteristics of the head pain (frequency, duration, location, quality, onset, associated symptoms, precipitating factors, relieving factors) are key points in the history. Table 3-2 uses these characteristics to differentiate the major causes of headaches. Note that, contrary to common belief, headaches are rarely caused by decreased visual acuity or oculomotor imbalances (Waters, 1970). Other aspects of the history include review of systems, past history, family history, and personal background data.

During the review of systems leading questions may be necessary. The practitioner should determine if the client has any specific problems that are known to cause headaches and involve the eyes, ears, nose, throat, teeth, or neck. For example glaucoma, tooth decay, sinusitis, otitis, or torticollis may be present. Additionally, specific questions should be asked about menses, ovulation, and pregnancy, and their connection to headaches. The menstrual-related migraine occurs just before, during, or after menses. It frequently occurs in menarchial females. It once was thought that progesterone was the triggering factor. However, it has been shown that the rise and fall of plasma estradiol levels before ovulation and menstruation seem to trigger the migraines. In one study it was noted that migraines began after the estradiol level fell below 20 μg after the preovulating peak and/or after the peak seen in the luteal phases before menstruation (Lance). Others support these findings (Kudrow, 1976). The prostaglandins, especially E_1, act on the uterus and may also have a role in triggering menstrual-related migraines. Carlson and associates (1968) showed that, when infused into normal subjects, prostaglandin E precipitated migraines. Oral contraceptives also have exacerbated migraine attacks and are contraindicated in clients having a migraine history. Lance and Anthony (1966) reported that 64% of the women who had migraine attacks linked with their menses became headache free during the time of their pregnancy.

During the review of systems the practitioner should search for organic problems, such as a space-occupying lesion. This cause can be suspected with recently developed headaches associated with symptoms of a progressive neurological deficit. Such symptoms are loss of consciousness, sensory or motor impairment, drowsiness, seizures, or vomiting.

The past history should include surgeries; allergies; head trauma; recurrent ear, nose, or throat problems; and serious or chronic illnesses. Also, migraine sufferers may report a life-long spectrum of symptoms related to migraines. This includes colic in infancy, childhood motion sickness and cyclic vomiting, common headaches, and occasionally cluster headaches. Migraine symptoms tend to occur at "milestones" in the client's life, such as going to school, puberty, graduation from school, first job, marriage, deaths, and family problems (Graham, 1979).

Key questions in the family history include known problems of cancer, heart disease, hypertension, past and present communicable diseases, neurological diseases, strokes, aneurysm, and headaches. About 70% of migraine sufferers report that another family member has similar headache problems. Studies on offspring of migraine subjects have led some to believe that migraine is probably inherited through a recessive gene (Wolff). Graham states that a negative family history for migraine should lead one to reconsider this diagnosis. Clients may be unaware of this history because no one has headaches as severe as theirs or because family members use the term "sick headaches" instead

Table 3-2. Differential diagnosis of headaches

	Tension headache	Sinus headache
Frequency	Variable	Varies with underlying cause, e.g., allergy season or upper respiratory tract infection
Duration	1 hr to "all day every day"	From morning or early afternoon to evening
Location	Usually bilateral	Over sinuses; may involve teeth, other facial structures
Quality	Steady, nonpulsatile, viselike, burning, pressing, drawing	Sustained diffuse, deep aching
Onset	Usually on rising	Gradual
Associated symptoms	Involved muscles may be tender, rigid; anxiety, e.g., clenched hands, nausea, fatigue	Pain by shaking or holding head in dependent posture
Precipitating factors	Sustained muscle contraction of head and neck; ischemia of cervical musculature 2° to stress	Barometric changes (weather, air travel); sensitivity to foods or inhalants; upper respiratory tract infection
Relieving factors	Emphasize analgesics; relaxation techniques; tranquilizers	Steamy shower; hot, moist compresses; analgesics, decongestants
Other	Abnormal electromyogram of frontalis muscle	Tenderness over affected sinus; possible positive transillumination and nasal-postnasal drainage

	Posttraumatic headache	Common migraine
Frequency	After head trauma	Variable, weekly to yearly
Duration	Hours to days; uncommon, 2 mo	Intermittent, lasting hours to days
Location	Usually bilateral	Usually unilateral frontotemporal; alternates sides
Quality	Severe aching	Throbbing, then severe and constant
Onset	Usually within hours after trauma	Gradual, usually starts on awakening
Associated symptoms	Giddiness, insomnia, nervousness, irritability, trembling, inability to concentrate	Photophobia, sweating, blurred vision, unilateral tearing, nausea/vomiting, blocked nasal passage, chilling, conjunctival injection, polyuria, hyperesthesia of scalp
Precipitating factors	Trauma; pain with mental or physical effort; noise, bright lights, confusion	Vasoactive amine foods; hypoglycemia, missed meals; abuse of vasoconstricting or vasodilating drugs; stress; hypertension; environmental stimuli
Relieving factors	Dark, quiet, restful environment; goes away with time; cautious use of analgesics	Rest in darkened room; rebreathing into paper bag to shorten vasoconstrictive phases; analgesics; ergotamine tartrate; pregnancy
Other	NA*	Birth control pills contraindicated

	Classic migraine	Cluster headache
Frequency	Variable	Usually in young men; sporadic with episodes of attacks in clusters of 20 per wk, then none for months or years; in spring and fall

*NA, not applicable.

Continued.

Table 3-2. Differential diagnosis of headaches—cont'd

	Classic migraine—cont'd	**Cluster headache—cont'd**
Duration	4-6 hr—usually less than common migraine	Few minutes to few hours; usual, 30-90 min
Location	Usually unilateral like common migraine	Unilateral behind one eye, extends to temple or maxilla; consistently same side of head during cluster of headaches
Quality	Same as common migraine but reaches its peak within an hour	Excruciating; steady or throbbing pain synchronous with pulse
Onset	Any time	May appear with clocklike regularity often during sleep or after relaxation and naps
Associated symptoms	Same as with common migraine	Blurred vision in ipsilateral eye, conjunctival injection, nasal congestion, lacrimation, perspiration especially on affected side of face, nausea at times
Precipitating factors	Stress; may be frequent during first few months of pregnancy	Vasodilating agents; strain or overwork; stress
Relieving factors	Same as for common migraine	Same as for common migraine (but there is sudden cessation of pain as well as sudden onset)
Other	Birth control pills contraindicated	Temporal vessels on affected side involved; salivation; ⅓ of time ptosis and miosis in ipsilateral eye; rhinorrhea from ipsilateral nostril

	Subdural hematoma	**Temporal arteritis**
Frequency	Increasing frequency over weeks or months after trauma	More frequent in women over 50; usually no previous symptoms
Duration	Variable	Days to weeks
Location	Unilateral or generalized	Unilateral or bilateral; localized over affected arteries
Quality	Deep seated and steady	Severe; pulsating, then constant
Onset	After trauma; variable onset of symptoms	Varies; pain over time with possible sudden blindness
Associated symptoms	Drowsiness at inappropriate times; hemiparesis usually on side opposite lesion	Weight loss; visual changes; night sweats; aching joints; low-grade fever; temporal artery tender and erythematous
Precipitating factors	NA	NA
Relieving factors	Initially responds to analgesics	Corticosteroids
Other	Exam may reveal neurological signs	Lab: ESR greatly increased, mild hypochromic anemia

	Viral or bacterial meningitis	**Brain tumor**
Frequency	NA	Intermittent; headache-free periods in early stage
Duration	Variable	Varies
Location	Bilateral, extends down neck	Usually localized, but not necessarily over tumor
Quality	Severe over time	Nonpulsatile, dull to constant and severe
Onset	Gradual over hours or days; rare, explosive onset	Sudden; progressive, often in morning

Table 3-2. Differential diagnosis of headaches—cont'd

	Viral or bacterial meningitis—cont'd	Brain tumor—cont'd
Associated symptoms	Photophobia; meningeal signs; fever; tachycardia	History of progressive neurological deficits (seizures, drowsiness, etc.)
Precipitating factors	NA	Sudden postural changes; exercise; straining or coughing
Relieving factors	Analgesics, but only for 3-4 hr	None
Other	Lab: abnormal findings in spinal fluid	NA

	Angiomas/aneurysms	Trigeminal neuralgia
Frequency	More sporadic than migraines	Sporadic; headaches come in quick succession; usually in woman aged 40-60
Duration	24 hr to days if bleeding occurs	Seconds to a few minutes
Location	Consistently same location; i.e., on side opposite neurological signs	Sensory distribution of trigeminal nerve root area
Quality	Severe; like subarachnoid hemorrhage when bleeding occurs	Stabbing or lancinating
Onset	Sudden, peaks within minutes	Sudden, usually related to triggering factors
Associated symptoms	Neurological disturbances start after last headache and last beyond headache	NA
Precipitating factors	Exertion, fever, genetic defect	Talking, chewing, swallowing; touching face or gums as in tooth brushing; touching trigger areas around nose and lips
Relieving factors	Ergotamine never relieves	Procaine (Novocaine) hydrochloride, alcoholic, or surgical blocks to trigeminal nerve; thermocoagulation of gasserian ganglion; carbamazepine (Tegretol) 200-400 mg t.i.d.
Other	NA	NA

	Subarachnoid hemorrhage*
Frequency	NA
Duration	Depends on amount of blood (days to weeks)
Location	Unilateral, then bilateral and spreads to back of head and neck
Quality	Severe, explosive
Onset	Sudden neurological signs develop rapidly
Associated symptoms	Photophobia; sometimes, loss of consciousness; stiff neck; back and leg pain
Precipitating factors	Trauma
Relieving factors	No relief by rest
Other	Retinal hemorrhages; fever; albuminuria and glucosuria; hypertension; ECG changes; bloody spinal fluid

*Represents a true emergency and must be diagnosed and treated quickly.

of migraine. Conversely, it is common for clients with any type of severe headache to label it "migraine."

Personal data may reveal precipitating or aggravating factors. Migraine headaches often occur *after* stressful periods, such as particularly difficult work or family situations (Graham). Clients are frequently unaware of the degree of stress they experience daily. A tool such as the Social Readjustment Rating Scale (see Chapter one) may facilitate an awareness of the stress. Parnell and Cooperstock (1979) found that many clients with migraines probably are not sensitized to looking for aggravating factors in their personal behavior. Thus misleading information may be obtained if the practitioner simply asks what factors precipitate or aggravate a headache.

The "migraine personality" is mentioned in various texts. They describe clients with migraines as being shy, obedient, reliable, and stubborn in childhood (Chusid, 1979). However, studies show that the "migraine personality" is an invalid belief (Bakal, 1975; Philips, 1976). Still, there is conflicting information about traits of clients with migraines.

Personal data also include use of tobacco, alcohol, medications, caffeine, and food patterns. The practitioner should ask whether any of these factors trigger headaches. Clients are often unaware of such connections until asked by the practitioner.

Physical examination

The physical examination focuses on identifying a lesion of the extracranial or intracranial structures (including nerves). When sophistocated laboratory or x-ray data are necessary, referral is indicated. Table 3-2 includes positive findings from more common tests (e.g., CBC, ESR).

CASE STUDY
Subjective

Mrs. Adams is a 29-year-old nurse. She has been "happily" married for 9 years to an Army captain. At age 18 the client began having severe headaches before menses. They were diagnosed as common migraines, a problem also experienced by her mother. The migraine attacks were infrequent, three to four times a year. They were relieved by codeine and rest in a dark room. She has taken no other medication for migraines. Otherwise, her past history and family history are negative.

The client is seeking care because her headaches are becoming more frequent and severe. She has had a severe migraine monthly for the past 3 months. The headaches do not relate to menses or ovulation. The pain begins as a mild earache, which gradually worsens and spreads to cover one side of her head from the temple to the ear. She experiences temporary relief from pain by compressing the affected temporal area with the palm of her hand. However, as the pain worsens, it becomes throbbing and spreads across her head. The pain remains move severe on the originating side. When the pain becomes this excruciating, the client goes to a darkened room, lies down, and applies pressure to the affected area with a pillow or her hand. She states, "When the pain gets so bad, it feels as if my head is going to burst."

The review of systems is noncontributory.

Personal data reveal several factors that may contribute to the present problem. Mrs. Adams works as a nurse in a medical-surgical unit. She has held this position for 4 months. During this time she has had to alternate shifts frequently. She likes her work but has not been able to sleep well when she works nights and must sleep during the day. She at times feels additional stress

Essential physical examination for the client with headaches

Sex _____ Age _____ Last completed grade in school _____
Vital signs: Temp. _____ Pulse _____ Resp. _____ BP _____
Height _____ Weight _____

General appearance: Posture, motor behavior, dress, personal hygiene, facial expression, emotional state

HEENT

Inspection: Texture of skin and hair distribution, scalp lesions, masses, contusions, abrasions, areas of ecchymosis or edema, café au lait patches, cutaneous fibroma, sinus transillumination

Palpation: Muscle tenderness, sinus tenderness, temporal arteries for firmness and tenderness, temporomandibular joint tenderness

Percussion: Sinuses and mastoid processes for tenderness

Auscultation: Over orbits of eyes, temples, and mastoid processes for bruits, muscle contraction sounds over frontal and temporal muscles producing constant noise

Eyes: Inspect lacrimal apparatus, conjunctiva, fundi; visual acuity 20/—, 20/—; visual fields, ocular movements, nystagmus, pupils equal and reactive to light and accommodation, tonometry

Ears: Inspect ear canals, tympanic membranes; auditory acuity; Weber's test, Rinne test

Nose: Sense of smell, drainage, mucosa, septum

Mouth: Condition and tenderness of teeth and gums, any dark pigmentation on lips and buccal mucosa, lesions

Pharynx: Postnasal drainage, exudate or injection

Neurological examination

Mental status: Coherent and relevant thought process; cognitive function, orientation, attention and concentration (serial 7s or serial 3s), memory (remote and recent); information (answering questions on well-known subjects), vocabulary (definition of selected words), abstract reasoning (explanation of proverbs), judgment, sensory perception and coordination

Cranial nerves: I-XII

Reflexes: Deep tendon (biceps, triceps, patellar, Achilles), superficial (abdominal, plantar)

Motor: Strength, any noted tremors, inability to relax muscles, muscle tone

Cerebellar: Gait; Romberg test; point-to-point testing, finger-to-nose testing; rapid alternating movements

Sensory: Light touch, pain, vibration, position

Speech: Quality (loudness, articulation inflection), quantity (pace and volume), organization (coherence, relevance, circumstantiality)

when she has a very busy day at work. She is unaware of any foods that trigger her attacks, although she eats irregularly when working evening shifts. She does not smoke or drink alcohol. The only medication she takes is codeine for her headaches.

Objective

The physical examination includes a thorough examination of the head, eyes, ears, nose, throat, and nervous system. There are no abnormal findings. There is no indication for laboratory studies.

Problems

1. Alteration in comfort
2. An increase in frequency and severity of migraine headaches
3. Ineffective rest-activity pattern
4. Alterations in diet—irregular mealtimes

Plan

Triggering factors. Although there are advances in therapy for migraines, there is no totally effective treatment for prevention of these headaches. Each client is a unique person, and the treatment regimen must be tailored to meet individual needs. Paramount in the management of migraines is elimination of triggering or precipitating factors. To aid in the identification and control of these stimuli, clients must become an active participant in planning their care. The headache attack diary sheet (Fig. 3-1) allows the client to focus on potential triggering stimuli and identify patterns of onset. The headache attack diary needs to be kept for 3 months to 1 year, depending on the frequency of the attacks. The client uses one diary sheet for each attack.

Graham thinks that combinations of factors or additive insults are most important in migraine induction. Psychological stimuli such as fear, anxiety, stress, and rage added to physiological stimuli such as menstruation, irregular sleep, or late meals are more likely to result in an attack than either alone. External stimuli such as hot, muggy days or changes in the weather may be unavoidable, but the client does not, for example, have to add the insult of alcohol or tyramine-containing foods.

The nurse pointed out factors that may contribute to Mrs. Adam's headaches. Among these were irregular sleep patterns, irregular meals, and stress at work. Mrs. Adams planned to discuss her work schedule with her supervisor to see if they could determine a more favorable plan.

Relaxation. There are multiple studies on the effectiveness of various relaxation techniques, such as biofeedback. Most authorities agree that these methods are effective for some clients. A 5-year retrospective study was performed to determine the long-term effects of relaxation exercises and physiological feedback on headache problems. The most successful biofeedback candidate was the woman under 30, with vascular headaches, who was not habituated to drugs, and had no symptoms of depression (Diamond and others, 1979a).

Autogenic training is another type of relaxation technique. The client gives himself such verbal commands as "I feel quiet . . ." and "I feel relaxed . . ." (Luther, 1969). Johannes and Schultz developed autogenic training and effectively used it to alleviate migraine attacks (Sargent and others, 1973). Drury and associates (1979) used a treatment package consisting of (1) instructions aimed at generating favorable therapeutic expectations, (2) modified relaxation training, (3) use of autogenic phrases, and (4) fingertip temperature feedback. The results from their treatment regimen included a decrease in the intensity of headache pain and a decrease in use of analgesics.

Physiological coping techniques that can be taught and practiced within a primary care setting include simple relaxation training exercises. Audiotapes or an instructor's voice gives the client commands to contract and relax specific muscle groups.

```
Name_____
Date_____Day of the week_____
Day of menstrual cycle_____Days before next menstruation_____
Time of onset_____ or ____How long did headache last?_____
Experience of any pre-warning symptoms [No] [Yes]  What were they?_____
```

Location: Darken in the areas affected by the headache

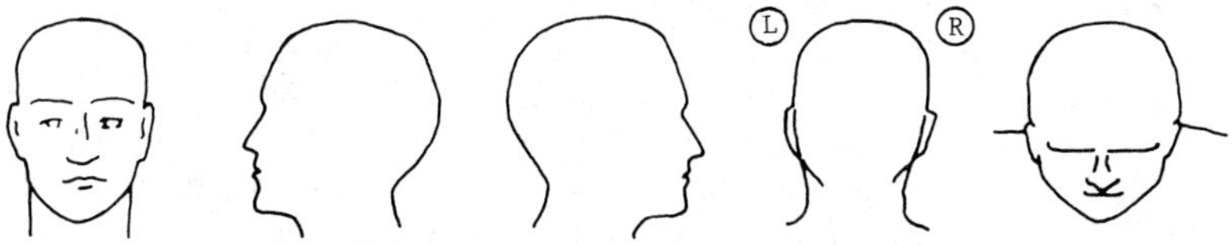

```
   Front         Left         Right      Back of head    Top of head
```

How long did it take the pain to reach its peak? _____min _____hr
or
[abruptly]   [gradually]

Nature of the pain_____ examples: burning, throbbing, dull, aching, constricting, band-like, stabbing, sharp, constant

Pain is made worse by:_____
Pain was relieved by:_____
Associated symptoms_____ examples: nausea, vomiting, dizziness, sweating, disturbed sense of smell, light sensitive, blurred vision, increased urination, slurred speech, runny nose, tearing eyes.

During the 24 hours before the attack
1) Did you have any special worry, overwork, shock or trauma?

2) What had you done during the day?   normal work?
                                             extra tired?
                                             unusual activity?
3) What food had you eaten and when?
   Breakfast _____ time _____

   Midmorning _____ time _____

   Lunch _____ time _____

   Midafternoon _____ time _____

   Supper _____ time _____

   Evening _____ time _____

   Bedtime _____ time _____

4) What do you think caused this attack?

Fig. 3-1. Headache attack diary sheet.

Relaxation training instructions

 I want you to sit comfortably in your chair and simply relax. To help you to learn to relax listen to my voice and I will give you directions that will help you learn how to deeply relax all of your muscles.

 Do not go to sleep but try to become deeply relaxed. And as you listen to the sound of my voice don't be too concerned about trying to *do* something, just allow yourself to relax and to flow with the directions. Now I would like you to focus your attention on the tips of your toes. Imagine for a moment that you have a band of relaxation, starting at the tips of your toes, and beginning to drift slowly and at its own rate up your body. Imagine that the band of relaxation is drifting slowly and comfortably. And as the muscles start to let go the band of relaxation drifts slowly and at its own rate as you control it. As it drifts slowly from the tips of your toes, drifting slowly, through your feet, the tops of your feet relax, the soles of your feet relax, and soon the band of relaxation has reached your ankles. Allow yourself to become even more relaxed as the band of relaxation drifts slowly upward. The band of relaxation now drifts slowly into your legs. Focus your attention and allow all of your muscles to let go. Drifting slowly upward and allowing the lower leg muscles to leg go and relaxed and comfortable. Drifting slowly upward and let all of the tension slide away. Drifting slowly upward and allowing the muscles at the tops of the legs to let go, and the feeling of relaxation becomes more and more profound. The imaginary band goes at your own rate, at your comfortable, relaxed, and easy rate, drifting slowly to the knees and allowing all of the tension to slide away. Drifting ever so gradually beyond the knees, and allowing your attention to focus on your thighs as you let the muscles go and they become limp, relaxed, and comfortable. The tension slides away and the band of relaxation spreads slowly at its own rate beyond your knees, allowing the tension to slip away, drifting into the thigh muscles, letting the muscles go and allowing yourself to drift into an easy and comfortable and relaxed state. And as the band of relaxation drifts slowly upward, as all of the tension slides away, you become more and more relaxed, easy and relaxed and comfortable. Very soon the band of relaxation has reached as far as your waist, as you focus your attention and allow the tension to slip away from the stomach muscles, letting all of the tension slide out. Allowing yourself to drift and become more and more relaxed. Allowing yourself to become more and more comfortably relaxed. And the band of relaxation has relaxed your stomach muscles and into the lower back, drifting slowly upward, allowing the tension to slide away, drifting into the chest, drawing more and more relaxed, allowing yourself to drift, grow relaxed, and easy and comfortable. Focusing your attention now, particularly on the back of your

From Masur, F.T.: A comparison of EMG biofeedback, relaxation instructions, and attention-placebo in the treatmen neck and your shoulders, allowing the tension to slide away at its own rate as the band of relaxation begins to drift, drift into your arms, allowing the muscles to become supple, and relaxed and comfortable. Drifting into the upper arms and soon reaching as far as the elbows. You become more and more relaxed, allowing the tension to slide away, allowing the band of relaxation, drifting at its own rate, to go beyond the elbows. And as the muscles let go and become very relaxed and supple the band of relaxation reaches as far as your lower arms. The band of relaxation continues to drift and moves slowly, and at its own rate into your wrists. And the wrists become relaxed, and supple and comfortable. The band of relaxation begins to go into the hands slowly and comfortably, each individual muscle letting go and becoming so relaxed and comfortable. Drifting into the fingers, slowly and comfortably, drifting into the fingers and letting the tension go. Drifting into the fingers and allowing the tension to seem to flow out of the fingertips, as you become more and more relaxed, and easy and comfortable. Allowing the tension now to drift slowly upward once more, drifting, drifting into the neck muscles, allowing the jaw muscles now to let go, allowing your teeth to part just slightly, and the feeling of relaxation spreads now into the face so that the area around the eyes becomes very relaxed and comfortable. Drifting slowly upward and allowing the tension all the way through the neck and the back and the front to become more and more relaxed. Drifting slowly upward, drifting up so that the area around the eyes is now very relaxed, and easy and comfortable, around the eyebrows, and into the forehead, and the top of the head. And that's very good. And you've allowed yourself to become very relaxed, very relaxed and easy and comfortable. And you've allowed your thoughts and feelings to drift. But we can increase your level of relaxation even more completely than it is now. I would like you to become conscious of your breathing. Your breathing is shallow and regular and comfortable. And as you breathe out, silently in your mind, I want you to count the number "one" and relax. And as you do this, you may notice that other thoughts intrude, that's fine, just continue to count, and during this time I'm going to stop talking for awhile. You continue to count and allow yourself to relax even more completely. And soon I'll start talking again. Allow yourself to become even more relaxed, and comfortable, and easy. Now begin counting the number "one" in your mind and become conscious of your breathing and relax even more completely (Silence: 4.5 minutes.) That's fine and you've allowed yourself to become very relaxed. You can go back now to your regular means of thinking but enjoy the feeling of relaxation. In a few more minutes this session will be over, but for the moment simply remain relaxed.

You can now turn off this tape recorder.

The practitioner discussed relaxation techniques to allow the client more control over her response to stress. Relaxation training instructions were provided (see pp. 80-81). It was suggested that the client tape-record the instructions and use the recording to assist with relaxation. The client was instructed to use the exercise when she was aware of increased stress or when she had difficulty sleeping. The use of biofeedback may be necessary at a future time to augment relaxation techniques.

Health habits. Mrs. Adams was instructed to practice good health habits as another coping technique. These habits include:
1. Three meals a day at regular times instead of snacking, avoiding large carbohydrate loads
2. Breakfast on arising every day
3. Moderate exercise (long walks, bike riding, swimming, gardening) two or three times a week
4. Seven or eight hours of sleep a night
5. No smoking
6. Maintaining a moderate weight
7. No alcohol

There is evidence that life expectancy and better health status are significantly related to the use and practice of these basic health habits (Belloc and Breslow, 1972). Also, many of these habits incorporate avoidance of possible triggering factors.

Medications. Pharmaceutical agents are often necessary. It is important that the client not perceive the use of analgesics or other medications as failure or weakness in self-care techniques. The use of pharmaceutical agents in the management of migraine depends on the nurse practitioner's scope of practice and setting. Physician consultation is desirable whenever the use of medications for migraines is initiated.

The client was given instructions for taking ergotamine (Gynergen) if another severe attack occurred. When aspirin or codeine does not provide pain relief, ergotamine may prove helpful in aborting an attack. This drug is a vasoconstrictor. It is most effective if taken at the onset of symptoms. Rest in a dark room may enhance the drug's effectiveness. The dosage is 2 to 3 mg at the onset of a headache. This may be followed by 1 to 2 mg every hour until the pain resolves. The total dose should not exceed 6 mg in 24 hours or 10 mg in 1 week. The drug is contraindicated in pregnancy, peripheral vascular disease, infectious states, or any other condition in which vasoconstriction is dangerous. It may produce a synergistic vasoconstrictive response in clients taking propranolol (Inderal).

There are many advances in drug therapy for migraines. These include the use of antiinflammatory drugs, antiplatelet drugs, anticonvulsants, antidepressants, antihistamines, β-adrenergic blockers, and antiserotonin drugs. The use of these drugs requires referral to a physician who prescribes these drugs routinely.

Mrs. Adams was asked to call the nurse if the severity or frequency of the headaches increased. Otherwise, she was to return for follow-up in 2 months.

Evaluation

Mrs. Adams returned as scheduled for follow-up. She had been headache free since her last visit. Her work schedule improved after talking with her supervisor. Also, she organized activities at home to allow more rest time when she did have to work evenings. She ate her meals at more consistent intervals and did not omit meals.

The client recorded the instructions for the relaxation exercise. While at home after each workday she played the tape and practiced this exercise. She was convinced of its relaxing effect. Also, she was encouraged by the headache-free months.

EVALUATION

The majority of clients with migraine headaches do not need constant supervision. Rather, follow-up should consist of return visits for increased frequency of headaches, nonresponse to therapy, medication refills, a change in the pattern of headaches, and wellness care. Since migraine headaches are a chronic problem, the nurse's role is to educate the client for self-care with the goal of preventing or lessening the number and severity of acute attacks. Clients should be able to:
1. State the definition of migraine
2. List factors that commonly trigger migraines in susceptable persons
3. List their specific trigger factors, if present
4. State the correct dosage, schedule, side effects, and any special instructions for medications
5. Describe their performance of relaxation techniques
6. State situations that require follow-up

Physician consultation is essential when headaches increase in severity or frequency, are refractory to treatment, or occur with new symptoms. In addition, physician consultation is preferable before selection of any drug regimen for migraines. In many cases drug therapy is the only treatment prescribed for the client with migraines; however, the nurse can play a vital role in management by educating the client toward knowledgeable self-care.

REFERENCES

Anderson, J.A., and others: Migraine and hypnotic therapy, Int. J. Clin. Exp. Hypn. **23**:48, 1975.
Anthony, M., and Lance, J.W.: The role of serotonin. In Pierce, J., editor: Modern topics in migraine, London, 1975, Heinemann.
Bakal, D.A.: Headache: a biopsychosocial perspective, Psychol. Bull. **82**:369, 1975.
Basmajian, J.V.: Biofeedback principles and practice for clinicians, Baltimore, 1979, The Williams & Wilkins Co.
Belloc, N.B., and Breslow, L.: Relationship of physical status and health practices, Prev. Med. **1**:409, 1972.
Benson, J., and others: The usefulness of the relaxation response in the therapy of headache, Headache **14**:49, 1974.
Carlson, L.A., and others: Clinical and metabolic effects of different doses of prostaglandin E in man, Acta Med. Scand. **183**:423, 1968.
Casey, R.L., and others: Quantitative study of recall of life events, J. Psychosom. Res. **11**:239, 1967.
Chusid, J.G.: Nervous system. In Chatton, M.F., and Knupp, M.A., editors: Medical diagnosis and treatment, Los Altos, Calif., 1979, Lange Medical Publications.
Dalessio, D.J.: Classification and mechanism of migraine, Headache **19**:114, 1979.
Dalton, K.: Migraine: avoiding trigger factors, Nurs. Mirror **145**:18, 1977.
Diamond, S.: Headache: its diagnosis and management, Headache **19**:113, 1979a.
Diamond, S.: Biofeedback and headache, Headache **19**:180, 1979b.
Diamond, S., and Medina, J.L.: Double-blind study of propanolol for migraine prophylaxis, Headache **16**:24, 1976.
Diamond, S., and others: The value of biofeedback in the treatment of chronic headache: a five-year retrospective study, Headache **19**:90, 1979a.
Diamond, S., and others: The use of analgesics in headache, Headache **19**:185, 1979b.
Drury, R.L., and others: Temperature biofeedback treatment for migraine headache: a controlled multiple baseline study, Headache **19**:278, 1979.
Edmeads, J.: Vascular headaches and the cranial circulation, Headache, April 1979, pp. 127-132.

Friedman, A., and others: When you suspect migraine in a child, Patient Care **13**:84-85, 88-89, 92-93, 96-99, 103-105, 109, 112-115, Sept. 30, 1979.
Friedman, A.P., and others: Classification of headache, Arch. Neurol. **6**:173, 1962.
Graham, J.R.: Migraine headache: diagnosis and management, Headache **19**:133, 1979.
Hannington, E.: Migraine, Westport, Conn., 1973, Techmomic Publishing Co.
Hannington, E.: Diagnosis of migraine, Nurs. Mirror **149**:14-16, Aug. 11, 1977.
Henry, K., and others: Psychological aspects of migraine, J. Psychosom. Res. **17**:141, 1973.
King, A.B., and Robinson, S.M.: Vascular headache of acute mountain sickness, Aerosp. Med. **43**:849, 1972.
Kudrow, K.: Hormones, pregnancy and migraine. In Appenseller, O., editor: Pathogenesis and treatment of headache, New York, 1976, Spectrum Publishers.
Kunkel, R.S.: Evaluating the headache patient: history and workup, Headache **19**:122, 1979.
Lance, J.W.: Mechanism and management of headache, ed. 3, Boston, 1978, Butterworth Publishers, Inc.
Lance, J.W., and Anthony, M.: Some clinical aspects of migraine, Arch. Neurol. **15**:356, 1966.
Luther, W., editor: Autogenic therapy, vols. 1 to 6, New York, 1969, Grune & Stratton, Inc.
Mason, J.W.: A review of psychoendocrine research on the sympathetic adrenal medullary system, Psychosom. Med. **30**:631, 1968.
Mitchell, K.R., and others: The prevention of self-management of anxiety, parts 1 and 2, Sidney, Australia, 1974, Psychological Behavior Associate Press.
Parnell, P., and Cooperstock, R.: Tranquilizers and mood elevators in the treatment of migraines: an analysis of the Migraine Foundation questionnaire, Headache **19**:78, 1979.
Philips, C.: Headache and personality, J. Psychosom. Res. **20**:535, 1976.
Pierson, L.B.: A protocol for the chief complaint of headache, Nurse Pract. **2**:12-16, Sept. 1976.
Sargent, J.D., and others: Preliminary report on the use of autogenic feedback techniques in the treatment of migraine and tension headaches, Psychosom. Med. **35**:129, 1973.
Waters, W.E.: Headache and the eye, Lancet **2**:1, 1970.
Wolff, H.G.: Headache and other head pain, ed. 3, New York, 1972, Oxford University Press, Inc.

SECTION TWO

Problems with body fluids

CHAPTER 4

Anemia in the adult client

Linda Lindsey Davis

Primary care nurse practitioners who work in ambulatory settings are frequently called on to assess and manage the problems of adults with vague somatic complaints such as fatigue, weakness, lassitude, headache, dizziness, shortness of breath, and chest pain. These symptoms are often the first subjective indicators of anemia in the adult. Occasionally, routine health screening identifies the asymptomatic adult with anemia. In these instances meticulous interviewing may reveal the presence of symptoms.

Estimates of the prevalance of anemia as a presenting problem among adults vary. Whitfield (1967) describes anemia as a presenting symptom in more than half of 100 consecutive hospital admissions to a medical service for indigent clients. In a review of patient problems seen in a general practice setting, Brown and co-workers (1971) describes the incidence of anemia among ambulatory patients as being on the order of 0.5% to 1% of all the patients seen. In a compilation of common asymptomatic diseases for inclusion in routine health screening, Frame and Carlson (1975) suggest an incidence of 2.5% of anemias in the general population. The most frequent occurrence involves pregnant women (10% to 60%) and aged women (15%).

Anemia in itself is not a disease. Rather it is a sign of a defect, deficiency, or disease process that results in an inadequate number of circulating red blood cells and a concomitant reduction in the oxygen-combining capacity of the blood.

PHYSIOLOGY OF RED BLOOD CELL PRODUCTION

The stem cells of the bone marrow form blood cells, which evolve through several states. The result is a mature red blood cell, or erythrocyte. Normally, a small percentage of one of the immature forms, reticulocytes, is present (Table 4-1). The percentage of circulating reticulocytes increases when the rate of red blood cell production is very rapid, as in response to rapid blood loss or iron therapy. The number, shape, size, and coloration of the red blood cells in a peripheral blood smear are indicative of bone marrow activity.

Hemoglobin accounts for approximately 95% of the dry weight of a red blood cell. Heme (an iron and porphyrin compound), globin (a protein substance), and oxygen form the hemoglobin molecule (Guyton, 1976). Normal production of the hemoglobin molecule depends on adequate stores of iron and protein-synthesizing amino acids.

Table 4-1. Differentiation of blood cells: a simplified model*

```
                              Stem cells
         ┌──────────────┬──────────────┬──────────────┐
    Normoblast     Lymphoblast     Monoblast      Megakaryocyte
         │              │              │              │
    Reticulocyte    Lymphocyte      Monocyte       Thrombocyte
         │
    Erythrocyte
```

*It is important to note that blood cells evolve from a common origin in undifferentiated reticuloendothelial tissue. Thus, when one is evaluating the client with anemia, it is important to look at the total hematopoietic picture.

The hormone erythropoietin regulates the rate of red blood cell production in response to tissue hypoxia. The kidney produces large amounts of erythropoietin. The liver and possibly other tissues produce lesser amounts (Guyton). Thus secondary anemias may occur as a result of chronic renal or hepatic disease.

The life span of a red blood cell is approximately 120 days. As the old red blood cells rupture, the released hemoglobin is almost immediately phagocytized and digested by reticuloendothelial cells. The majority of the iron thus liberated returns to the marrow for use in the synthesis of new hemoglobin. The porphyrin converts to bile pigments. The protein globin reduces to simple amino acids for utilization in the synthesis of new proteins.

Adequate amounts of iron, folic acid, and vitamin B_{12} are necessary for the normal production of red blood cells. Anemias result from insufficient or defective production of red blood cells or from their increased loss or destruction.

In order to support the production of sufficient numbers of red blood cells, the healthy adult needs approximately 0.5 to 1.0 mg of iron daily. There are two notable exceptions to this rule. First, the menstruating woman loses about 17.0 mg of iron per monthly cycle and requires 1.5 mg of iron daily. Second, the pregnant woman, who experiences a significant hypervolemia in the later stages of pregnancy, requires at least 2.5 mg of iron daily (Lee and others, 1977). The average American diet supplies approximately 6.0 mg of iron per kcal or a total of about 10 to 20 mg of iron per day. However, the body absorbs only about 10% of dietary iron. Thus individuals must ingest approximately 10 times the daily iron requirement to maintain adequate iron stores.

The iron deficiency anemias are those most frequently encountered in the primary care setting. Causes of iron deficiency anemia in the adult include increased loss of red blood cells through frank or occult bleeding; insufficient intake of iron as a result of poor or inadequate diet or pica; and increased metabolic demands, such as those experienced during the later stages of pregnancy.

Folic acid deficiency results when the diet lacks fruits and vegetables high in folate. Additionally, this deficiency may result from situations involving increased metabolic demands, such as pregnancy. Some authorities indicate that folate deficiency may be very common among low income people. Disturbances in the absorption of folate in the gastrointestinal tract may occur as a result of taking substances such as barbiturates, alcohol, or other drugs.

Vitamin B_{12} is found chiefly in dairy products and red meat. Individuals who eat a strict vegetarian diet may develop a vitamin B_{12} deficiency anemia. Vitamin B_{12} deficiency may also result from decreased absorption in the ileum caused by some pathological condition (such as ileal resection or infection).

Vitamin B_{12} must combine with the intrinsic factor produced by the parietal cells of the stomach. Individuals who lose a significant amount of gastric musosa as a result of aging or gastric surgery are unable to produce sufficient amounts of intrinsic factor to ensure absorption of vitamin B_{12}. The resulting condition is called pernicious anemia. This anemia is a possible predisposing factor in the development of gastric cancer (McDonald and Rubin, 1977).

ASSESSMENT

Factors that may cause or contribute to the development of anemia receive special attention in the history (see p. 90). Assessment includes family history; social history; nutrition history, including pica; elimination habits; rest-activity patterns; prescription and over-the-counter drug use; and alcohol, tobacco, and substance use. In addition, review of body systems (particularly a search for blood loss), physical examination, and laboratory studies are included. Clues from the history often minimize the need for multiple invasive and frequently expensive laboratory studies. An example is the adult who gives a history of pica.

There is no typical clinical picture of a client with anemia. The signs and symptoms of the anemia depend on the causative defect, disease, or deficiency. The symptoms of anemia—fatigue, weakness, headache, dizziness, shortness of breath, and chest pain—generally occur as a result of tissue hypoxia. These symptoms usually are absent until hemoglobin levels approach 7 to 8 g/dl (Elmwood and others, 1969). However, sudden reductions in hemoglobin levels, as in rapid blood loss, may result in earlier, more pronounced symptoms.

Two factors account for the signs commonly associated with anemia. Decreased perfusion of peripheral tissues shunts blood toward the brain, heart, and skeletal muscle. This results in pallor of the skin and mucous membranes. A compensatory increase in heart rate increases cardiac output. This accounts for the clinical findings of tachycardia, systolic flow murmurs, and bruits (Ersley, 1972).

The anemias are classified according to the size and relative color of the red blood cells. These two indices are measured through assessment of (1) the size of the cell, that is, the mean corpuscular volume (MCV); and (2) the color of the cell, that is, the mean corpuscular hemoglobin concentration (MCHC). Thus red blood cells may be normocytic, microcytic, or macrocytic, and normochromic, hypochromic, or hyperchromic. Mean corpuscular hemoglobin (MCH) is the content of hemoglobin in the average red blood cell. Since hemoglobin normally varies slightly from cell to cell, MCH is of less clinical value than MCHC. Also, these indices are based on an average red blood cell volume and hemoglobin concentration. As averages they are subject to misinterpretation. Furthermore, anemias of mixed types occur, with varied cell sizes and coloration. The practi-

Risk factors for anemia in adults

A. Adults at risk
  1. Menstruating women
  2. Women with intrauterine devices and resultant heavy menses
  3. Individuals with malignancy involving the gastrointestinal or genitourinary tract
  4. Individuals receiving anticoagulant therapy
B. Nutritional factors
  1. Strict vegetarians
  2. Food faddists
  3. Alcoholics
  4. Individuals with history of gastrointestinal surgery
  5. Dieters
C. Long-term drug therapy
  1. Acetylsalicylic acid
  2. Phenytoin
  3. Barbiturates
  4. Methyldopa
  5. Chloramphenicol
  6. Para-aminosalicylic acid
  7. Penicillin
  8. Sulfonamides
  9. Dapsone
  10. Griseofulvin
  11. Oral contraceptives
D. Chronic illness
  1. Rheumatoid arthritis
  2. Hiatal hernia
  3. Chronic liver disease
  4. Chronic renal disease
  5. Hypothyroidism or hyperthyroidism
  6. Leukemia
  7. Lead poisoning
  8. Hereditary anemias, such as sickle cell anemia or thalassemia
E. Increased metabolic demand
  1. Pregnant women
  2. Adolescents

Table 4-2. Normal hematological values in the adult

Test	Normal values
Hemoglobin (Hb)	
Male	13-18 gm/dl
Female	12-16 gm/dl
Hematocrit (Hct)	
Male	40-54%
Female	37-48%
RBC	4.2-6.2 million/mm^3
MCV	80-94 μm^3
MCHC	33-38%
MCH	27-31 $\mu\mu g$
Reticulocyte count	0.5-1.5%
Serum iron	50-150 mg/dl
Total iron-binding capacity (TIBC)	250-450 mg/dl
Iron saturation	20-55%
Serum folate	5-25 ng/ml

tioner determines red blood cell indices by using the following simple formulas (Barry, 1974):

$$\text{MCV} = \frac{\text{Hematocrit (\%)} \times 10}{\text{RBC (millions/mm}^3)}$$

$$\text{MCHC} = \frac{\text{Hemoglobin} \times 100}{\text{Hematocrit (\%)}}$$

Table 4-2 gives the range of normal hematological values for adults.

The peripheral blood smears should always be reviewed with someone who has recognized expertise in the interpretation of red blood cell morphology. The peripheral smear is evaluated for the presence of any abnormal or atypical cells. Some atypical red blood cells include:

microcytes —Cells having diameters of less than 5 μm, usually seen in iron deficiency anemia.
macrocytes —Cells having diameters greater than 10 μm, usually seen in vitamin B_{12} and folic acid deficiency anemias, occasionally in liver disease, the hemolytic anemias, and sickle cell disease.
target cells —Cells that stain in a characteristic "bull's eye" pattern. The center stains darkly and is surrounded by a lightly stained ring and then a darker-stained periphery. These cells are found in obstructive jaundice, after splenectomy, in hypochromic states (especially thalassemia), and in hemoglobin C disease.
burr cells —Normal-sized red blood cells with many spiny projections, seen in situations involving hemolysis or sometimes in ulcer disease and uremia. Do not confuse burr cells with crenated red blood cells (small red blood cells with prickly points seen in improperly prepared blood smears).
spherocytes —Small red blood cells that stain well, show little or no central pallor, and are found in hemolytic anemias.
sickle cells —Crescent-shaped red blood cells associated with sickle cell disease (Whitfield).

Many clinicians consider the reticulocyte count an excellent indirect measure of bone marrow activity. The percentage of circulating reticulocytes increases when the rate of red blood cell production is greatly accelerated. This occurs in response to rapid blood loss, red blood cell destruction, and iron therapy. Examples of loss or destruction are bleeding from the gastrointestinal, genitourinary, or respiratory tract; and hemolysis of healthy red blood cells, which occurs with some drug reactions. In rapid blood loss, the initial response is one of brisk reticulocytosis. As iron stores become depleted, the reticulocyte count begins to decrease. A low reticulocyte count in an anemic state reflects depressed bone marrow activity, which is caused by mechanisms such as iron or vitamin deficiency or a chronic disease state (Whitfield).

The anemia commonly seen in chronic disease is a hypoproliferative one in which a peripheral blood smear shows normocytic and hypochromic or normochromic red blood cells. The total iron-binding capacity is often normal or decreased, and the serum iron level is low.

Two processes that contribute to the development of anemia occur on a cellular level in the presence of a chronic inflammatory disease, such as rheumatoid arthritis. First, the rate of red blood cell destruction increases, which places a greater demand on the bone marrow for a more rapid erythrocyte production. Second, inflammatory changes

Table 4-3. Assessment factors in simple anemias

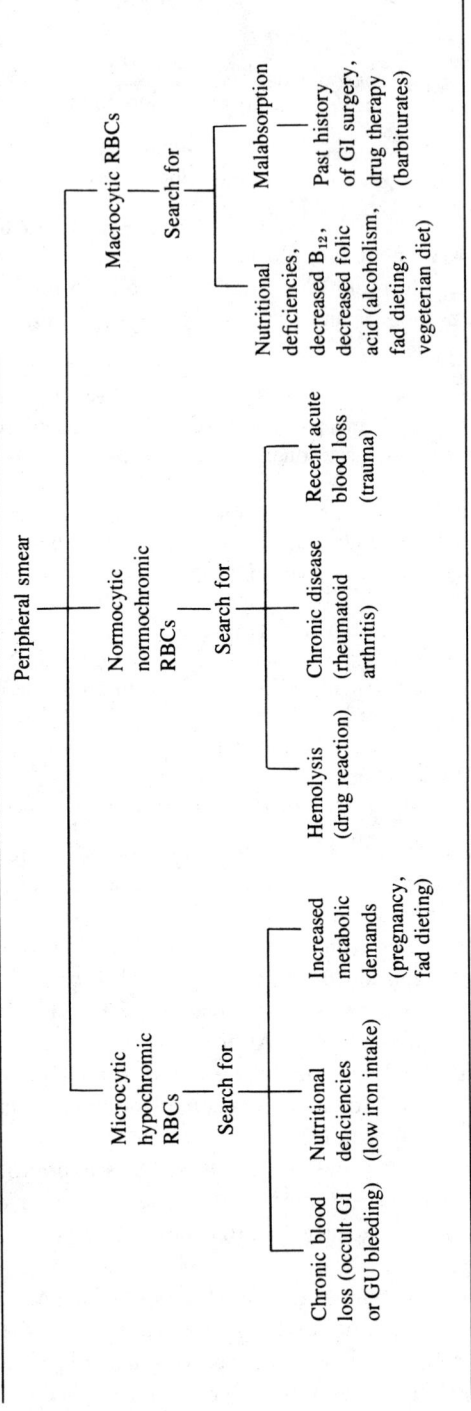

block the orderly release of iron by reticuloendothelial cells. This iron is trapped in the reticuloendothelial cell and causes a rise in the serum ferritin level. Iron stores in the marrow are normal or increased. Ellin and co-workers (1977) showed that 2 or more weeks are necessary to reestablish normal body iron levels after even a brief period of systemic inflammation.

Since the diagnosis of anemia depends on laboratory findings, excluding the possibility of testing error is essential. An initial repeat of the hematocrit and hemoglobin may prevent unnecessary procedures. Next, the anemia should be classified according to morphology. Then, the possible causes of anemia can be determined according to this classification (Table 4-3). Findings from the history and physical examination aid in this last step.

PLAN AND EVALUATION
CASE STUDY 1: MICROCYTIC, HYPOCHROMIC ANEMIA

David is a 53-year-old chief accountant with a mortgage company. He lives with his wife and two teenage daughters. David describes himself as one who "worries about everything." For the past 3 years he sporadically attended a family practice clinic for treatment of mild uncomplicated essential hypertension.

Subjective

Chief complaint. "Always tired for the last 2 months."

History of present illness. David has a 2- to 3-month history of increasing fatigue, which is present when he awakens and worsens in the afternoon and evening. He further describes this fatigue as reduced ability to do physical work and a decreased capacity to think and make decisions. Sleep and increased rest periods do not relieve the symptoms. In the last 2 months he also noted a 5-pound weight loss not attributable to changes in his appetite or dietary pattern. His last physical examination was 3 years ago, when his wife gave him a "hard time" about needing a checkup.

Social history. David has a master's degree in accounting. He and his wife are much involved in raising their two daughters (ages 13 and 15). They spend their spare time in activities related to the junior high school band boosters club. David's widowed mother died 4 months ago after a lengthy illness from breast cancer. His sister lives in a small town nearby, and the two families get together frequently.

Nutrition. David follows a 2-g sodium diet except for an "occasional lapse" (beer and pretzels while watching Monday night football). He eats three meals a day and an evening snack while watching television. A usual day's meals are:
Breakfast: coffee, cooked cereal, scrambled eggs
Lunch: sandwich, cookies, iced tea
Dinner: meat, vegetables, salad, coffee
Snack: Jell-O, fruit, or cookies
He uses a potassium salt substitute.

Elimination. He has a bowel movement every other day. Constipation and hemorrhoids are problems for which he takes Metamucil daily. The stool is dark brown, hard, and formed.

Rest and activity. David sleeps 8 to 10 hours a night and takes a 30-minute nap after he gets home from work. His work is sedentary, being at a desk 5 days a week. He formerly played racquetball at lunch daily, but he discontinued this a month ago because of fatigue. He plays golf once or twice a month. He spends evening hours watching television and being with his family.

Substance use. He drinks two to three cocktails in an evening, usually limited to weekends while entertaining friends. He gave up cigarettes last year after smoking one pack per day for 20 years. Medications include hydrochlorothiazide, 50 mg b.i.d.; Metamucil, one teaspoon dissolved in water in the morning and evening; and aspirin, grains x "one to two times a month for headache."

Review of systems. This is noncontributory except for the gastrointestinal system. He has had blood mixed with stool one to three times a month over the past "couple" of years. He attributes this to hemorrhoids.

Objective

General. Ht, 5 ft 8 in; wt, 152 lb; BP, 140/88; T, 98.8; P, 94; R, 22. The physical examination is unremarkable except for:
  1. A I/VI midsystolic murmur heard at the apex.
  2. Stool benzidine test: mildly positive for occult blood; heart rate, 94.
  3. Rectal examination: small external hemorrhoids, no masses palpable; prostate not enlarged and without nodules.

Laboratory data

RBC: 3.8 million/mm^3	Reticulocytes: 1.7%
Hct: 28.0%	WBC: normal
Hb: 9.0 gm/dl	Platelets: low normal
MCV: 73.6 μm^3	Serum iron: 34 mg/dl
MCHC: 32.1%	TIBC: 480 mg/dl

David has not had a complete physical examination in 7 years. He has not been evaluated for his periodic rectal bleeding in more than 3 years. At that time he was told the bleeding was due to hemorrhoids, since a barium enema and upper GI x-ray findings were normal.

David's fatigue and history of rectal bleeding are suggestive of a blood loss anemia. The red blood cell indices show a microcytic and hypochromic process, typical of iron deficiency. The reduced serum iron level and the increased serum iron-binding capacity also indicate an iron deficiency. The midsystolic murmur reflects increased flow across a valve and is an occasional finding in a high-output state such as anemia.

Problems

  1. Hypochromic, microcytic anemia
  2. Alteration in bowel elimination—rectal bleeding
  3. Lack of knowledge about preventive care

Plan

Clients followed for a chronic disease are also at risk for other potentially serious diseases. Regular, periodic screening is as much a part of primary health care as routine maintenance for chronic disease states. While many clinicians perform routine screening for asymptomatic diseases, they often do not provide the necessary health education and advice regarding screening and follow-up. All men and nonpregnant women who have an iron deficiency anemia must be evaluated for blood loss. David's sporadic clinic visits are typical of the middle-aged wage earner who places the needs and responsibility for health care on other family members. In David's situation, the identification of an iron deficiency anemia warranted screening for conditions resulting in a blood loss.

Both the Geller tables (Robbins and Geller, 1972) and the American Cancer Society health statistics (Silverberg and Holleb, 1973) place men in David's age group at particular risk for gastrointestinal malignancies, a causative agent in occult rectal bleeding. Carcinoma of the colon and rectum is one of the most frequently occurring cancers in 50- to 60-year-old men.

In a review of colorectal cancer research, Frame and Carlson (1975) found that 70% of these cancers occur in the distal 25 cm of the bowel. More than 80% of persons with rectal cancer had complaints of bloody stools before diagnosis. This disease has a much better prognosis if identified and treated early. The simple, noninvasive testing of stools for occult bleeding, especially consecutive stools while the client is eating a no-meat, high-residue diet, has a high yield of early detection of gastrointestinal tract bleeding.

Rheingold and co-workers (1979) recommend guaiac-impregnated slides as the most accurate method for screening stools for occult bleeding. Specimens taken from two different parts of stool are placed on slides for evaluation. Three separate stools are collected on consecutive days, for a total of six specimens, while the individual is eating a high-roughage, meatless diet. A positive reaction in any one of the six slides warrants further evaluation. Randon guaiac tests may show false positive results in individuals who consume diets with even small amounts of meat. Thus, the test results should be interpreted with discretion. False positive tests are a likelihood with improper preparation, but false negative tests are rare.

Evaluation

Physician referral was needed because of the severe anemia and history of rectal bleeding.

David was prescribed a restrictive diet and over 1 week demonstrated occult gastrointestinal bleeding on two out of three occasions. Subsequently, a proctosigmoidoscopy revealed carcinoma in the left descending colon. Surgical intervention and colon resection were essential. The surgery was successful and David's recovery uneventful. A careful assessment of his subjective symptom, "fatigue," and subsequent microcytic, hypochromic anemia revealed a potentially life-threatening cancer.

CASE STUDY 2: MACROCYTIC, NORMOCHROMIC ANEMIA
Subjective

Susan is a 20-year-old college junior who works part-time as a department store clerk. Her only prior contact in the Student Health Clinic was for an upper respiratory tract infection. Also, Susan attended one of the evening health education sessions given in the dormitory by a nurse practitioner. This time she is coming to the clinic for a routine pelvic examination and Pap test. She is requesting these tests because she wants to use some form of contraception in the near future. She expresses interest in "the pill" for contraception.

Social history. Susan shares a room in the dormitory with another student. Susan's family lives 100 miles away in a small town. Until recently Susan lived at home and attended the local junior college. Her job as a part-time clerk in a department store requires 3 hours every evening and all day Saturday. Susan describes herself as a "worrier"; she is concerned about money, keeping up with classes, and, until recently, minimal involvement with members of the opposite sex.

Nutrition. Susan has no history of pica. She has lost 24 lb in the last 9 weeks by fasting one day each week. Her diet for the remainder of each week is:
Breakfast: coffee, skim milk
Lunch: two hard-boiled eggs, diet soda
Dinner: large piece of chicken, fish, or cheese and iced tea

Elimination. She has had three loose stools per day over the last 2 weeks.

Rest and activity. Susan sleeps 7 to 8 hours each night and is "always on the go" with classes or her part-time job. She plans no time for hobbies or other recreation.

Substance use. She denies use of alcohol, tobacco, or medications. She takes no over-the-counter drugs.

Review of systems. This is noncontributory except for "cracks" in the corner of her mouth, which have not healed since their onset 2 weeks ago. She has used alcohol to dry these lesions, but there has been no perceptible improvement.

Objective

General. Ht, 5 ft 4 in; wt, 114 lb; BP, 108/72; T, 98.4; P, 72; R, 18. The physical examination is unremarkable except for:
1. Decreased skin tone on the thighs, abdomen, and upper arms
2. Ulcerated areas at right corner of the mouth and under the tongue

Laboratory data

RBC: 3.4 million/mm^3
WBC: 4,600/mm^3, 3 to 5 multisegmented neutrophils/high-power field
Hct: 34%
Hb: 12 gm/dl

MCV: 100 μm^3
MCHC: 35.2%
Serum iron: 50 mg/dl
Reticulocytes: 0.5%
Serum folate: 3 ng/ml

Problems

1. Macrocytic, hypochromic anemia—folic acid deficiency
2. Alteration in nutrition
3. Lack of knowledge about contraception
4. Impairment of skin integrity

Plan

Susan had devised and followed her own reducing diet for more than 2 months. The diet severely restricted B complex vitamins as well as folic acid. Susan's diet history coupled with the macrocytic, normochromic anemia and the presence of multisegmented neutrophils on the peripheral smear was indicative of a folic acid deficiency anemia. A serum folate test showed that the level was lower than normal. The persistent diarrhea and development of lesions involving the tongue and mouth are common clinical occurrences in this type of anemia.

A nutritional anemia is one in which there is inadequate intake, impaired absorption, or chronic loss of iron, folate, and/or vitamin B$_{12}$. The adult with a nutritional anemia typically has subjective complaints of fatigue and weakness and possibly headache and shortness of breath. Young women of childbearing age may complain of menorrhagia or amenorrhea. A blood smear may show microcytic and hypochromic red blood cells, indicating an iron deficiency anemia. In contrast, a folate or vitamin B$_{12}$ deficiency produces macrocytic, normochromic red blood cells (Tilkian and others, 1975). Pernicious anemia is associated with a classic triad of symptoms: numbness and tingling in the extremities, sore tongue, and a feeling of weakness or lassitude (Bunn, 1977). These symptoms may precede the hematological picture of pernicious anemia.

Susan was given 1.0 mg of folate supplement daily. In addition, the nurse practitioner discussed the need for raw vegetables and fruits to supply essential vitamins and minerals. Together they developed a well-balanced diet to include foods from the necessary food groups. Susan was discouraged from applying alcohol to her skin lesions. The nurse practitioner stressed keeping the area clean with mild soap and water and applying a mild emollient until the cracks resolved.

Susan was also given Modicon 28, a low-dosage estrogen-progestin birth control pill. Oral contraceptives may slightly lower the serum and red blood cell folate levels. In young women who eat a nutritionally balanced diet, with adequate amounts of uncooked vegetables and fruits, there is ordinarily little indication for additional folate supplements.

A PARADIGM FOR REFERRAL OF ADULTS WITH ANEMIA

The importance of identifying individuals at risk for the development of anemia or in whom anemia is indicative of a serious condition cannot be overemphasized. The outline on p. 90 gives a partial listing of individuals to evaluate carefully for the presence or potential development of anemia.

Many primary care nurse practitioners treat the referral process as a bipolar phenomenon. That is, either they refer every adult they see who has a new symptom, or they refer no one until they have tried a treatment approach without success. Neither strategy is sound or cost effective. Decisions to refer an adult with an anemia should be based on a systematic assessment process. This approach is based on the following four concepts:
1. Anemia is always a secondary manifestation of some other disease process, defect, or deficiency. A careful, comprehensive history and a thorough physical examination help define the underlying cause.
2. With iron deficiency anemia in adults, the nurse practitioner should evaluate for possible occult bleeding. Bleeding sites may be discovered by rectal examination, pelvic examination, urinalysis, and the presence of petechiae.
3. Red blood cell indices give only average values for corpuscular volume and hemoglobin concentration and, although necessary, are subject to misinterpretation. A peripheral blood smear and a reticulocyte count are the most definitive indirect measurements of bone marrow activity. The nurse practitioner should always review the peripheral blood smears of an adult suspected of having an anemia.
4. Vitamin and mineral supplements are not a cure for anemia in adults. Iron preparations may cause an initial improvement in the red blood cell indices of an individual with occult bleeding, but the improvement should not obscure the need to find the source of the bleeding. Vitamin B_{12} preparations may alleviate some of the symptoms of a pernicious anemia, but they will not cure the gastric carcinoma that may have preceded the anemia. Also, injudicious use of vitamin B_{12} injections may mask pernicious anemia while neurological damage continues.

The nurse in primary care practice should refer adults with anemia for a more extensive clinical evaluation when:
1. The cause is undetermined from the history, physical examination, and routine diagnostic studies.
2. Malignancy is suspected to be the cause.
3. Unexplained occult bleeding or frank hemorrhage occurs.
4. Current drug therapy may be the cause of anemia.
5. An anemia secondary to vitamin or mineral deficiency does not respond to the appropriate therapy in 1 month.
6. The anemia is present with abnormal white blood cells and platelet production, indicating a significant bone marrow problem.

REFERENCES

Barry, W.: Evaluation of the patient with anemia, Primary Care **1:**109, 1974.
Brain, M.: Hemolytic anemia, Postgrad. Med. **64:**127, Oct. 1978.
Brown, J., and others: A study of general practice in Massachusetts, J.A.M.A. **216:**301, 1971.
Bunn, J.: Approach to the patient with anemia. In Harrison, T.R., editor: Harrison's principles of internal medicine, ed. 8, New York, 1977, McGraw-Hill, Inc.
Disler, P.B., and others: The mechanism of inhibition of iron absorption by tea, S. Afr. J. Med. Sci. **40:**109, 1975.
Ellin, R.J., and others: Effects of induced fever on serum iron and ferritin concentration in man, Blood **49:**147, 1977.
Elmwood, P.C., and others: Symptoms and circulating hemoglobin level, J. Chron. Dis. **21:**615, 1969.

Ersley, A.: General effects of anemia. In Williams, W.J., and others, editors: Hematology, New York, 1972, McGraw-Hill, Inc.
Finch, C.: Anemia of chronic disease, Postgrad. Med. **64:**107, Oct. 1978.
Flynn, K.T.: Iron deficiency anemia among the elderly, Nurse Pract. **3:**20, Nov.-Dec. 1978.
Frame, P., and Carlson, S.: A critical review of periodic health screening using specific screening criteria, J. Fam. Pract. **2:**123 (part 2); 283 (part 4), 1975.
Guyton, A.C.: Textbook of medical physiology, ed. 5, Philadelphia, 1976, W.B. Saunders Co.
Hillman, R.: Blood-loss anemia, Postgrad. Med. **64:**88, Oct. 1978.
Lee, R.G., and others: Iron-deficiency anemia and the sideroblastic anemias. In Harrison, T.R., editor: Harrison's principles of internal medicine, ed. 8, New York, 1977, McGraw-Hill, Inc.
McDonald, W., and Rubin, C.: Cancer, benign tumors, gastritis and gastric diseases. In Harrison, T.R., editor: Harrison's principles of internal medicine, ed. 8, New York, 1977, McGraw-Hill, Inc.
Rheingold, D., and others: Carcinoma of the colon, Postgrad. Med. **66:**201, Nov. 1979.
Robbins, L.C., and Geller, H.: Probability tables of deaths in the next ten years from specific causes. In Health hazard appraisal, Indianapolis, 1972, Methodist Hospital of Indiana.
Silverberg, E., and Holleb, A.: Cancer statistics 1973, CA **23:**2, 1973.
Tilkian, S., and others: Clinical implications of laboratory tests, ed. 2, St. Louis, 1979, The C.V. Mosby Co.
Whitfield, C.: The patient with anemia: diagnosis, New Phys. **4:**184, July 1967.

SECTION THREE

Problems with family coping

CHAPTER 5

Sexuality during puberty

Suzy H. Fletcher

In reviewing adolescent sexuality and developing recommendations for action, the Wingspread Conference on Early Adolescent Sexuality and Health Care in April 1974 identified four underlying issues that reflect the problems associated with adolescent sexuality. First, adolescents are second-class citizens in our society. Second, society maintains a conspiracy of silence about the lack of accurate information regarding human sexuality. Third, health care is inaccessible especially for contraceptive services. Finally, the impact of a sex-negative society is profound on potential adults (Scales, 1979).

Many of these issues remain current and vitally important in preparing sex education information for adolescents and their families. In reviewing the current literature on adolescents and human sexuality, one notices commonly discussed topics. One frequent subject is the pregnant adolescent and the consequences for the adolescent girl and the father of the child, and the effects on the adolescents' families. The assumption is that the majority of adolescent girls become pregnant. Another common subject is the statistical incidence of venereal disease. A third topic is physiological changes, including those of the endocrine and reproductive systems during puberty, an area in which J.M. Tanner has demonstrated expertise throughout his many years of work. Other subjects include contraception information, its incidence of use and failure rates, and related developmental tasks for the adolescent and family. However, by far most information still conveys the message: "These are all the bad things that can and will happen to you if you engage in sexual intercourse before . . ." (whenever the magic time is).

The purpose of this chapter is to present briefly the developmental and physiological information in the literature and to provide a bibliography for further study in these areas. The nurse practitioner should use the two as a basis for dealing with adolescents who are or may become sexually active during the adolescent years. This chapter does not emphasize the adolescent who is pregnant, has been pregnant, or has venereal disease, since this information is available elsewhere. Therefore, the primary focus is the "normal" adolescent and the changes and subsequent concerns that take place during this period. The goals for the reader are to:
  1. Utilize the steps of the nursing process (that is, assessment, planning, and implementation) to meet the sex education needs of the adolescent and family.
  2. Devise an evaluation procedure for the strategies used in meeting sex education needs.

3. Assist the adolescent and family in understanding the anatomy, physiology, and developmental tasks of normal adolescents.
4. Help the family develop and implement coping strategies that aid everyday living with adolescents and that assist the adolescent in completing developmental tasks.

Any text in psychiatric nursing, medicine, or the behavioral sciences provides a list of general counseling principles and skills necessary to obtain an assessment of problems and the client's readiness and ability to deal with them. The reader is referred to these texts for general counseling guidelines. The following information on developmental tasks, anatomical and physiological changes during puberty, and some behavioral characteristics of the adolescent and family provide the framework for counseling normal adolescents and their families in the area of human sexuality.

LEGAL ASPECTS IN NURSING CARE OF ADOLESCENTS

It is impossible to address adolescent sexuality without including legal aspects of rendering care. The age of consent changed in a number of states when the legal age was lowered to 18. In addition, in 1973, 14 states (California, Colorado, Florida, Georgia, Illinois, Kentucky, Maryland, Mississippi, Oregon, South Carolina, Tennessee, Virginia, West Virginia, Wyoming) and Washington, D.C., had statutes allowing minors to receive contraceptive information without parental consent. Since then, others have followed suit. Individual state statutes should be checked before one provides health care to adolescents.

"Emancipation" is another way to interpret the legal status of minors. According to Chow (1979), the requirements for emancipation include one or more of the following:

Away from home with and in some cases without parental consent
Earning own support
Married minors
Minor parents
Minors in the service
Fifteen years or older depending on individual state statutes

The term "mature minor" is also an important one. It indicates that the adolescent is "sufficiently intelligent to understand and appreciate the nature and consequences of a proposed medical treatment for his own benefit" (Kelly, 1977). Therefore, minors can consent and sign for their own health care.

The law may be more restrictive than popular opinion. A Gallup poll of personal interviews of 1,518 Americans over 17 states indicated that 56% of those interviewed favored making "birth control devices available to teenage boys and girls" (Kelly, 1978). Seventy-seven percent said that sex education should be taught in schools, and 69% supported inclusion of contraceptive information.

ANATOMICAL, PHYSIOLOGICAL, AND BEHAVIORAL CHANGES DURING PUBERTY

Puberty is that period of time when the individual attains the physical capacity to reproduce. Adolescence, on the other hand, is the chronological age span from approximately 12 to 18. Tanner developed the most widely used sequence of pubertal events for

Table 5-1. Range of development for various indicators for girls during adolescence

Indicator	Onset (years)	End (years)
Height spurt	9½	14
Menarche	10	16½
Breast development	8	13
Pubic hair	8	14

Modified from Tanner, J.M.: Growth at adolescence, ed. 2, Oxford, 1962, Blackwell Scientific Publication, Ltd.

Table 5-2. Range of development for various indicators for boys during adolescence

Indicator	Onset (years)	End (years)
Height spurt	10½-16	13-17½
Penis	11-14½	13½-17
Testis	10-13½	14½-18
Pubic hair	10-15	14-18

Modified from Tanner, J.M.: Growth at adolescence, ed. 2, Oxford, 1962, Blackwell Scientific Publication, Ltd.

adolescent boys and girls (Tables 5-1 and 5-2). The underlying cause of these physical changes is a complicated endocrine process, which differs in specific outcomes for girls and boys.

Endocrine process in the female

The hypothalamus is the "master gland" which controls the development of secondary sex characteristics. It also controls both the anterior and posterior portions of the pituitary gland. The anterior part of the pituitary gland produces two hormones related to sexual development: follicle-stimulating hormone and luteinizing hormone. These two hormones are responsible for the following changes at puberty (Chow):
1. An increase in the overall size of the ovaries.
2. An increase in the production of estrogen (generally considered the female sex hormone). This causes growth changes that include:
    a. Skeletal system: increased height and weight, including increased growth rate of the long bones; increased overall pelvic dimension; and closing of the epiphysis of the long bones.
    b. Sexual organs: increased length and width of the vagina; increased uterine size; increased size of the fallopian tubes; development of the menstrual cycle; and enlargement of external genitalia, including the addition of adipose tissue.
    c. Breasts: enlargement of the nipples and increased breast size, which initially is asymmetrical.

d. Skin: increased sebaceous gland production and increased adipose tissue, especially over the pelvis, hips, and thighs.
  e. Hair: increased generalized body hair, especially axillary and pubic areas, including the inner thighs.
3. Secretion of progesterone after maturation of the ovaries. This prepares the uterus for egg implantation during the proliferative phase of the menstrual cycle. It also aids in development of milk ducts in the breast.

Endocrine process in the male

In boys the pituitary gland secretes interstitial cell–stimulating hormone, which is chemically similar to luteinizing hormone in the female. It is responsible for stimulating production of estrogen and testosterone in the gonads. Testosterone is primarily responsible for the following changes at puberty (Chow):
1. Skeletal system: a marked increase in height and weight, including increased growth rate of the long bones.
2. Muscles: increased muscle mass, especially in the shoulders and chest.
3. Sexual organs: increased penis size and length and increased size of scrotum and testes.
4. Skin: increased sebaceous gland production.
5. Hair: increased generalized body hair, including an abundance over the lower half of the face.
6. Voice: change in vocal cords, which allows for voice deepening.
7. Libido: increased sexual desire.

In addition to these physical characteristics, the changes in hormone production lead to behavioral changes that evoke a response by the adolescent and his family.

Behavioral characteristics of the adolescent and family

Certain behavioral characteristics are related directly and indirectly to hormonal activity. The adolescent demonstrates:
1. Extreme moodiness such that behavior may change from rage to sweetness over a few seconds.
2. Strong need for peer approval, which is more important than the approval of parents.
3. Need for exploration and experimentation with himself or herself and the world, which helps develop a sense of sexual identity.
4. Ambivalence toward parents, in which the adolescent sees them as acceptable one minute and the worst parents in the world the next.
5. Hostility and verbal aggression toward parents and others.

In response the parents demonstrate:
1. Ambivalence toward the adolescent, wanting them to grow up on the one hand, and wanting them to remain children on the other.
2. Guilt, anger, and sometimes unreasonable punitive actions as responses to the adolescent's hostility and verbal aggression.
3. Feelings of failure when the adolescent does not live up to parental expectations.

FAMILY TASKS DURING ADOLESCENCE

The adolescent and family also have developmental tasks associated with this period of rapid changes. Many subdivisions of developmental tasks for adolescents exist; however, the following five are representative of those found in the literature:
1. Development of a comfortable sexual identity.
2. Emancipation (physical and financial) from parents and other adults.
3. Beginning a career.
4. Utilization of a personal value system.
5. Realistic acceptance of personal strengths and limitations.

As described by Duvall (1971), family developmental tasks during adolescence are to:
1. Provide household facilities that allow for differences between the adolescent and other family members.
2. Develop a realistic financial system that considers the needs of the adolescent and other family members.
3. Develop a family-oriented sharing of responsibilities.
4. Renew the marital relationship.
5. Develop an effective communication system.
6. Expose adolescents to interactions with relatives, especially older ones.
7. Develop individual interests of all family members.
8. Promote a philosophy of family life.

Duvall's list of family developmental tasks is helpful for several reasons. It helps the family keep perspective. All the above tasks can readily be applied to today's concerns. As the practitioner deals with adolescents and their families, the list of tasks helps reinforce the fact that they are not alone or very different from others in their concerns. Finally, this list correlates well with the adolescent's behavioral characteristics and developmental tasks. It helps adolescents and families realize that many changes are occurring simultaneously and that it is important to keep communication open and allow for individual needs.

ASSESSMENT
History

In establishing a relationship with adolescents and their families, the practitioner should assess each available family member. Some agencies do not have a standard form; use of the guidelines provided here may be helpful. The interview should begin with all family members present and with a discussion of the agency, its policies, services, confidentiality, and what to expect during the appointment. Family members should state their goal for using the agency and what they expect during this and other appointments. The practitioner should inquire about previous experiences with health care agencies and correct any misconceptions. Reinforcing the importance of each family member in this and subsequent appointments is valuable. The practitioner should also stress that what each of them has to say helps her formulate a plan of care. Regarding confidentiality, the family needs to understand that information will become part of the health care record and as such is available to other members of the health team involved with the care of the family.

During this initial conversation the family should understand that the nurse will see the adolescent and parents separately, maintaining confidentiality for both. This should apply to anyone over the age of 12 years. Confidentiality is encouraged by an explanation of the necessity of building rapport with the adolescent, which will gain information to help the adolescent and family in solving their current problems. It is helpful to bring both adolescents and their families together at the end of the appointment to discuss any questions. My experience suggests that many adolescents want their parents to know what is transpiring in their lives (including sexuality). They merely need an intermediary to facilitate communication.

The structured interview. A questionnaire may be useful to gain information from adolescents. In order to use the questionnaire, the adolescent must be able to read. The provider should observe if there is difficulty filling out identifying data initially in her presence. Then, if necessary, the questions can be read aloud. The questionnaire itself provides a good opportunity to build rapport, as it is a focus for discussion.

The following are sample "yes" and "no" questions from which a questionnaire could be developed:

Do you like being a male/female?
Do you have questions about sexual behavior with your friends of the same sex?
Are you interested in birth control information?
Are you able to discuss sexual matters with your parents?
Are you currently using a regular method of birth control?
Do you have questions about venereal disease?
Do you have questions about your sexual activities?
Do you think your body is normal?
Do you sometimes have sexual feelings that you think might not be normal?
Are you having any trouble with your sexual organs?

Some adolescents may not initially give correct identifying data, because they fear the nurse may not be trusted. Initially the nurse should not pressure or confront the client but address him as though he were telling the truth. The client usually becomes comfortable enough by the end of the first appointment to tell the truth. However, it is important to let the adolescent know when he is not giving accurate information, since this also builds rapport. Honesty, regardless of personal beliefs, values, or differences, is more effective than offering practiced communication skills or services.

During the interview, questions about human sexuality may arise: the male and female reproductive system, male and female sexual response cycles, masturbation, menstruation, nocturnal emissions, intercourse, reproduction, contraception, same-sex behavior, venereal diseases, and terminology. Any other areas that need inclusion should also be introduced. Other assessment areas include previous sex education, level of cognitive understanding of information previously given, body image, motivation, level of maturity, current support system, drug history (including street drugs), outside interests, school experience, current and past health, and level of current sexual activity. Areas to explore with parents include their views regarding normal sexual behavior for adolescents, how they have provided and plan to provide sex education, and at what level of sexual functioning they believe their adolescent to be.

The unstructured interview. If the provider prefers a nondirective method rather than or in addition to a printed questionnaire, the following guidelines can be used:

1. Ask questions that assume the normalcy of a behavior, and indicate that most people have experienced it; for example, "Most adolescents experience some concerns about their sexual development. What are your concerns?" Use words and phrases such as "When did you . . . ?" "Where did you . . . ?" "How did you . . . ?" Less preferable are "why" questions or those that need a simple "yes" or "no" answer, because they do not promote dialogue.

2. Help the adolescent describe sexual behavior or concerns in words that mean the same to both of you. For example, use "love making" instead of intercourse, "sleeping together" instead of coitus.

3. Structure the interview to proceed from less sensitive to more sensitive areas. For example, begin the assessment with an adolescent girl by asking questions about menstruation. "How old were you when you began having your menstrual periods?" End with questions about masturbation or same-sex behavior.

4. Use correct terms in a simple way. Use more difficult adjectives with words commonly understood to describe sexual functioning, such as the word "menstrual" preceding "period."

5. Let the adolescent decide on the "goodness" or "badness" of a particular sexual behavior. However, convey the idea that each person has responsibility not to harm another physically or emotionally. In addition, there is a great deal of variation in human sexual behavior. It is important to convey to the adolescent that it is perfectly acceptable to say "no" to a particular sexual activity at any time even if he or she responded "yes" at a previous time.

6. End the interview by asking if there is anything else the adolescent thinks you need to know to help him or her understand sexuality. This question is an excellent technique for obtaining additional information.

Physical examination

During the physical examination signs of sexual maturation should be pointed out and their normalcy emphasized. The physical examination for the adolescent includes all components of any routine physical examination, along with the following appropriate to sexual development:

General: Height, weight, blood pressure.
Skin: Body hair growth and distribution in axilla and pubis, external genital development, acne and oily skin.
Neck: Thyroid.
Breast: Teach breast self-examination; discuss gynecomastia in males, if present.
Female genitalia: A pelvic exam is not usually done unless the girl is menstrual, sexually active, or requesting contraceptive information. Then describe the procedure. Show a movie or pictures of the examination, and provide reinforcement during the examination.
Male genitalia: Descended testes; teach testicular self-examination.
Laboratory procedures: Pap smear, gonorrhea culture, hematocrit, urinalysis, rubella titer, VDRL test, and test for sickle cell, if needed.

PLAN
Counseling methods

Sexuality begins with conception and ends with death. The nurse must know the biological, psychological, and sociological stages of adolescent development to understand the importance of sexuality during this time. It might prove helpful to stay with one particular developmental framework in terms of counseling. Money and Musaph (1978) have divided human sexuality into four categories: (1) biological sex (the external and internal physical sexual structure), (2) sex gender (who the person feels he or she is sexually, that is, male or female), (3) sex role (the part the individual chooses to play in society), and (4) sex object choice (the person with whom one becomes involved). Biological sex is a fact of birth, and sex gender usually is apparent by school age. Sex role and sex object choice partially comprise the developmental tasks during adolescence.

Counseling adolescents in the area of human sexuality takes time and patience. First, the nurse must be able to assure the adolescent that confidentiality will be respected. One approach is to make a general statement that the nurse will hold in confidence whatever the adolescent discloses, provided that the information does not harm the adolescent or others.

From the assessment, priorities can be made of the areas with which adolescents and their families are having difficulties. Some adolescents and their families can clearly identify why they came; others seem to have a vague idea but cannot state it. One of the best ways for the nurse to deal with the first group is to provide the service they request, then together deal with other issues. An example commonly seen in practice is the adolescent girl who wants a quick pregnancy test and nothing else, especially not counseling. It is difficult to do, but the nurse should simply perform the pregnancy test and let the girl go, after providing information on other available services. My experience is that the girl not only returns but brings her friends, because she has some control over one aspect of her life and can begin to demonstrate more responsible behavior.

Some specific interventions for common areas of concern follow.

Contracts. One way of working with adolescents in counseling is the use of verbal or written contracts. The term "contract" as used here refers to two people (the nurse and the adolescent) forming an agreement in which each of them will do certain things.

The contract between the adolescent and nurse contains four basic components. The first component is the goal. Both the adolescent and the nurse should have a mutually agreed upon goal. This allows the adolescents' active involvement in working out their own behavior. It allows the nurse to reinforce responsible behavior and provide guidance in decision making.

The second component is usefulness. Frequently individuals use the word "helpful"; however, adolescents may not find the relationship particularly helpful initially, especially as it involves taking responsibility for their own behavior and actions. Both adolescent and nurse should feel that the relationship can be useful.

The third component is duration. Both parties should decide on frequency of visits, length of visits, and possible duration of the contract. The usual duration is six visits of about 45 minutes each. Obviously, the duration depends on the goal.

The fourth component involves conditions. One condition involves the adolescent's understanding the limits of confidentiality. Additionally, each participant in the relationship has specific behavioral tasks to achieve the goal. The consequences of noncompliance should also be clear. For example, if both parties decide that a certain number of missed appointments negates the contract, the nurse and adolescent must understand that at the outset.

Examples of contracts made with adolescents in the area of sexuality include:

Adolescent:
1. Using foam and condoms until the next menstrual period before starting contraceptive pills.
2. Calling the practitioner to report the start of the next menstrual period.
3. Coming into the office within 48 hours after an abortion or calling if problems arise earlier.
4. Calling before attempting any harm to oneself or to others.

Practitioner:
1. Being on call 24 hours a day.
2. Making special appointment times for an adolescent in school or needing to come while the parents are at work.
3. Providing special payment arrangements, if necessary.

Co-counseling. Education and counseling in human sexuality can be provided by male and female co-counselors to groups of adolescents. Ideally, the adolescents in each group should be about the same age. It is not useful to have a 14-year-old and a 17-year-old in the same group, since developmentally they are at different stages and will compete with each other for attention. They also may have different needs. Co-counseling also works well with parents.

Transactional analysis. Transactional analysis is also a useful theoretical framework for counseling. It is assumed that the "adult" is the part of our ego that protects us when we are playing and having fun; and, if it is assumed that sexuality is fun, it seems logical to strengthen the "adult" by educational methods. Obviously, fun takes place only after we make a responsible decision to participate. The reader is referred to *Games People Play* by Eric Berne for further information.

Values clarification. Values clarification is another method of counseling that works well with adolescents, either in the classroom or individually. First, the adolescents are provided information regarding their sexuality, such as: (1) physiological knowledge of how the body works; (2) developmental tasks of adolescents and their parents; (3) financial aspects of marriage, childbearing, and childrearing; (4) physical and emotional responsibilities of marriage and childrearing; and (5) legal status of adolescents. Next, they are given exercises, such as role-playing, which enable them to use this information and to make responsible decisions. The exercises allow adolescents to practice skills necessary in adulthood and provide them with knowledge necessary for responsible decision making. The key point of values clarification is the knowledge base on which the exercises rest. The reader is referred to *Values Clarification* by Sidney Simon and his colleagues for further information.

Media material. Providing reading material for the adolescent to check out is an excellent method of education on a one-to-one or group basis. (See the adolescent reading list at the end of this chapter.) It is of utmost importance for the nurse to read the recommended material before giving it to the adolescent. In addition, the nurse must provide follow-up of the material by reviewing it with the adolescent on a subsequent visit. One way for the nurse to begin the follow-up session is to take the material, turn to a particular section that the adolescent may have questions about (as indicated by the assessment), and begin a discussion of that area. This allows the adolescent the opportunity to ask questions. If asked for questions, the typical adolescent will respond in the negative. Using the printed material in conversation allows the adolescent to focus on something concrete, because sexuality is a difficult area to discuss. It also prevents the adolescent from appearing uneducated in this area.

Managing problems of adolescents

Physical and emotional changes. Using graphs or diagrams, the nurse should focus intervention on the variability of sexual maturity. The genetic relationship to menstruation, the ability to get pregnant, sexual urges, sexual fantasies, nocturnal emissions, and erratic behavior should also be emphasized. It is important for adolescents and their families to understand that erratic behavior is normal. It is not always predictable or controllable and will decrease with time. Parents may react with occasional or consistent expressions of anger, resentment, or punishment. It is important for parents to maintain a consistent and nonpunitive environment in which adolescents can "try out their wings." Parents can be helped to accept the fact that adolescents will soon leave home; the parents can be encouraged to develop interests and hobbies outside the family.

There are many rules that families might apply during this period of constant changes. However, only two seem appropriate for the essentially well-adjusted family. First, the family should continue doing at home whatever has been done with sexuality. For example, if the family is relatively immodest and the adolescent suddenly becomes very modest, the adolescent's need for privacy should be respected; however, changing long-established family habits should *not* be recommended. This change would only reinforce the negative feelings the adolescent is experiencing. Second, parents should not be encouraged to suddenly want to share all parts of the adolescent's life and to discuss previously unmentionable subjects, such as sexuality. Adolescents need consistency during this time in their lives. If parents wish to change their own behavior, the change should be made gradually.

Still another problem is the rapid growth of the body and external sexual organs, which forces adolescents to be acutely aware of their bodies. This awareness frequently focuses on what adolescents see as a defect, whether it be real or imagined. Examples are being too fat, having breasts that are too large or too small or unequal, or having a penis that is too small. It is, therefore, important to show acceptance of the adolescent's body and help the client to develop respect for it. This can be facilitated by focusing realistically on positive aspects and building on personal strengths. The family can be very helpful by assisting the adolescent in developing interests and in becoming involved in sports or other groups and by providing positive feedback when the adolescent succeeds in any way.

Autoerotic stimuli and accompanying fantasies. Masturbation, or manipulation of the genitals for the purpose of pleasure, is a widespread practice during adolescence and adulthood. Masturbation is a very difficult subject for adolescents and most adults to discuss. Adolescents frequently can talk about masturbation when a general discussion has taken place about its normalcy and general practice among adolescents and adults. Before personal disclosure of the experience, they most often relate that some of their friends masturbate. The majority of adolescent girls know that their boyfriends masturbate; this common knowledge can be an excellent way to promote discussion.

The most frequently asked question regarding masturbation is "How often is too often?" The answer is that, if the person is able to perform activities of everyday life without interference, then he or she is not masturbating too often. This answer avoids the numbers game, as it is common to find many adolescents who masturbate several times daily.

Another question that arises about masturbation and its usual accompanying fantasies is "What kind of fantasies are normal?" The practitioner can stress that there is a difference between fantasy in everyday life and what really happens. This is true about sexual fantasies, also; but most important, the practitioner can stress that the client has a clear choice and can exercise control of that part of his or her life. In other words, the fantasy can come true only if the individual lets or helps it happen. This answer usually produces a great deal of relief, especially when common fantasies include those of same-sex activity and violence.

In a general sense, I promote masturbation as a viable and realistic alternative to sexual intercourse for adolescents who indicate much sexual desire but feel that they are not ready for intercourse. In a discussion with the adolescent, the practitioner can also include the idea that mutual masturbation may be an alternative to intercourse. This is especially helpful for sexually active adolescents as protection against unwanted pregnancy, if they use only the rhythm method of contraception.

Orgasm. Another frequently asked question is "What is orgasm or climax?" Most authorities use these words interchangeably, although some people use the term orgasm for females and climax for males. The nurse can explain that orgasm or climax is a series of muscular contractions in the genital area, which produces a pleasurable sensation. In males it is accompanied by ejaculation, which is release of semen from the penis. In males or females orgasm results from erotic dreams, masturbation, or psychological or physical stimulation of body areas. The client should be told that orgasm can be different for different people. The differences may be the physical feelings experienced, the duration of the feelings, and the experience of pleasure. More scientific explanations are not helpful, because the adolescent simply wants to know what the experience is like.

Contraception. Counseling for birth control of course includes all the various methods available as well as statistical safety, failure rates, and complications. Because adolescents vacillate between childhood and adult behaviors and demonstrate inconsistent responsibility, choosing the most appropriate contraceptive may be difficult. Other important information to include is the rate of pregnancy among adolescents. "One in five adolescents has had sexual intercourse by age 15, and more than half by 19. More than 1.3 million 10- to 19-year-olds became pregnant in 1977. Over one-third of 14-year-olds will have at least one pregnancy by the age of 20" (Scales).

A summary of articles by Card and Wise (1978) and Trussell and Menken (1978) indicates that childbearing before 15 years of age, regardless of marital status or education, produces alarming morbidity. When compared with peers 15 years later, these adolescents show (1) an increased likelihood of illegitimate births, (2) an increased number of total children, (3) increased job dissatisfaction for females, (4) decreased total schooling, (5) decreased occupational attainment, (6) decreased socioeconomic status, (7) increased unstable marriages, and (8) an increase in the number of total marriages per person. These conclusions hold within various racial, educational, and religious subgroups.

Same-sex behavior. Normally, most individuals progress through sexuality on a continuum, beginning with autosexuality (masturbation), next same-sex behavior, then heterosexuality. The relative normalcy of this behavior needs reinforcement. Obviously, the nurse must provide a climate in which the adolescent feels comfortable in sharing information about same-sex behavior. Intervention focuses on explaining developmental stages and discussing what interpretation the adolescent gives to the behavior. Of utmost importance is to stress that same-sex fantasies or one or more same-sex experiences do not "make" one a homosexual. The term "same sex" rather than homosexual or lesbian should be used, since these terms commonly have negative connotations in American society. In addition, adolescents may label themselves or others who have few or no same-sex experiences as homosexuals, or even use the term for adolescents who date little.

Venereal disease. In 1979 minors in all 50 states were guaranteed confidential diagnosis and treatment of venereal disease (Scales). However, the incidence of venereal diseases is skyrocketing, partially because of the increase in sexual intercourse among the population in general and among adolescents specifically. Although the right to treatment is established, access to treatment remains a problem. There is a great need to increase access through adolescent clinics, hot lines, education and referral services in schools, and media advertisement, which include the signs, symptoms, and need for and location of treatment.

Guidelines for parents of teens

1. Keep open communication lines by giving sexual information in a nonthreatening manner.
2. Include a regular discussion time in the family structure.
3. Show approval of developing sexuality.
4. Reinforce previous sex education.
5. Attend and promote appropriate sex education programs in schools and churches.
6. Discuss changes in the body and in emotions anticipated during puberty.
7. Ask for assistance in providing sex education to your adolescents.
8. Use correct terms when discussing body parts and functions.
9. Include both parents when discussing sexuality.
10. Model normal and open sexuality by touching, warmth, and conversation.
11. Avoid double messages, such as on the one hand referring to your adolescent as "well stacked" or a "stud" and then complaining about his or her level of sexual activity.
12. Above all, be honest about your own level of knowledge and comfort. Adolescents always *know!*

Guidelines for parents

As previously stated, parents need to be consistent in dealing with adolescents and sexuality. Some general guidelines for parents are included on the opposite page (Gadpaille, 1975).

EVALUATION

When evaluating sexuality during puberty, the practitioner should avoid a focus on frequency or absence of sexual behavior. Through the development of rapport the adolescent client should begin to ask questions about general sexual behavior in adolescents and adults. Gradually the client may be able to share personal insight or seek answers to more personal questions. This may not always be true, as the adolescent may be working through the role transition necessary for future adult adjustment. Dealing with feelings about sexuality may take months to years before the adolescent feels comfortable with his own working rules for sexual behavior.

The adolescent client who needs referral is one who (1) threatens harm to self or others, (2) exhibits extreme withdrawal even after multiple visits, or (3) desires a different provider for counseling. These situations are rare because most adolescents who seek counseling honestly want to have their questions answered.

SUMMARY

Of all age groups, adolescence is probably the developmental level that is the key to healthy adult human sexual functioning. The nurue who cares for the adolescent needs to be cognizant of the physiological and developmental changes that the young person undergoes. In addition to the personal upheaval experienced, changes probably occur in the family structure and function which are an expected part of the developmental stages of family life. With no other problems, these stresses alone exert significant pressure on an individual striving for a sense of personal identity and independence.

The nursing process is readily applied to the health supervision of adolescents. Initially the assessment process, which involves both strategic interviewing and appropriate physical examination, seeks to gather data to confirm the individual's passage into puberty. Honesty and confidentiality, while always important in client assessment, are essential and often must be stated clearly to establish the trust necessary for an ongoing relationship. The physical examination, in addition to observation of the function of all body systems, should pinpoint evidence of physical sexual maturity and correlate with the developmental level revealed in the interview.

Specific concerns during the interview with the adolescent include information about contraception, venereal disease, masturbation, opposite and same-sex relationships, family communications, and the person's perceptions of inappropriate personal growth and development. In addition, breast self-examination and testicular self-examination are taught as part of personal hygiene routine, a habit adolescents should maintain for the rest of their lives.

Nurses need to consider the paucity of sound research providing a background for care of the adolescent. Research on adolescence now comes from the social and behavioral sciences. Nursing care of the adolescent requires nursing research to support recommendations for specific care of this age group.

ADOLESCENT READING LIST

The Boston Women's Health Book Collective: Our bodies ourselves, ed. 2, New York, 1976, Simon & Schuster, Inc.
The Diagram Group: Man's body: an owner's manual, New York, 1976, Paddington Press.
The Diagram Group: Woman's body: an owner's manual, New York, 1977, Paddington Press.
Jones, K.L., and others: Sex, New York, 1973, Harper & Row, Publishers, Inc.
Race, A.R., and others: The sex scene, New York, 1975, Harper & Row, Publishers, Inc.

REFERENCES

Barnard, U., and others: Human sexuality for health professionals, Philadelphia, 1978, W.B. Saunders Co.
Berne, E.: Games people play, New York, 1964, Ballantine Books, Inc.
Card, J.J., and Wise, L.L.: Teenage mothers and teenage fathers: the impact of early childbearing on the parents' personal and professional lives, Fam. Plann. Perspect. **10:**199, 1978.
Chinn, P.L., and Leitch, C.J.: Child health maintenance: a guide to clinical assessment, ed. 2, St. Louis, 1979, The C.V. Mosby Co.
Chow, M.P. and others, editors: Handbook of pediatric primary care, New York, 1979, John Wiley & Sons, Inc.
Creighton, H.: Law every nurse should know, Philadelphia, 1975, W.B. Saunders Co.
Duvall, E.M.: Family development, Philadelphia, 1971, J.B. Lippincott Co.
Gadpaille, W.J.: The cycles of sex, New York, 1975, Charles Scribner's Sons.
Gordon, S.: The sexual adolescent, North Scituate, Mass. 1973, Duxbury Press.
Kelly, L.S.: The rights of young people in health care, Nurse Pract. **2:**10, Nov.-Dec. 1977.
Kelly, L.S.: Large majority of Americans favor legal abortion, sex education and contraceptive services for teens, Fam. Plann. Perspect. **10:**159, 1978.
Marshall, W.A., and Tanner, J.M.: variations in the patterns of pubertal changes in boys, Arch. Dis. Child. **45:**22, 1970.
Mercer, R.T.: Perspectives on adolescent health care, Philadelphia, 1979, J.B. Lippincott Co.
Money, J., and Musaph, H., editors: Handbook of sexology, New York, 1978, American Elsevier Publishers, Inc.
Morrison, E.S., and Price, M.U.: Values in sexuality: a new approach to sex education, New York, 1974, Hart Publishing Co., Inc.
Murray, R.B., and Zentner, J.P.: Nursing assessment and health promotion through the life span, ed. 2, Englewood Cliffs, N.J., 1979, Prentice-Hall, Inc.
Nakashima, I.I.: Teenage pregnancy—its causes, costs and consequences, Nurse Pract. **2:**10, Sept.-Oct. 1977.
Pierson, E.C. and D'Antonio, W.V.; Female and male: dimensions of human sexuality, Philadelphia, 1974, J.B. Lippincott Co.
Poole, C.: Contraception and the adolescent female, J. Sch. Health. **46:**475, 1976.
Scales, P.: Preparing today's youth for tomorrow's family, Impact **1:**2, 1979.
Simon, S.B., and others: Values clarification, New York, 1978, Hart Publishing Co., Inc.
Sutterly, D.C., and Donnelly, G.F.: Perspectives in human development: nursing throughout the life cycle, Philadelphia, 1973, J.B. Lippincott Co.
Tanner, J.M.: Growth at adolescence, ed. 2, Oxford, 1962, Blackwell Scientific Publications, Ltd.
Trussell, J., and Menken, J.: Early childbearing and subsequent fertility, Fam. Plann. Perspect. **10:**209, 1978.
Wilson, S., and others: Human sexuality: a text with readings, St. Paul, Minn. 1977, West Publishing Co.

CHAPTER 6

Divorce: potential for growth

Barbara Conway-Rutkowski

Where do ideas arise convincing contemporary Western civilization that love, marriage, and happiness thereafter are inextricably interwoven? Along with the values transmitted to the young during socialization, the media and the advertising industry have a tremendous impact on shaping ideas about marriage. The idea of matrimony for beautiful, successful, and happy young lovers is a popular one. Thus couples often lack realistic preparation for entry into the lifetime relationship inherent in the marriage vows. Additional marital stress occurs if the couple's roles change from those of their traditional models. The ever-quickening pace of life-styles in Western society places additional demands on the marriage.

Prevention of divorce by facilitating suitable mate selection and marital adjustment is an important goal. However, when this is impossible, the practitioner is in a position to assist the divorcing couple. Thus the couple may achieve a successful divorce rather than one locked in angry battles and unsatisfactory adjustment. This chapter presents factors that may interfere with marital adjustment, an assessment of the adults' and children's responses to divorce, and a plan for assisting the family members through the complexities of divorce.

A number of alternative family groups exist for individuals who select life-styles outside of traditional marriage. Dissolution of these relationships frequently includes the same emotional responses as in divorce. In subsequent paragraphs divorce often refers to the ramifications of separation in traditional or nontraditional relationships. However, legal obligations differ for marital dissolution and the severance of alternative relationships.

BACKGROUND FOR DIVORCE
Early influences on the adult

The most rudimentary threads of divorce may be evident many years before marriage occurs. In childhood there often exists an inadequate capacity to love and to adjust to life's circumstances and challenges. Many authorities trace such personal maladjustment to the previous generation, in which significant individuals neither fully accepted nor unconditionally loved the child. Moreover, the child frequently lacks the opportunity to identify with one or both parents through honest sharing and witnessing the realities of the adult role. Thus the child has an inadequate and inaccurate concept of adulthood on which to pattern subsequent years. There is no model for acceptance of the rules and disciplinary constraints of adulthood. In short, there is an inadequate emotional climate in childhood based on poor parent-child relationships. The adult in question emerges with significant emotional immaturity and instability, albeit well masked at times. This instability often remains buried during the early years of marriage. It surfaces as the demands of living increase. Stresses such as major illness, job pressures, and the presence of children try one's patience, and even the marriage. Ineffective behaviors continue until the two parties feel hopelessly deadlocked in patterns of hostility, hurt, and bitterness. When this occurs they seek a means of escape.

Child's perspective

As the end of a marriage nears, the children sense problems between the adults. Children may awaken at night to hear arguments, may overhear phone conversations, or may detect differences in parental behaviors toward them. Frequently children feel guilty because they think they are accountable for the family situation. Children believe they are the ones at fault and "bad" because they view parents as omnipotent and infallible. As the adults separate, a child's anxiety increases if parents make denials or offer explanations that are incongruent with the distraught behavior they convey. The adult often feels satisfied that everything possible has been done to calm the child during the trauma of divorce. Still the child may feel intense grief for the absent parent and a mixture of love and hate for the custodial parent. To regain the comforts of the old relationship, the child may manifest a number of somatic problems or may regress to become the focus of parental attention.

ASSESSMENT
Adult's response

When the practitioner assesses a client experiencing marital difficulties, the history reveals several factors. First, the clients may be oblivious to their major problems. They frequently seek help for minor problems, while being unaware of the underlying concern. Second, divorce may exist with emotional ties broken but legal connections remaining. When this state exists, the home front deteriorates into both a covert and an overt battlefield. Hostilities destroy portions of each family member, particularly the children, who are innocent bystanders. Third, a careful total assessment may reveal a lack of positive comments, or as a defense the client may excessively flatter the spouse. Fourth, careful interviewing elicits some resentment about childhood. The client may either accept or boldly deny the relevance of these events to the present situation. Fifth, the client may be aware of anxiety, depression, or some dissatisfaction with his or her pattern of living. Sixth, comments of dissatisfaction are common as the practitioner carefully queries the client on matters of sex and finance. Sexual communications and financial operations of the marital unit often mirror general incompatibility and communication patterns. Negative feelings and responses in these areas cause one to assess further. Seventh, physical manifestations of emotional dissatisfactions are common. Client history frequently reveals multiple concerns. Examples are diarrhea, constipation, changes in dietary patterns, complaints of digestive disturbances, alterations in sleeping, disinterest in daily activities, fatigue, fears of being "anemic," focus on being old, headaches, or complaints of disorganization and unhappiness. One of these problems may be the reason for the client's initial visit. Eighth, asking the client about the health, growth, and development of the children may elicit useful information. Such comments are:

1. The child seems nervous and irritable.
2. The child has difficulty sleeping and has frequent nightmares.
3. The child shows a recent change in eating patterns.
4. The child has difficulty in school or with peers.
5. The child shows regressive behavior such as resuming bedwetting or physically clinging to the other parent.
6. The child exhibits recent behaviors that seem atypical; for example, temper tantrums are a new problem or the child is more withdrawn or outspoken. Parents often attribute these manifestations of the child's insecurity and emotional turmoil to normal stages of maturation rather than to protest against disquieting home events.

Child's response

While all children react to divorce in some way, much more definitive data are necessary to understand age-specific responses. However, responses of children may be grouped in three categories. These include the preschool child, the elementary school child, and the adolescent. Knowledge of the typical responses aids in assessment.

The early years. When parents separate it is important for the practitioner to know the arrangements for child custody and to assess the responses of the child and the adults. The practitioner must also determine what explanations the child receives. If the child is under 5 years old the mother frequently receives custody. The child is often "tied to the mother's apron strings" because of age-related dependency. Consequently, some fathers reject the child along with the mother in the early emotional responses following a divorce. Optimally, the young child receives the truthful, simple explanation that both parents are still parents but must live in separate households to ensure happiness for everyone involved. The practitioner must determine if the mother supports an ongoing father-child relationship. This support is important to the child's welfare.

When the mother becomes the absent parent, it is important to present the mother's departure as resulting from her own unhappiness. Because the mother-child relationship carries great importance at this age, the child must understand that the mother's leaving is not an outcome of his behavior.

Elementary school years. The world of elementary school children is ever-broadening. Their perceptions of a parental breakup may include a greater awareness of antecedent events as well as the actual divorce. School-aged children may seem independent. However, they normally feel a sense of great dependency on both parents. As parental strife increases, the child may express few overt signs of despair. However, accurate assessment demands a closer look. Clues to the presence of an underlying problem are changed interest in peer play; problems with eating, sleeping, or elimination; new complaints of abdominal pains or headaches; and changes in study habits and school performance.

Even though the school-aged child seems disinterested in knowing the facts or in discussing the divorce, there are numerous gnawing, unexpressed fears and questions. For example, the child often fears desertion and wonders who will provide for his care. The practitioner should support the parents in encouraging the child to openly express feelings and concerns. When the situation is not ideal, the practitioner may meet with the child or the parent(s) or both. During this time the practitioner should facilitate the transition from one pattern of living to another by encouraging a positive approach to exploration of alternatives and acceptance of new patterns of living. In some children responses are overtly hostile. Again, parental honesty is essential. A parent's tactful admissions about the unpleasant events occurring around the time of the divorce can open and strengthen the lines of family communication.

Some anger and hostility are inevitable in a divorce. One parent frequently has difficulty restraining negative comments about the other. In offering a positive approach beneficial to the child, the practitioner should emphasize that although the two adults were incompatible in their relationship, they probably have some good parenting qualities. Each parent may find it easier and more honest to describe these specific attributes than to feign affirmation of general qualities in the other party.

Touch remains as important to school-aged children as it is to children under 5. Children at this age require great amounts of understanding, love, and emotional support to endure the hurt and anguish. They may compare their situation with the perceived happiness of a friend in a two-parent family. One needs to remind the child that outward impressions are not always accurate.

Beyond the elementary years. The movement into preadolescence and adolescence is tumultuous. It is characterized by a number of maturational stages. These primarily involve family, peers, and matters of identity as they relate to the gradual attainment of independence. The child in this period has the advantage of increased mobility and independence. He has activities, friends, and resources beyond the family unit. Damage to an adolescent is often not readily apparent; long-term repercussions may occur if the adolescent develops a jaded view of adult male-female relationships. The success of any future relationships depends on a positive view of the self and members of the opposite sex. Feelings about the parent of the same sex and the parent of the opposite sex contribute to this view. The practitioner may be vital in preventing one parent from trying to prejudice the adolescent against the other parent. Also, if parents mistake the intelligent behavior of an adolescent for emotional maturity, they may transfer too great a burden onto the adolescent.

There are several goals of intervention: (1) to fortify the adolescent's relationship with each parent; (2) to assist the parents and child in handling emotion surrounding divorce; and (3) to aid the adolescent in forming new patterns of living, healthy interpersonal relations, and positive attitudes about oneself and members of the opposite sex. To assess progress, the practitioner should monitor key areas, including changes in physical health, peer relations, school, extracurricular activities, and attitudinal and emotional responses. Parental reports, self-report from the adolescent, reports or interviews with interested others (with permission), and observation by the practitioner provide important sources for continued assessment.

PLAN
Intervention in early stages

The stage at which signs indicate that the marriage is very weak but the parties deny this reality warrants that the practitioner proceed with caution. If subtle questions cause defensive responses about the integrity of the marriage, the practitioner must not press. The adults may not be ready for confrontation and realistic dissection of their problems, concerns, and behaviors. During return visits the practitioner should continue to assess the family situation and the need for support systems. The parents must be assisted in correctly identifying any of their child's behaviors that may reflect a problem. If the child is experiencing difficulty, one must approach the problem without making the child the focus of the parents' conflict. By maintaining contact and stressing availability for consultation, the practitioner remains accessible when problems increase or when support is necessary during the actual process of divorce. In some cases the practitioner helps the couple resolve marital conflicts. This resolution often strengthens the marriage.

Assisting the child

The practitioner may intervene to assist the child in coping with the realities of divorce and the distance from one parent. The goal of therapeutic intervention is to minimize the child's negative thoughts about parents, oneself, and the situation. This is done while teaching the child to maximize the positive aspects of the relationship with each parent. Structured therapeutic play is a tool used to unveil anxieties and to alleviate feelings of guilt brought on by belief in adult infallibility. If the practitioner knows of a pending divorce, it is possible to discuss ways that parents might present the situation to the child. When necessary, the practitioner may speak to a child alone (with parental permission) or with the parents. Interventions during discussion and therapeutic play help cushion the blow of divorce.

It is important to reduce the child's anxieties about separation. If the father is the absent parent, he should be encouraged to demonstrate his feelings of love for the child through touch and discussion of common interests. Truthful remarks about future events to be shared cement the ongoing father-child relationship. The father must be reminded that empty promises cause the child concern about relying on the father's love. The practitioner should encourage the parent with custody to help make the absent parent's visits positive experiences. For example, the mother may suggest to the absent father activities that interest a young child.

One should remember that carrying out ideal suggestions is not always possible. The involved adults undergo extreme emotional reactions to their negative experiences and the situational turmoil. They must begin new life patterns, voyage into self-discovery, and face the realities of both their assets and limitations. As one parent leaves the home, the other parent faces the conflict of maintaining a positive attitude with the child in the face of great distress. There is concern related to financial matters, added responsibility, possible full-time employment, and too often a lower material standard of living. Hostile attacks against the absent parent do little good. The parental client should be encouraged to express feelings in therapeutic sessions while seeking realistic solutions to situational problems. Also, the practitioner should encourage positive thinking and emphasize positive aspects of living to the child, who is now a member of a single-parent family.

Commonly experienced feelings

Life-styles change suddenly for those involved in divorce. The practitioner often provides a vital support system for family members experiencing the extreme feelings of grief, loss, and anger. Even when one adult is glad to see the other spouse go, a sense of dissolved routines, uncertainty, and anxiety about change is apparent. These often are in relation to job acquisition and finance, caretakers for children, possible relocation, and the dissolution of friendships. The adult experiences emotional upheaval during this crucial decision period. One should intervene at this point by helping the family identify situational alternatives and arrive at the best decisions within these constraints. The parental clients should be encouraged to delay as many final decisions and precipitous moves as possible. Decision with long-range outcomes and those that are hard to revoke are better left to a time of greater emotional stability. The practitioner should help the client identify other support systems. Many clients choose to move in with supportive relatives during the immediate period surrounding a divorce; this allows them to settle down before making serious decisions. It is probably helpful to many individuals to make as few changes as possible until they feel more stable.

The nurse must be aware that each client has highly personalized thoughts and feelings about divorce. It is a difficult experience for most to endure. Practitioners observing divorced individuals for the first year after divorce frequently recognize the classic stages of grief. Clients need assistance through these stages. The practitioner should help them accept normal and common reactions to loss. Success in the new life depends on how well an individual undergoes, resolves, and grows from the experience.

Other emotions commonly take place in newly divorced individuals. A couple without children may feel great remorse about being childless. They must be helped to identify realistic options for parenthood. Adults also express concern about disappointing their relatives and friends because of the failure of the marriage. They often require assistance in presenting the divorce to those significant individuals. Paternal and maternal parents may need assistance in accepting the divorce and supporting their children. Unfortunately, although their grief and guilt remain intense the individuals often receive little actual assistance with resolving these negative feelings. Another common experience is dismay and surprise to discover some friends are not loyal or dependable. Reasons for the lack of support include a breakdown in common interest, discomfort with one who is divorced, or loyalty to the other involved party. These are additional losses that add to the pain of divorce. The practitioner should provide support to the client by stressing that such losses are common and unavoidable. The client must be encouraged to seek and ally with others who have common interests and are potential friends.

The newly divorced individual usually feels overwhelmed at the task of reorganizing life and is distressed about the myriad of changes. Anxiety about coping with the change is apparent in general behavior and in comments made during the assessment interview. Feelings of failure, guilt, and low self-esteem may be evident in the individual's appearance and self-care. Individuals express a lack of interest in activities outside of those meeting immediate needs. They lack the desire to look into a mirror or have a photograph taken, and they constantly desire to think about or verbalize negative aspects of the divorce or its outcomes. Other emotions are extreme anger, resentment, self-pity, frustration, and fear of future failure. Expression of these feelings should be encouraged. The knowledge that such feelings are commonly experienced during divorce makes the situation more tolerable. While listening to the client's concerns, one can glean positive capabilities that the individual may have. The practitioner should continue to foster hope and encourage realistic action while the client works through the phases of divorce.

Postive outcomes of successful divorce should be stressed. An unhappy marital state is destructive and devastating, but divorce need not be a continuation of the same patterns. Instead, divorce may be the first step in a maturing process wherein involved individuals benefit from prior mistakes and improve their quality of living. When such a positive step occurs, both the involved adults and children improve their quality of life.

When children are present in the family, the parent has great guilt and concern and worries about preventing emotional damage to and providing care for the children. For the parent without custody, there may be a mixture of worry and resentment about providing financial support and being relegated to the role of a visitor. For the parent with custody, concerns center around reliance on the ex-spouse for monetary aid, problems in arranging visitation, and the strain of assuming the role that society assigns to two people. Again, the practitioner should encourage the expression of feelings.

When feelings are voiced and not confronted, spouses often wage war by placing the child in the middle. Thus they make decisions to "get back" at the other adult rather than to work together to achieve the best outcome for the child. When this happens the practitioner should meet with the parents to help break this destructive pattern. The parents may be unaware of their actions. Counseling the child is also necessary when the child has extreme hostility toward one parent. The most important factor in rendering advice is to carefully evaluate all aspects of each situation. One should help the parents look at options.

Some clients may seek pharmacological methods of dealing with the crisis. The use of tranquilizers or sedatives may limit the clients' successful adaptation and may promote drug dependence. A clear explanation of the problems associated with psychotropic medications should be given to those special clients.

First year after divorce

The first year after divorce is the most difficult for both parties. It is a time for relinquishing the old life and forming new patterns. As negative feelings subside, the individual commonly makes a visible change. One notices a change in hair style, a change in dress, or acquisition of new material goods. These changes might be a surprise if the individual was formerly more retiring. The individual may also experience a return of thoughts, feelings, and issues dormant since adolescence. Facing the prospect of being single once again may cause some clients to be concerned about the adequacy of their total sexuality. If as an adolescent a client had low self-esteem or felt inadequate to compete with peers, the client may resume these same concerns. Resolution is necessary for the adult to achieve mature self-acceptance and an understanding of personal assets and liabilities. Thus successful participation in future adult relationships becomes possible.

Fatigue. During the first year fatigue is a common problem. Knowledge of contributing factors assists intervention. Adjusting to a lower standard of living brings pressures that add to fatigue. When immediate improvement of financial resources is impossible, the services of a financial counselor are helpful. These counselors analyze the family budget and make suggestions for changes. It is important for some clients to receive a vocational analysis. Vocational rehabilitation counselors who receive compensation on a sliding scale are available in most communities. A realistic plan for career development is possible after evaluation of aptitude, interest, and preparation. The practitioner should assist the client by providing encouragement and information concerning resources for funds for education.

Difficulty in setting priorities and budgeting time results in fatigue, anxiety, and frustration. The client can be taught to analyze the problem by assessing the tasks and the time limits. The practitioner should outline a concrete plan with methods for accomplishing these tasks within the time frame and help the client evaluate the reasons for not meeting deadlines. Inappropriate steps or unrealistic deadlines should be modified according to the evaluation. In this way the client learns to correct any disorganization.

The daily care of children is a major source of concern and energy expenditure. To provide normal experiences for the child, the parent may attend some of the child's school, religious, or community functions. While this is important to the child, the adult may sense a distance between himself and married parents. This feeling usually occurs because of guilt and self-consciousness on the part of the single parent, lack of commonality between married and single parents, or the threat that the single parent poses to an insecure married parent.

Irritability. Irritability may increase insidiously in the single parent. Children frequently become targets for the irritability, since they are defenseless and offer no threat to the adult's position in the social or work world. The adult should be encouraged to develop better ways to vent frustration. Adult-oriented extracurricular activities provide outlets for this energy. The practitioner should assist in planning solutions to questions of time, money, and child care that may be obstacles to this necessary pleasure. Counseling the client about the importance of self-improvement, relaxation, self-reward, and adult socialization may be necessary to allay client concerns about "taking time and money away from the children." A satisfied adult is better equipped to provide quality involvement with the children and in other areas of life.

Loneliness. As the adult copes with the multiplicity of issues and problems that comprise daily living, the day becomes busy with activity. Even so, an intense feeling of loneliness sets in. As the single parent looks around at work, in the grocery store, or in other public places, it seems that everyone has someone and has a place to go. The single parent may feel isolated from others, especially those of the opposite sex. Evenings, weekends, and holidays in particular are hard to cope with. Close friends or relatives can offer some support for these periods, but they cannot relieve the single adult from all lonely moments.

As loneliness intensifies, the adult thinks about himself, interpersonal relationships, and the future. Movement into new relationships may take a number of directions. A potential problem during this period is that an intense desire for sex may lead to early commitments based on insufficient information or lowered standards. In these cases outcomes are often less than desirable. Relationships with both sexes tend to be sounder when the adult proceeds slowly while continuing personal growth.

How can the client meet new friends? The practitioner can offer suggestions such as informal arrangements, singles clubs, place of employment, avocational interest groups, introductions through family or friends, introductions through participation in children's activities, housing selection, and religious groups. A key point for the client to realize is that one cannot remain reclusive and meet others. The practitioner may aid the client and children in analyzing life patterns and interests to maximize socialization and development of desired relationships.

Informal arrangements such as sharing babysitting duties with a parent in the same situation may lead to a new relationship. Some individuals decrease expenses and make friends by sharing meals on a regular basis. These people may include other singles who live in close proximity and are in the situation of cooking alone or dining without other adults.

Singles clubs form around a variety of themes and interests. An example of a group that combines socialization for single adults and children with educational programs is Parents without Partners. Some groups are exclusive to sailing enthusiasts, travelers, college graduates, or to others with shared interests. For some, such groups provide reassurance and emotional support; the adults discover they are not alone. Opportunities may exist for discussing problems and concerns with a variety of people who offer alternative solutions. In addition, the client observes that others progress through the difficult postdivorce period. A potential problem is clients involvement with individuals who remain locked into negative or immature patterns. Those persons repeat their past mistakes.

There are some advantages when friendships arise from introduction by friends and relatives. First, each individual has an endorser known by the other party. Some background information is therefore available. Second, the circumstances of meeting are quite socially acceptable.

As the client moves into the arena of dating, many of the rules, issues, joys, and concerns of the adolescent dating period reappear. This is often a painful realization for an adult. For example, many presume that the divorced woman is sexually promiscuous. Consequently, the divorced woman again faces the issue of reestablishing her moral code and reputation. The divorced male has different concerns resulting from the usual situation of living alone coupled with society's concept of maleness. While the moral questions may or may not be the same, men and women both have feelings and concerns about past hurts and future involvements.

As establishment of new patterns for male-female relationships begins, the adults in a relationship must carefully consider their needs and the needs of their children. This is essential before making decisions regarding the scope of the relationship, living together, or other long-range plans. The practitioner may be of great assistance in helping adult clients make decisions about dating behaviors.

EVALUATION OF ADJUSTMENT

During the first year it is expected that routines of living, working, and child care fall into place. The adult begins to accept the self as a divorced person. Patterns of socialization begin to develop. Life continues.

After the first year one notes that the divorced individual is more stable. Patterns of living and working are evident. Some of the frequent emotional highs and lows obvious during the first year occur less often and for shorter periods. Awareness of other divorced individuals and of their situational concerns is common. Such information provides the divorced individual with a yardstick for measuring the degree of personal adjustment. Progress in relationships with both males and females is usually obvious. Moreover, interests and concerns frequently reveal thoughts and actions that encompass more than the individual's immediate or basic needs.

Interruption of the orderly progression of adjustment for single parents commonly is related to issues of custody, support, and visitation. When ex-spouses continue arguing over these issues, such sessions become upsetting to the adults and the children. Practitioners may work with one or both adults to resolve angry feelings and establish a mutually agreeable plan for visitation. If destructive behaviors continue, they impede progress and the establishment of positive patterns of living. Expert counseling may be necessary.

There are multiple reasons why some individuals are unable to move beyond grief and to establish a new life. If the client remains in this unhappy stage, expert counseling may be necessary to resolve grief and promote growth.

By touching on the numerous outcomes that result from divorce one can see that each issue is complex. The practitioner with formal education in counseling, personal growth and development, and family dynamics is a valuable support either to clients working to stabilize a marriage or to clients in the process of divorce.

SUGGESTED READINGS

Africano, L.: Dating and the single parent, Women's Day, Feb. 20, 1979.
Blackwood, C.: The stepdaughter, New York, 1976, Charles Scribner's Sons.
Edwards, M., and Hoover, E.: The challenge of being single, New York, 1974, The New American Library, Inc.
Eisler, R.T.: Dissolution: no-fault divorce, marriage, and the future of women, New York, 1977, McGraw-Hill, Inc.
Erickson, M.L.: Assessment and management of developmental changes in children, St. Louis, 1976, The C.V. Mosby Co.
Erikson, E.H.: Childhood and society, ed. 2, New York, 1963, W.W. Norton & Co., Inc.
Gersh, M.J.: How to raise children at home in your spare time, Greenwich, Conn., 1966, Fawcett Books: Crest, Gold Medal, Premier & Popular Library.
Hoeffer, B.M.: Single mothers and their children: challenging traditional concepts of the American family. In Brandt, B., and others, editors: Current practice in pediatric nursing, vol. II, St. Louis, 1978, The C.V. Mosby Co.
Krantzler, M.: Creative divorce, New York, 1974, The New American Library, Inc.
Levine, J.A.: Who will raise the children? New York, 1977, Bantam Books, Inc.
McGinnis, M.: Single, Old Tappan, N.J., 1976, Fleming H. Revell Co.
Montague, L.: A new life plan: a guide for the divorced woman, New York, 1978, Doubleday & Co., Inc.
Moustakas, C.: The child's discovery of himself, New York, 1966, Ballantine Books, Inc.
Napolitane, C., and Pellegrino, V.: Living and loving after divorce, New York, 1977, The New American Library, Inc.
Newman, M., and Berkowitz, B.: How to be your own best friend, New York, 1971, Ballantine Books.
O'Neill, N.: The marriage premise, New York, 1978, Bantam Books Inc.
O'Neill, N., and O'Neill, G.: Shifting gears, New York, 1974, Avon Books.
Petri, D.: The hurt and healing of divorce, Elgin, Ill., 1976, David C. Cook Publishing Co.
Stone, L.J. and Church, J.: Childhood and adolescence, ed. 3, New York, 1973, Random House, Inc.
Sutterley, D.C., and Donnelly, G.F.: Perspectives in human development: nursing throughout the life cycle, Philadelphia, 1973, J.B. Lippincott Co.
Whipple, D.V.: Dynamics of development: euthenic pediatrics, New York, 1966, McGraw-Hill, Inc.

FILMS

Felt, H., and Felt, M., producers and directors: Mothers after divorce. 20 min., color, rental $30, purchase $285, Boston, 1979, Polymorph Films.
Felt, H., and Felt, M., producers and directors: Stepparenting: new families, old ties. 25 min., color, rental $35, purchase $345, Boston, 1979, Polymorph Films.
Fiering, A., producer and director: Memories of family. 24 min., color, rental $35, purchase $345, Boston, 1979, Polymorph Films.
Fiering, A., producer, and Weinstein, M., director: Not together now. 25 min., color, rental $30, purchase $325, Boston, 1979, Polymorph Films.

CHAPTER 7

Caring for women during the climacteric

Patricia E. Brisley

The climacteric is one of the least understood phases in a woman's life. No two women perceive or proceed through this particular developmental stage identically. Since the experience is highly variable, making assumptions about its effects on an individual is of questionable value. The purpose of this chapter is twofold: to review current knowledge about the climacteric as it relates to women's health needs and to provide a reference for the primary care practitioner who cares for women in this age group.

The climacteric, interchangeably labeled the menopause or "change of life," is that midlife period when women undergo changes in the menstrual cycle which lead to cessation of menses. Specifically, menopause is the actual cessation of menses and is complete when menstrual bleeding is absent for at least 12 months. Afterwards, authorities use the term postmenopausal (Jazzman and others, 1969). The climacteric is the time immediately preceding, during, and following natural cessation of menses (Timiras and Meisami, 1972). Many refer to this often broad span of time as perimenopausal or, in lay terms, "the change of life."

For some women menses ceases abruptly; for others surgical intervention produces what clinicians call artificial menopause. Menopause usually occurs between 45 and 55 years of age, with the average being 50 years of age. It takes between 2 and 4 years to complete menopause, with hot flushes becoming more noticeable during the last year of menstruating life. The most common physical sign of onset is menstrual irregularity. Some women experience a gradual lengthening of menstrual cycle with 1 or 2 missed menses. Menses may then occur at regular intervals followed again by periods of amenorrhea. Other women may experience diminished time between cycles or a change in duration or amount of bleeding, with menstrual flow becoming either lighter or heavier (Mantz and Schwabb, 1978).

PHYSIOLOGY

The physiological basis for changes associated with cessation of menses is unknown. The cessation of ovarian follicular activity after menopause leads to changes in androgen, progesterone, gonadotropin, and estrogen secretion. Changes in androgen metabolism include (1) decreased ovarian secretion of androgen, (2) increased ovarian secretion of testosterone, and (3) decreased adrenal secretion of androgen (Benson, 1980).

Progesterone, produced primarily by the corpus luteum after ovulation, becomes decreased in postmenopausal women. Since the ovaries do not contain functional follicles after menopause, many authorities feel this to be the cause of decreased progesterone. Small amounts of this hormone are present after menopause, although the source is unknown.

There is a marked increase of circulating gonadotropins with menopause. Follicle-stimulating hormone (FSH) levels are usually much higher than luteinizing hormone (LH) levels. It is believed that increased gonadotropins are a response to the absence of ovarian steroids. However, authorities believe that the ovaries secrete less estrogen because of inability to respond to pituitary gonadotropin stimulation. When this occurs, the hypothalamus responds to the hormonal imbalance by secreting large quantities of releasing factors in an attempt to increase circulating estrogen. Thus during early climacteric, the characteristic hormone pattern is decreased amounts of estrogen and progesterone and increased amounts of pituitary gonadotropins. The blood levels of FSH and LH start to rise about a year before menstruation ceases and peak 2 or 3 years after menopause. In 70% of women this elevated FSH level remains for 20 to 30 years after menopause (Chakravarti and others, 1976).

Erratic estrogen production causes irregular uterine bleeding. When the ovary secretes insufficient amounts of estrogen, endometrial proliferation decreases, menstruation ceases, and menopause has occurred (Willson and Carrington, 1979). The decline of estrogen levels is gradual, and some estrogen continues to circulate in the bloodstream of the postmenopausal woman albeit in highly variable amounts. In general, the overall production of exogenous estrogen is reduced with a greater decrease in estradiol. The source of postmenopausal estradiol appears to be the adrenal glands rather than the ovary. The ovary and adrenal glands produce androstenedione, a weak androgen that converts to estrone, a weak estrogen. Estrone and testosterone are converted to estradiol in peripheral tissue. After menopause there are higher amounts of estrone than estradiol. The specific clinical signs produced by the alteration of hormones are discussed in the section on assessment.

PSYCHOSOCIAL ASPECTS
Societal expectations of menopausal women

Although the general public often views menopause negatively, most women consider it a nontraumatic event and handle it more easily than expected. Approximately 10% to 25% of women seek medical advice for symptoms attributed to the climacteric (McKenzie, 1978). However, this area has been inadequately studied, and it is unclear if the problems presented are attributable to menopause or to other medical causes. Additionally, researchers of menopause have collected data only in the last 20 or 30 years, with a focus primarily on women who seek medical care. In terms of predicting which women will have more complaints during menopause, the literature cites the following differences. Women with the fewest complaints are more likely to be single, have professional careers, be nulliparous, or have a final pregnancy at an older age. They also have higher incomes and educational levels; see menopause as associated with increased stature, respect, and freedom of activity; and do not suffer from premenstrual depression. Women with more menopausal complaints are more likely to be married, have been pregnant, or have a final pregnancy at a younger age. They have lower incomes and educational levels and place much emphasis on sex, youth, and glamour. They also have premenstrual depression with marked dysmenorrhea, have low self-esteem, and have "overintegrated" into the motherhood role (Tucker, 1977).

Traditionally, Americans perceive menopause as a stressful experience that all women who live to middle age must endure. Nonetheless, a paucity of research exists that accurately describes this phenomenon or provides information to assist these women. To date there is little agreement on why and how menopause occurs, what symptoms and body changes directly relate to menopause, or how to manage problems resulting from these physiological changes. Lack of investigation before 1900 exists because a woman's life expectancy was less than 50 years, leaving few women to experience the climacteric (Cali, 1972). Additionally, in a male-oriented culture females were expected to cope with "women's problems," which were considered unimportant. Investigators are now evolving a body of knowledge about the climacteric because of the changing view of women's place in society, the expanding knowledge of human physiology, and the developing sophistication of research in the past 50 years.

Generally, women who have adapted well during previous developmental stages cope with individual limitations as they grow older. As in any other major developmental stage, many changes influence adjustment and satisfaction during the midlife years. Conditioning and social beliefs greatly influence the individual meaning a woman ascribes to menopause. This includes the ramifications of becoming old. Regardless of how well she is, looks, and feels, others constantly remind her of her changing status. She may notice that men attend to younger women and that hot flushes and the resultant need to regulate room temperatures produce jokes. When she is nervous or angry as a legitimate response to real-life situations, others may attribute her mental state to menopause and dismiss it lightly (Fuchs, 1978).

American culture emphasizes youth and vitality. American society views the aging female as losing her femininity and becoming unattractive, sexually inept, and useless as a bearer of children in a culture that stresses fertility and procreation. Coping with physical changes associated with aging is distressing for most women. They dread the signs of advancing age, such as wrinkles, sagging breasts, and flabby muscles. They are often gullible about products or promotions that claim to guarantee, prolong, or restore youthful appearance and energy. It is noteworthy that the past decade reveals an upsurge in women who question what they have been taught. Women are emerging as capable, intelligent, worthwhile individuals who make valuable contributions to society. As a result, the older woman views herself favorably as someone who is attractive and accordingly demonstrates confidence in herself and her abilities. Very recently the mass media have attempted to portray the older female as an attractive sexual being. Women's magazines include articles on the advantages of being older. The fashion sections are beginning to use models in the 40- to 60-year age group. One is no longer expected to be dowdy if over 30 or a grandmother.

Menopause receives the blame for a multitude of undesirable occurrences and behaviors. For example, younger women or men can be irritable, forgetful, or have disintegrating marriages. If these problems occur during middle age, menopause is a frequent explanation. Menopause can be used as an excuse or reason for almost anything that goes wrong physically or emotionally with a woman during those years. Consequently men and women often endure problems that might be alleviated if put in proper perspective.

The threat of mental instability presumed to accompany menopause may be another source of stress to many women. It is a common belief that women have little control over their emotions because of unpredictable hormonal influences. Nonetheless, cessation of menstruation at midlife does not seem to alter that opinion. Many consider menopause a time of emotional lability when women become nervous and depressed, possibly lose their sanity, or require institutionalization (Feeley and Pyne, 1975). An individual's personal experience may reinforce generalizations about the emotional state during the climacteric. For example, a woman's own mother, relative, or family friend may have experienced depressive illness or attempted suicide during this particular time of life. This may arouse fear of mental instability in the offspring or friend. There are no data to confirm that depression in women is more prevalent during the climacteric or that involutional melancholia is directly associated with menopause (Winokur, 1973). Authorities estimate that about 6 in 100,000 menopausal-aged women experience the mental disorder involutional melancholia (Rosenthal, 1968).

With the advent of family planning, women gained control over their procreative function. However, some women view procreation as the only purpose for sex. Some women look forward to menopause so they will not have "to put up with sex anymore." This supports certain cultural expectations or myths that sexual desire and activity decrease significantly or cease to exist with advancing age (Gruis and Wagner, 1979). Although this trend is changing, many young people still recoil at the thought of older people participating in and enjoying sex.

Unfortunately, professional attitudes about the female climacteric do not lag far behind the predominantly negative one portrayed by the general public. To quote one: "A girl becomes a woman when estrogen and progesterone arrive; when they depart, she is a woman by courtesy only, in reality a castrate" (Wilson and Wilson, 1963). Health care providers often approach middle age and older women with a paternalistic attitude. They see her as a "crocky" demanding individual, someone to palliate or ply with medicine to keep happy. Drugs such as diazepam substitute for discussion or preparation for referral to a mental health provider. Some women receive reassurance and support, while others receive high doses of estrogen.

In addition, women from all age groups complain that their doctors are insensitive, sexist, dictatorial, and convey a demeaning attitude during pelvic examination (Glass, 1976). The difference in gynecological care provided by various types of health providers has not been well studied, although this area is ripe for research. If the nurse practitioner views her role as more "cure" oriented than "care" oriented it is much easier to lose sensitivity. Without attentiviness to the unified person the practitioner may overlook the menopausal woman's expression of need.

Effects of recent role changes on menopausal women

Working women. Traditionally, married women have had difficulty coping with role changes in the family as they became older. Some women still experience the "empty nest syndrome" during menopause, but the increased number of working mothers outside the home has helped ease this transitional period when children leave. The trend in activity patterns in women is due to a number of factors: federal law now regulates hiring practices for women and minorities; esteem of the traditional housewife role has declined; divorce rates are increasing; and more families desire a better standard of living. By the time many women reach menopause, they do not have children under 18 living at home. However, current trends in education and career goals for women may postpone pregnancy and alter this pattern in the future. What might become more significant to the middle-aged woman is child rearing later in life or caring for the physical and financial needs of aging parents. The smaller, more mobile family may alter support systems so that fewer children are able to share the responsibility for the care of aging parents (Fuchs).

Married women. Marital relationships can also pose conflict and often produce a reassessment of roles during the climacteric. Couples may realize they no longer have a common bond after the children leave home. Either partner may feel trapped and dissatisfied with life and individual accomplishments. If sexual needs are unmet, the wife may seek an extramarital affair despite lack of societal sanction of this. Should the husband be involved in adultery, the discovery can be shattering, although many women expect male infidelity. This is particularly painful if the wife feels less attractive and desirable than her younger counterparts. If the husband is involved with work and outside activities, the mother without children at home may become bored or feel useless because of failure to promote personal growth. Another source of frustration for the married woman is coping with her sexual needs if her spouse is physically incapacitated or shows waning sexual potency.

Recently there has been a sharp rise in divorces initiated by women wishing to sever the relationship (Kaluger and Kaluger, 1974). An increase in the number of runaway wives also reflects this trend. Whatever the reason for separation—be it divorce, runaway, or widowhood—the woman encounters loneliness and must learn to be independent and self-sufficient. Although pregnancy may not concern the menopausal woman, it may be difficult to discard religious or societal conventions to maintain an active sexual life. In addition, there are more older women than men. This implies competition with younger women for male affections. If she becomes involved with a younger man, she may have to cope with rejection from family members or friends.

Single women. Society generally views the climacteric as a dramatic and difficult time for the single or childless woman. A review of the literature shows almost nonexistent research regarding the effects of the climacteric on this group. While some women may feel unfulfilled without bearing and raising children, it is not emotionally devastating for everyone. Today women find it less difficult to admit even when married that they do not want to have children. In the past, verbalizing these feelings encouraged labels of being antimotherhood, selfish, or abnormal. On the other hand, more single women are having children as natural mothers or through single-parent adoptions. Single women who grow older and do not chose parenthood may find parental desires waning as they become fulfilled in other ways. Relationships that enhance one's feelings of contributing to future generations without childbearing are important alternatives. Women who enjoy having children as a part of their lives may seek involvement with children of family members, friends, church organizations, or volunteer agencies. A profession that enables contact with children may also meet this desire.

ASSESSMENT

Involvement in the health care of women during the climacteric can be challenging and rewarding to the nurse practitioner. A woman may have nonspecific problems that can frustrate both client and provider. Since these problems may occur during menopause, it is easy to attribute vague signs and symptoms to menopause. Any middle-aged woman, whether or not she exhibits menopausal symptoms, deserves a careful assessment attending to specific risks for her age group. Since climacteric symptoms can shield organic disease, a thorough assessment is essential before any attempt to manage nonspecific symptoms. Table 7-1 lists symptoms ascribed to menopause that may signal the presence of organic disease.

Table 7-1. Examples of symptoms often ascribed to menopause that may signal the presence of organic disease or other health concerns

Symptom	Differential consideration
Alteration in menstrual bleeding patterns	Uterine or cervical cancer Tuberculosis Fibroids Diabetes Thyroid imbalance Early pregnancy Emotional disturbances
Anxiety/depression	Thyroid imbalance Drug use (Aldomet, reserpine, oral contraceptives) Hypertension Psychiatric disorders
Sweating	Tuberculosis Bacterial infections (urinary tract infection, pneumonia) Hypertension Thyroid imbalance
Fatigue	Anemia Congestive heart failure Arthritis Depression Urinary tract infection Thyroid imbalance Diabetes
Headache	Hypertension Cervical arthritis Migraine Muscular tension Dental problems
Low backache	Renal disease Postmenopausal osteoporosis Herniated vertebral disc Acute back strain Obesity Metastatic cancer

History

There is no consistent agreement about what constitutes the menopausal syndrome except the presence of hot flushes (Jazzman and others). Authorities attribute sweats and chills accompanied by hot flushes, nervousness, irritability, depression, and headaches to estrogen withdrawal. However, social, environmental, and emotional factors may influence development of these symptoms independent of estrogen deficiency (Yen, 1977). Although a comprehensive history is essential, those areas particularly relevant to menopause are discussed in the following sections.

Menses. Changes in regularity, duration, amount, and character of flow should be documented to assess the existence of abnormal bleeding. General criteria for making this determination include (Kemmann and Jones, 1979):
1. Prolonged bleeding more than 8 days' duration
2. Excessive bleeding, more than two pads over normal daily pad count
3. Polymenorrhea with frequency more often than every 21 days
4. Intermenstrual bleeding or spotting
5. Bleeding after absence of menses for 12 months
6. Continuation of menses after age 54

One should keep in mind that some women accept gynecological problems and menstrual irregularities without question. They are unaware of risks related to changes and of the importance of seeking care. Schneider (1974) tabulated the reasons most mentioned by patients with carcinoma of the vulva who delayed seeking relief for symptoms such as pruritus, discharge, and irritation for 2 to 8 years before consultation. One half of these patients expressed a sense of embarrassment and modesty, and lack of a sense of urgency or desire for therapy. Some of these findings may also apply to women with menstrual irregularities and so pose a challenge to the primary care provider. Elderly clients may exhibit minimal symptoms of invasive carcinoma of the cervix. A watery discharge may be the initial symptom before the appearance of increasingly bloody discharge (Schneider). Many clients appear surprised when the provider explains that bleeding after menopause is abnormal.

Dyspareunia. A complete assessment of the menopausal client must include a sexual history. The practitioner should interview the client while obtaining information related to the genitourinary system or when doing the pelvic examination. Some practitioners view initiating a discussion about the client's sexual experiences or problems as prying. The nurse may initially feel awkward when approaching the subject, but it is my experience that clients are less reluctant to discuss sexual matters than expected. One needs to discuss such intimate matters of importance without passing value judgments or expressing shock. The practitioner should keep in mind that sex terminology connotes various meanings. Common problems that women express during menopause include dyspareunia lasting for hours afterward and postcoital bleeding. These may be a result of thinning vaginal walls, decreased ability for vaginal expansion, and decreased vaginal lubrication during coitus (Gruis and Wagner). However, vaginal bleeding can also signify neoplastic disease. Clients may also report changes in sexual frequency. Some women experience decreased sex drives, while others experience increased sex drives. Both are normal.

Occasionally a client prefers not to discuss sexual matters. If this occurs, the practitioner should inform her that sexual functioning is an appropriate health concern and convey availability should she wish to discuss this at a later time. She may be more willing to share personal information after a relationship of trust develops. Occasionally an anxious client may reveal only part of the problem because of past rebuffs or unavailability of a concerned listener. An openness and willingness to discuss both feelings and identified problems may improve the client's ability to communicate. Other less threatening topics to initiate a discussion might include general education about aging and sexuality and sexual response changes related to aging or chronic disease.

Vaginal secretions. Vaginal pruritus and leukorrhea may result from local bacterial invasion of traumatized skin. The color, amount, frequency, and odor of vaginal discharge should be noted. In contrast, cervical mucous secretion may decrease during menopause and lead to excessive dryness of the vagina and dyspareunia.

Urinary symptoms. Declining estrogen levels may produce genitourinary problems such as thinning of the urethra and bladder neck and make the urethra susceptible to irritation. Most genitourinary complaints occur after menopause after vasomotor symptoms subside (Seiler, 1977). Increased residual urine in the bladder is a common explanation for urinary complaints. Although dysuria is common, the incidence of proven urinary tract infections increases only after age 65 (Brown, 1977). Another problem, nocturnal urinary frequency, increases progressively with age. Authorities speculate that cerebral deterioration rather than bladder inflammation is responsible for this age-related finding. In addition, stress incontinence is common in postmenopausal women because of loss of tone in structures supporting the bladder and uterus.

Vasomotor symptoms. Vasomotor disturbances such as hot flushes, headaches, and palpitations occur in varying degrees in approximately 40% to 75% of women (Dyer, 1979). True vasomotor symptoms are unlikely during early climacteric years if menstruation is regular. Although the precise physiological mechanism of flushing is unknown, hormones may mediate the response, particularly reduction of ovarian estrogen secretion or increase of gonadotropins. Exercise, eating, and excitement, stress, or other emotions may also precipitate or aggravate it (Seiler). One source suggests that declining estrogen levels alter the ability of subcutaneous small blood vessels to dilate and constrict as before. After a flushing response, constriction reduces the blood supply and produces dizziness or cold hands and feet (Mantz and Schwabb). However, some investigators question this hormonal cause. A double blind study using clonidine, a drug that does not effect hormonal balance, was found to produce a highly significant improvement in hot flushes (Clayden and others, 1974). Of those who experience flushing, 25% to 50% will complain of this symptom for more than 5 years (Benson, 1980).

Hot flushes, occasionally termed flashes, usually occur above the waist and start at the neck and face. Many women describe flushing experiences as sensations of extreme heat. One individual may have flushes that last a second; another, a few minutes or half an hour. Flushes can occur once or twice a week, or they can occur many times daily. There may be visible flushing or beads of perspiration. Occasionally formication, a crawling sensation on the skin, occurs. Weakness, fatigue, faintness, and vertigo are less commonly associated symptoms. Perspiration of the scalp may complicate hairstyle upkeep, and profuse underarm wetness can be embarrassing and uncomfortable. With severe flushing and perspiration, women may have to change bed linens and clothes during the night, which also can interrupt sleep and rest.

Somatic and emotional symptoms. There is no causal relationship between the incidence of subjective or emotional symptoms and menopause. Many middle-aged women experience emotional changes; however, the role of ovarian failure in the initiation of psychiatric disorders is unclear (Benson). Other stresses during middle adulthood may coincidentally contribute to psychological disturbances. However, the practitioner should note complaints of irritability, anxiety, insomnia, headaches, and depression and its attendant symptoms. Although few women exhibit all or even any symptoms, the vagueness of their presentation challenges the practitioner who evaluates such individuals.

Musculoskeletal symptoms. Skeletal problems during the climacteric become evident in numerous ways. Some clients may complain of vague joint pains, especially of the hands, feet, and back. Low back pain, the most common skeletal complaint, may be caused by obesity, chronic postural problems, insidious menopausal bone resorption, or systemic and local disease. A common first symptom of osteoporosis of the spine may be sudden severe back pain. It often follows muscular effort or trauma and lasts 3 to 4 weeks. The client may interpret this as a "lumbago" (Krone, 1974). The condition becomes chronic with increased bone loss from the vertebrae because of subsequent compression fractures. Occasionally the pain of vertebral compression is similar to that of gastric ulcer, pyelonephritis, pancreatis or herniated intervertebral disc (Benson).

Physical examination

Physical examination of the woman during climacteric should include height, weight, vital signs, and complete examination including pelvic with gonorrhea culture and Pap smear. The following are pertinent areas for observation.

Height. Accurate baseline measurement determines the height-weight ratio and aids in the gross evaluation of height loss because of vertebral crush fractures from osteoporosis. Authorities calculate that each fracture reduces one's height by about 1 cm. To assure accurate measurement, the practitioner should use a metal or plastic tape measure attached to the wall and a book rather than upright scales. The client should be measured without shoes, with heels placed together, knees straight, and head level. A difference of more than 2.5 cm from previous normal height suggests exploration of pathological causes.

Weight. Obesity, a prevalent health problem in the United States, may afflict the middle-aged and older woman as a preexisting problem or as age increases. Menopause appears to have little effect on obesity in comparison to socioeconomic and cultural variables. Decreased caloric requirements coupled with insufficient exercise can contribute to or compound the problem. Insidious weight gain needs to be carefully monitored.

Hair and integument. The aging female notices hair beginning to thin and turn gray. Pubic and axillary hair may also thin. Occasionally hirsutism develops, but the appearance of a few extra chin hairs is common. The skin and connective tissues become less elastic, with subsequent wrinkling and hyperkeratotic lesions. Nasal mucous membranes thin, and paranasal sinuses may become dry, producing signs and symptoms of atrophic rhinitis (Overstreet, 1976).

Breasts. As the female ages, the breasts begin to sag and generally diminish in size. The nipples become smaller and the erectile response diminishes (Mantz and Schwabb). Because of increased incidence of breast cancer with advancing age, it is imperative that the breasts be examined carefully. The examination should be performed with the client upright, leaning forward, and supine.

Genitourinary system. Urogenital atrophy increases with age. However, many women will not develop significant atrophy until many years after menopause (Botella-Llusia and van Keep, 1977). Some clinicians believe continued sexual activity delays problems associated with vaginal atrophy. A gradual decrease in subcutaneous fat of the genital labia may lead to ulcerations. A gaping vaginal introitus may be present with severe atrophy. Generally the vagina begins to shorten, narrow, and lose elasticity. Examination reveals increasingly pale vaginal walls, decreased rugosity, and a surface that erodes easily (Notelovitz, Aug. 1978). As the vaginal mucosa thins, the percentage of parabasal cells increases (Greenblatt, 1974). This change may lead to local irritation. The practitioner should note if slight trauma during insertion of the vaginal speculum or performance of a Pap smear creates some bleeding. The presence of any active bleeding site or the location of any lesions must be documented. Even though the mucosa may be too dry to obtain the usual amount of specimen, it is possible to obtain sufficient cells for testing.

Notelovitz (Aug. 1978) supports the idea that decreased estrogen leads to decreased glycogen in the vaginal epithelium. This may alter vaginal pH after menopause so that the atrophic vaginal mucosa becomes more susceptible to vaginitis. However, Gregoire and others (1971) were unable to demonstrate a statistical difference in vaginal glycogen levels between pre- and postmenopausal women. When inflammation occurs in the older client, the discharge is usually watery, whitish gray, and possibly blood tinged. Burning at the urethra during micturition, a burning sensation in the vagina, or excoriated skin may also accompany the discharge. Whenever a menopausal woman has vaginal discharge, it is essential to consider all possibilities rather than to assume that estrogen decline is the sole cause. Other underlying causes may be a fungus, diabetes, or gonorrhea. One should remember that gonorrhea may be atypical in appearance or asymptomatic in many women. Bimanual examination should reveal decreased uterine size. Tubes and ovaries may become impalpable. Any palpable ovary in a postmenopausal woman should alert the practitioner to the possibility of neoplasm, which requires referral and consultation.

Caruncles may develop at the urethral meatus. It is imperative that the practitioner refer patients with any mass, ulceration, or persistently tender area of the vulva or vagina to a gynecologist. Topical therapy is appropriate only after excluding malignancy; attempting a therapeutic trial may waste valuable time and give false reassurance to the client.

Laboratory data

The availability of resources and the cost-benefit ratio are the major issues to consider in diagnostic testing. If a women is healthy and without need of estrogen replacement therapy according to history and physical examination, then minimum baseline data include Pap smear, gonorrhea culture, urinalysis, VDRL, and complete blood count. Additional tests depending on age, family history, or preexisting disease include a chest film, bone x-ray examination, ECG, and blood chemistries, including lipid studies.

Endometrial biopsy is an important procedure used to rule out uterine disease. Authorities recommend it particularly for women at high risk for endometrial cancer. If the practitioner considers estrogen replacement therapy for a woman who is menstruating or who is obese, diabetic, hypertensive, or nulliparous, a referral is mandatory. Before making a referral, the practitioner should be sure the physician includes endometrial biopsy as a regular part of his practice.

Studies of *vaginal smears* demonstrate that an estrogenic effect persists for 10 or more years beyond menopause in 80% of women (Masukawa, 1960). A common test used to evaluate this effect is the maturation index (MI), which is obtained from vaginal smears. The practitioner scrapes the vaginal side walls and posterior fornix with an Ayre spatula, places the specimen on a slide, and applies a fixative. A cytologist then determines the percentage of superficial squamous cells expressed as percentages of parabasal, intermediate, and superficial cells. As amounts of circulating estrogen decrease, the number of parabasal cells increases. However, the MI is a reflection of numerous hormones, including estrogen, progesterone, and androgens. Not all practitioners agree that vaginal cytology can be reliably used to evaluate estrogenic activity or to estimate hormonal needs of postmenopausal women (Liu, 1965; Charles and others, 1966).

The most reliable test used to determine if the ovaries still secrete estrogen is a *serum FSH level* (Kemmann and Jones). After menopause, FSH levels rise significantly. However, a serum FSH level is more expensive than the MI and therefore is not always a practical choice. Plasma estradiol determinations may be helpful because a fall in this hormone is the last change that occurs with loss of ovarian function. It also may be impractical for clinical use.

PLAN

Women with families spend the bulk of their time in nurturing activities. These include pregnancy and attending to the welfare of others, such as children or the acutely ill. Self-care activities usually receive little thought or effort. As a result, women often approach middle age and the climacteric years with little preparation other than comments from family, friends, and the mass media. Data have revealed that middle-aged women seldom discuss the topic of menopause with other women. However, they are aware of old wives' tales and are eager to obtain more information about menopause (Neugarten and others, 1975).

The climacteric is an important transitional period for a woman. Her social, psychological, and physiological integrity reflects the quality of life during this time. Support from an understanding and knowledgeable nurse can be crucial for the individual who finds this a difficult time of life. If one believes that preventive care enhances quality of life, then care of the woman entering the climacteric years really begins during infancy. Unfortunately, in our mobile society individual cradle-to-grave care by one provider is rarely possible, but it is important to remember that health patterns and ideas established in childhood often carry over into adulthood. Young children are eager to learn and nurses are ideal teachers to influence health patterns, since nurses interact with children in a variety of health care settings.

This eagerness has much significance for the nursing care of the adult female. Nursing traditionally encompasses a comprehensive approach to care that emphasizes preventive care and teaching. Since women seek care more often in the middle years, when chronic diseases become evident and require attention, the nurse can use those contacts to discuss individual needs as well as those of the family. Other appropriate situations arise during well child visits or when the husband or parents seek care.

Nurses need to take a more active role in helping women identify and plan for their health needs. Teaching women to accept the importance of caring for themselves is also a vital function. Women generally put their family's needs before their own. However, when women's basic needs are met they can better cope with daily family problems. Women should learn to view themselves as important individuals and not merely extensions of others. This requires the nurse to be sensitive to and cognizant of the family as a functioning unit. Nurses must also be aware of developmental needs of women and be prepared to ask key questions at appropriate times.

Counseling

The nurse's contribution to the counseling needs of women can make a significant difference in psychological and physical comfort during menopause. The following are broad topics that need discussion with the client either before or during this time of life.

Diet. Good nutrition is as important to the physical and mental well-being of the older adult as to the younger person. Obesity is a major health problem for all age groups in the United States. It becomes increasingly difficult for the aging female to maintain a normal height-weight ratio when physical activity and the subsequent caloric demand decrease. Each woman needs instruction about adjustments in caloric requirements that maintain both a well-balanced diet and personal preferences. Stringent restrictions or a long list of "cannots" rarely produce desired results. However, most clients accept gradual diet modifications that control total dietary fat and carbohydrate intake and increase protein and calcium. It should be stressed that maintenance of weight within a normal range reduces stress to weight-bearing joints and the lower back, promotes higher energy levels, assists in preventing selected diseases, and helps maintain self-esteem.

A well-balanced diet should include sufficient bulk such as salad greens and fluids to maintain adequate bowel regulation. Insufficient fluid intake, especially water, is a frequent problem. With limited-income families any medications prescribed should be taken with water, juices, fruit, or bran cereal to ensure their inclusion in the diet. The client should be questioned about any long-standing laxative habits. Use of mineral oil inhibits absorption of fat-soluble vitamins A, D, K, and carotene and should be discouraged. There is increasing evidence that subclinical vitamin D deficiency may contribute to skeletal rarefaction in postmenopausal women. Therefore the aging female needs adequate exposure to sunlight to meet vitamin D requirements essential for the utilization of calcium (Henley and Martin, 1978). Although advocated by some individuals, the use of oral calcium supplements does not significantly increase bone mass (Aitken, 1976).

There are no documented frank nutrient deficiencies in postmenopausal women resulting from estrogen replacement therapy. The use of some drugs, however, may interfere with nutrient absorption and metabolism. For example, antacids, often used without discretion, may deplete phosphate levels.

Exercise. A feasible exercise program assists weight control, promotes a feeling of general well-being, and maintains the integrity of joints and body tone. Walking is an excellent form of exercise. Clients generally report feeling more alert and note improved sleeping habits. Some studies indicate a relationship between decreased activity and loss of muscle and bone mass (Henley and Martin). Additional studies need to address the value of exercise after osteoporosis has become clinically apparent (Aloia and others, 1978). The benefits of exercise in the prevention of bone demineralization are also largely unknown and merit further study (Cohn, 1978).

Breast self-examination. The client should know the technique for breast self-examination. Periodic follow-up demonstrations will determine if she is performing the examination correctly. The practitioner should request a return demonstration initially and at two subsequent visits to reinforce the importance and correct performance of this skill. As a means to promote and stress the importance of individual involvement, the client may be requested to teach someone else, such as a family member or a friend. If the client no longer menstruates, it may be recommended that she do the examination monthly at a time when it is easy for her to remember to do so.

Postmenopausal bleeding. In some cases, slight trauma during insertion of the vaginal speculum or performance of a Pap smear may create some bleeding. The client should be informed that spotting may occur after the vaginal examination, but otherwise it is abnormal and should be reported to the provider. The client should avoid douching 2 to 3 days before obtaining a Pap test. Many women are unaware of the significance of bleeding after menopause and need to be reminded that any bleeding after cessation of menstruation needs evaluation. Therefore it is important to stress the need for periodic gynecological examination and to encourage women to inform their friends and relatives that any vaginal bleeding or vulvar lesions after menopause need attention.

Personal hygiene. The use of vaginal sprays should be discouraged because they promote vulvar irritation. The practitioner should recommend that a woman douche only when it is prescribed for a particular problem. If she insists that she douche, a douche with one tablespoon of vinegar to a quart of water is the least likely to produce chemical irritations. In addition, a gravity flow douche apparatus held no higher than 18 to 24 inches above the perineum may produce less trauma than a bulb douche apparatus. The tip should have multiple openings, since a single-hole tip may produce physical trauma at the site of placement in the vagina.

Although toilet habits seem elemental, the client should be instructed to wipe from front to back, to urinate when she has the urge rather than to retain urine, and to empty the bladder when voiding.

Hot flushes pose a dressing problem for some women. Clothing choices can affect comfort. The practitioner should encourage layered clothing, which allows for frequent discreet changes when necessary. Daily use of nylon or polyester panties, panty hose, and slacks increases body heat and moisture retention. Cotton undergarments should be recommended because cotton allows better air circulation and absorbs moisture without chilling. If excess perspiration keeps panties wet and uncomfortable, the client should carry an extra pair in a small plastic bag so that she can change when necessary. Soft underwear will decrease irritation to exposed and sensitive urethral and vaginal tissues for the occasional woman who suffers from advanced labial atrophy. Apart from practical considerations, attractive lingerie can enhance the psychological well-being of the aging female.

Dry skin can present problems for any age group but is annoying to the older individual if pruritus also occurs. Depending on individual preferences, the practitioner may deemphasize complete daily bathing that can contribute to dry skin. Frequent use of lotions to retain moisture can alleviate some symptoms associated with dry skin.

Sexual counseling. Women in the middle years frequently have questions and concerns about their sexuality and sexual functioning although they may not initiate discussion. Some may even complain of depression or somatic problems. An atmosphere of openness may allow the client to discuss her concerns. It may also allow an opportunity to prepare her for the physiological and psychological changes that will occur. Contrary to what some may think, postmenopausal women do not lose the ability to respond sexually (Cali). While some women consider masturbation taboo, it is nevertheless a source of sexual release for some women who are without any other outlet for their sexual need. According to Masters and Johnson (1970), the masturbatory rate increases in women 50 through 70 years of age. If the practitioner suspects that such activity creates anxiety or feelings of guilt, the subject should be opened for discussion. It is important to stress that strong sexual desires do not imply that the client is oversexed.

Sexual intercourse is a prime measure to maintain vaginal lubrication and expansion (Masters and Johnson, 1966). Increasing frequency of intercourse will promote vaginal expansion and lubrication and prevent dyspareunia. Those individuals who express complaints of inadequate lubrication may need to lengthen foreplay and use K-Y jelly as a lubricant. The practitioner should stress communication and touching needs and suggest, if indicated, positional changes for improving sexual interaction. For example, if dyspareunia is a problem, side-by-side or rear entry may be recommended because it decreases complete penetration. Voiding before sexual activity may lessen the need to void during coitus (McKenzie).

Although some women's sexual frequency increases with menopause, the man's frequency may decrease with age. Many women do not know this and may misinterpret this as rejection. In addition, the client should be informed that penile erections take longer to achieve with age and can be maintained for longer periods without ejaculation. After ejaculation the refractory phase, or period when erection and ejaculation can occur again, may increase to 24 hours or longer. Anticipatory guidance in this area may alleviate many concerns.

Contraception. Many women are unaware that they can become pregnant just before menopause. Although fertility is less likely, the possibility of pregnancy is still present, and sexually active women need counseling (Fuchs; Stone, 1976). Most authorities advise the sexually active woman to use contraception for 1 year after the last menses (Curtis, 1969). The high incidence of complications with oral contraceptive use in this age group encourages the use of mechanical methods of contraception. However, a high degree of client motivation is necessary; and insertion of a diaphragm may be too uncomfortable. Tubal ligation, partner vasectomy, or an intrauterine device is another possible alternative. Another fairly successful option is the foam/condom method, but this also requires client and partner motivation.

Birth control pills are not a substitute for "hormones," because they contain excessive amounts of estrogen and progestin (Yen, 1977). Although some women can take birth control pills up to age 50 without problems, their use over age 40 greatly increases the prevalence of venous thrombosis and myocardial infarction (Notelovitz, Aug. 1978). Using a predominantly progesterone agent or minipill may produce variable bleeding and mask signs of cancer in this age group. It is difficult to establish the onset of menopause if the woman still uses oral contraceptives. If the provider desires to establish menopausal status, the pills can be discontinued for 6 weeks while the client uses nonsteroidal contraception such as foam, condom, or diaphragm. If ovarian failure is present, the level of plasma gonadotropins rises, especially FSH. Additional evidence is the development of hot flushes (Stone).

Safety measures. The aging adult who is prone to falls, fractures, and instability of leg and hip joints may need instruction on improving safety. The middle-aged woman should be counseled about the hazards of loose scatter rugs, poorly illuminated halls and stairs, and inadequately secured stair rails or steps. The practitioner should observe shoe style and fit and recommend lower heels and textured soles if necessary. The client should be taught to get out of bed or chairs slowly, particularly if she demonstrates postural hypotension. The client with osteoporosis should avoid lifting heavy objects or jammed windows and avoid riding in a car on rough roads. The use of a cane may be necessary. It is important that the practitioner know if the client visits a chiropractor; if so, it is important to inform him of the woman's condition (Peck and others, 1977).

Smoking. The practitioner should review the client's smoking habits and discuss their relationship to heart and lung disease. This is of prime importance if the client takes estrogens.

Planning for retirement. An often neglected aspect of counseling is planning for postretirement needs or alterations in role, life-style, and activities in later years. This type of intervention ideally occurs before the menopausal years. However, it is never too late for the client who perhaps consciously has not anticipated the personal implications of these changes. Referral to appropriate financial counselors or social workers may be necessary.

Estrogen replacement therapy

The nurse practitioner should collaborate with a physician to evaluate and manage women who need estrogen replacement therapy (ERT) when indications exist for the administration of estrogens. They may decide that ERT is beneficial for women with relative risk conditions, and the nurse may cojointly manage and counsel these women. Before initiating therapy the practitioner should obtain a history, physical examination, and laboratory data and investigate any nonspecific complaints. Unfortunately, some women view aging negatively and believe it is their right to receive estrogens to preserve youth and vitality and to help them through the climacteric. Because some practitioners advocate routine estrogen administration and some advertisements allude to the youth and happiness of women who take estrogens, the nurse practitioner may encounter inappropriate or unjustified client demands.

Debate exists over the appropriate use of ERT. Research on the subject is replete with inconsistencies, and current data on definitive usage are sketchy. Much of the disagreement is related to insufficient information about ERT's effects on the body. In addition, general knowledge is poor about normal aging as well as the actual physical alterations that occur during menopause. However, there is general agreement that estrogen production declines in many postmenopausal women. The level of decline is variable, and estrogen production continues from extraglandular sources (Yen). This situation poses problems for the practitioner when counseling women during the climacteric. I believe that clients need information on current thinking and the risk-to-benefit ratio before therapy is instituted.

Vasomotor symptoms. The use of estrogen to suppress problematic vasomotor symptoms is the one area where authorities recommend ERT. Some also advocate it to alleviate problematic atrophic vaginitis and cystotrigonitis (Cohn). This should be a consideration only after exclusion of all other causes for the presenting symptoms.

Osteoporosis. Age, sex, and race are three variables that affect the development of osteoporosis. It is uncertain if osteoporosis is a disease of aging or of estrogen deficiency. Men are less affected than women, presumably because of their greater initial bone density and reduced ability for bone loss in later years. Although both men and women lose bone mass after 40, women lose it 3 times faster than men (Aitken). Ethnic studies also reveal that osteoporosis and fractures are rare in black women (Grodin and others, 1973).

The use of estrogens to prevent or retard development of osteoporosis is unclear. Most clinicians use ERT for osteoporosis in women over 45 who have documented evidence of osteoporosis or fracture. This poses a dilemma for the practitioner who wishes to prevent rather than treat osteoporosis. Investigators believe that exogenous estrogens function by inhibiting bone resorption (Utian, 1976, 1977). Thus ERT may be more useful for prevention rather than for treatment of osteoporosis. However, the risks related to taking ERT and the inability to predict which women will develop osteoporosis raise questions about the justification of its prophylactic use.

Another problem is the lack of reliable predictors for women who will develop osteoporosis and subsequent fractures. All women with osteoporosis do not necessarily sustain fractures (Aitken). The trend is for the slim, nulliparous, Caucasian woman with a history of smoking and early ovariectomy to develop a greater degree of spinal osteoporosis rather than her obese parous counterpart. A possible explanation is that obese women die from cardiovascular disease before osteoporosis is obvious. The ability of adipose tissue to synthesize estrogens from androstenedione may also play a role here (Schindler and others, 1972).

Wallach and Henneman (1959) produced strong evidence that prophylactic ERT retards osteoporotic changes. However, once a woman developed height loss, they could not demonstrate radiological improvement although further deterioration was prevented. Other investigators have achieved similar results if clients start long-term cyclic ERT in "modest doses" within a few years after menopause and before development of osteoporosis (Nachtigall and others, 1979). Presently, clinical assessment of the minimum effective dose of estrogen needed to suppress bone resorption is unreliable. Evaluation of fasting plasma calcium levels may be helpful. An increased calcium level indicates increased bone resorption so that maintaining a normal fasting level of plasma calcium may be a fairly reliable method of monitoring estrogen response (Notelovitz, Sept. 1978).

Cardiovascular problems. The relationship between the effects of ERT and the incidence of cardiovascular problems in older women is complex. Risk factors such as obesity, smoking, and sedentary life-style further complicate this association. Current

ERT may enhance the increased prevalence of coronary heart disease that occurs in menopausal women (Benson). Clinicians should not use estrogens to prevent heart disease or acceleration of arteriosclerosis (Rosenberg and others, 1976). Some questions still remain about the relationship between estrogens and thromboembolic risk. Research data indicate a link between the use of synthetic estrogens such as ethinyl estradiol or mestranol and thromboembolic phenomena. This is chiefly because of the drugs' alterations and clotting mechanism (Dugdale and Masi, 1971; Coope and others, 1975). Specific contraindications for ERT include a previous history of thromboembolic disease or regular smoking. Obese and hypertensive women are also at greater risk, and physician consultation is mandatory. Mild essential hypertension is not an absolute contraindication to ERT. However, ERT rapidly increases plasma aldosterone levels so that monitoring of blood pressure in these women should be done monthly. If hypertension appears or worsens, ERT may be withdrawn, with physician consultation (Utian, 1977).

The association between exogenous estrogen and lipids is variable. It mildly increases blood cholesterol levels and produces a marked rise in serum triglycerides, a known risk factor for coronary artery disease. Exogenous estrogen can also exacerbate preexisting hyperlipidemias (Feldman, 1974). However, menopause alone does not influence triglycerides, which otherwise are affected by dietary habits and body weight (Beard, 1976). In general, those clients with abnormal lipid values should not receive exogenous estrogens without just cause.

Glucose tolerance. Exogenous estrogens mildly and reversibly impair glucose tolerance in some normal women (Segaloff, 1979). Mild estrogenic diabetic states do not appear to predict future onset of clinical diabetes unless the woman has a strong family history of diabetes or obesity. Although some clinicians prescribe ERT for menopausal women with latent or overt diabetes, Bransome (1974) considers ERT potentially detrimental until proven otherwise.

Hepatobiliary influence. Changes occur in the hepatic function of women taking estrogens, but data are insufficient to support true hepatocellular damage (Aitken). In addition, the incidence of gallstones requiring surgical intervention is 2½ times more frequent in women taking estrogens after menopause (Boston CDSP, 1974). The use of estrogens in women with a history of hepatitis or cholestatic jaundice is generally unadvisable, although some clinicians may use very low physiological replacement doses in these clients. If the physician prescribes ERT, management should include teaching the woman who receives therapy to immediately report any upper abdominal pain, dark urine, or jaundice.

Cancer risk. Much disagreement currently exists about the true risk or relationship between estrogen therapy and endometrial cancer (Ziel and Finkle, 1975, 1976). Those women at high risk for uterine cancer are nulliparous, obese, diabetic, or have a history of menstrual irregularities. The irregularities consist of frequent or irregular menses; for example, two to three menses monthly several years before menopause (Rutledge, 1977). There are increasing data to support an association between endometrial carcinoma and the continuous intake of estrogens. Some clinicians prefer to label this "unopposed estrogen" intake. This implies that a substance that investigators usually think is progesterone counteracts or opposes the effects of continuous estrogens on the body. The

Criteria for postmenopausal estrogen replacement therapy

A. Amenorrhea for at least 6 months
B. Normal history and physical examination to include breast and pelvic examination and Pap smear
C. Documented evidence of estrogen deficiency, for example
   1. Elevated plasma FSH level
   2. Presence of problematic atrophic vaginitis
   3. Reduced urinary estrogen and/or plasma estradiol levels
   4. Vaginal cytology (MI) congruent with estrogen deficiency
   5. History of frequent flushing that is problematic
   6. Osteoporosis
D. Absence of the following contraindications to ERT
   1. Undiagnosed vaginal bleeding
   2. Acute liver disease
   3. Chronic impaired renal function
   4. Acute vascular thrombosis
   5. Endometrial cancer
   6. Breast cancer
   7. Neuroophthalmological disease
   8. Pregnancy

---

most publicized effect of unopposed estrogen is endometrial proliferation, which can predispose the client to endometrial adenocarcinoma. Some authorities believe that using progesterone for women with intact uteri during the third or fourth week of monthly estrogen therapy may counteract the stimulation of unopposed estrogen on the endometrium (Cohn; Notelovitz, Sept. 1978).

Present studies do not report significant increases in breast cancer in women treated with estrogens (Burch and others, 1974). However, there are current concerns about the effect of estrogen on estrogen-dependent types of breast cancer. Clinicians should avoid estrogens if the client has a previous history of breast cancer, a strong family history of breast cancer, chronic recurrent cystic mastitis, or abnormal mammograms (Bransome).

Anxiety and depression. There is no empirical evidence to support administration of estrogens to relieve anxiety or depression (Utian, 1976). However, a recent crossover study used estrogen and placebo therapies. The findings suggest that estrogen has a significantly superior effect in producing a feeling of "well-being" (Utian, 1972).

Indications. For a summary of those criteria that determine eligibility for ERT in menopausal aged women and guidelines for administering ERT, see the above boxes. For the first few months, some clinicians prescribe conjugated estrogen, 0.3 to 1.25 mg daily for 3 weeks, followed by 5 to 10 mg progesterone daily for 1 week. Since a goal of therapy is to maintain a client on the smallest therapeutic dose, many clinicians reduce daily estrogen and evaluate the response. One side effect for some women is the breakthrough bleeding that occurs during progesterone administration. Since hyperplastic endometrium can develop with this therapy, some authorities recommend serial endometrial biopsy during ERT. The duration of therapy is extremely variable. The trend, however, is to

---

Guidelines for administration of estrogen replacement therapy

A. Prescribe the smallest dose to produce a satisfactory response. This depends on the type of estrogen used and individual client response.
B. Use estrogen cyclically, 3 weeks on and 1 week off. Add a progestational agent during the 1 week off.
C. Take medications at night or after meals if they produce GI upset.
D. Be aware of overdose signs or untoward effects
   1. Engorged tender breasts
   2. Excessive weight gain without change in eating and exercise habits
   3. Leukorrhea
   4. Asymptomatic elevations in blood pressure
   5. Abnormal uterine bleeding
   6. Alterations in coagulation, lipid, and glucose tolerance
E. Suspect any abnormal uterine bleeding and refer for evaluation. Do not assume that periodic bleeding protects against cancer.
F. Do not prescribe ERT as a treatment for "nerves."
G. Evaluate vaginal lesions and treat any infections before using estrogen vaginal creams.
H. Screen for hypertriglyceridemia shortly after initiating therapy in women with diabetes, history of glucose intolerance, family history of premature MIs, or arteriosclerotic disease.

---

discontinue ERT after 1 year and reevaluate the client. When atrophic vaginitis is a problem, a local preparation is appropriate because it is absorbed systemically. It also carries the same contraindications as oral preparations.

A possible alternative for the menopausal woman with hot flushes who cannot take estrogens is a combination drug such as Bellergal. This drug may correct imbalances of the autonomic nervous system. While some women express relief with this drug, autonomic depressants and sedatives are less effective than estrogens. They are not helpful to all women and are ineffective at night because sedation of the hypothalamus is ineffective during an unconscious state. Also, the practitioner must consider the relative contraindications and potential for abuse when using this type of medication with some individuals (Seiler).

EVALUATION

There is no standard schedule of follow-up care for women during the climacteric. A joint plan should take into consideration the individual's health needs. For the woman who has no overriding health problems and is not receiving ERT, an annual review with a pelvic examination, including Pap smear, and breast examination is sufficient. In addition, the practitioner should evaluate health status, observe for emergence of chronic disease, and discuss preventive health care needs. With ERT, returns should be scheduled every 3 months initially and every 6 months thereafter. Further instructions include additional return appointments if problems occur during the intervening time.

A comprehensive approach to the care of women during the climacteric requires the ability to synthesize a triad of complex medical, psychological, and sociological information. In addition, the provider must translate that information into health care that will enable women to experience midlife and later years positively. Nurses as person-oriented care providers need to take full advantage of this vital role.

REFERENCES

Aitken, J.M.: Bone metabolism in postmenopausal women. In Beard, R.J., editor: The menopause: a guide to current research and practice, Baltimore, 1976, University Park Press.

Aloia, J.F., and others: Prevention of involutional bone loss by exercise, Ann. Intern. Med. **89:**356, 1978.

Beard, R.J.: Estrogens and the cardiovascular system. In Beard, R.J., editor: The menopause: a guide to current research and practice, Baltimore, 1976, University Park Press.

Benson, R.C.: Current obstetric and gynecological diagnosis and treatment, ed. 3, Los Altos, Calif., 1980, Lange Medical Publications.

Boston Collaborative Drug Surveillance Program, N. Engl. J. Med. **290:**15, 1974.

Botella-Llusiá, J., and van Keep, P.A.: Vaginal cytology in the post-menopause: a study into some correlates, Acta Cytol. (Baltimore) **21:**18, 1977.

Bransome, E.D.: Medical complications of estrogens and oral contraceptives. In Greenblatt, R.B., and others, editors: The menopausal syndrome, New York, 1974, Medcom, Inc.

Brown, A.D.G.: Postmenopausal urinary problems, Clin. Obstet. Gynecol. **4:**181, 1977.

Burch, J.C., and others: The effect of long-term estrogen on hysterectomized women, Am. J. Obstet. Gynecol. **118:**778, 1974.

Butler, R.N., and Lewis, M.I.: Aging and mental health: positive psychosocial approaches, St. Louis, 1973, The C.V. Mosby Co.

Cali, R.W.: Management of the climacteric and postmenopausal woman, Med. Clin. North Am. **56:**789, 1972.

Centaro, A., and others: Epidemiologic studies of postmenopausal endometrial adenocarcinoma. In Greenblatt, R.B., and others, editors: The menopausal syndrome, New York, 1974, Medcom, Inc.

Chakravarti, S., and others: Hormonal profiles after the menopause, Br. Med. J. **2:**784, 1976.

Charles, D., and others: Significance of cornified cells in the vaginal smears of postmenopausal females, Am. J. Obstet. Gynecol. **94:**527, 1966.

Cherry, S.H.: The menopause myth, New York, 1976, Ballantine Books.

Christie-Brown, J.R.W., and Christie-Brown, M.E.: Psychiatric disorders associated with the menopause. In Beard, R.J., editor: The menopause: a guide to current research and practice, Baltimore, 1976, University Park Press.

Clayden, J.R., and others: Menopausal flushing: a double-blind trial of a non-hormonal medication, Br. Med. J. **1:**409, 1974.

Cohn, F.L.: The menopause and replacement estrogen therapy, Iss. Health Care Women **1:**2, 1978.

Coope, J., and others: Effects of "natural oestrogen" replacement therapy on menopausal symptoms and blood clotting, Br. Med. J. **4:**139, 1975.

Curtis, L.R.: The menopause, Bristol., Tenn. 1969, S.E. Massengill Co.

Dugdale, M., and Masi, A.T.: Hormonal contraception and thromboembolic disease: effects of oral contraceptives on hemostatic mechanisms, J. Chron. Dis. **23:**775, 1971.

Dyer, R.M.: Menopause—a closer look for nurses. In Kjervik, D.K., and Martinson, I.M., editors: Women in stress: a nursing perspective, New York, 1979, Appleton-Century-Crofts.

Feeley, E., and Pyne, H.: The menopause: facts and misconceptions, Nurs. Forum **14:**74, 1975.

Feldman, E.B.: Sex steroids and lipoproteins. In Greenblatt, R.B., and others, editors: The menopausal syndrome, New York, 1974, Medcom, Inc.

Fuchs, E.: The second season: life, love, and sex for women in the middle years, New York, 1978, Doubleday Publishing Co.

Glass, R.H.: Office gynecology, Baltimore, 1976, The Williams & Wilkins Co.

Gordon, G.S.: Role of estrogens in osteoporosis, Geriatrics, Sept., 1977, pp. 42-48.

Greenblatt, R.B.: Reprise. In Greenblatt, R.B., and others, editors: The menopausal syndrome, New York, 1974, Medcom, Inc.

Gregoire, A.T., and others: The glycogen content of human vaginal epithelium tissue, Fertil. Steril. **22:**64, 1971.

Grodin, J.M., and others: Source of estrogen production in postmenopausal women, J. Clin. Endocrinol. Metab. **36:**207, 1973.

Gruis, M.L., and Wagner, N.N.: Sexuality during the climacteric, Postgrad. Med. **65:**197, 1979.
Henley, E.C., and Martin, J.B.: Nutrition: a holistic approach for the older woman, Iss. Health Care Women **1:**13, 1978.
Jazzman, L., and others: The perimenopausal symptoms, Med. Gynecol. Sociol. **4:**268, 1969.
Kaluger, G., and Kaluger, M.F.: Human development: the span of life, St. Louis, 1974, The C.V. Mosby Co.
Kemmann, E., and Jones, J.R.: The female climacteric, Am. Fam. Phys. **20:**140, 1979.
Krone, S.M.: Osteoporosis. In Wintrobe, M.M., and others, editors: Harrison's principles of internal medicine, ed. 7, New York, 1974, McGraw-Hill, Inc.
Liu, W.: Continued estrogen throughout menopause, Acta Cytol. (Baltimore) **9:**400, 1965.
Mantz, M.L., and Schwabb, R.B.: Early menopause. Iss. Health Care Women **2:**45, 1978.
Masters, W.H., and Johnson, V.E.: Human sexual response, Boston, 1966, Little, Brown & Co.
Masters, W.H., and Johnson, V.E.: Human sexual inadequacy, Boston, 1970, Little, Brown & Co.
Masukawa, T.: Vaginal smears in women past 40 years of age with emphasis on their remaining hormonal activity, Obstet. Gynecol. **16:**407, 1960.
McKenzie, C.A.M.: Sexuality and the menopausal woman, Iss. Health Care Women, **1:**37, 1978.
McKinlay, S.M., and Jefferys, M.: The menopausal syndrome, Br. J. Prev. Soc. Med. **28:**108, 1974.
Nachtigall, L.E., and others: Estrogen replacement therapy. I. A 10-year prospective study in the relationship to osteoporosis, Obstet. Gynecol. **53:**277, 1979.
Neugarten, B.L., and Kraines, R.J.: Menopausal symptoms in women of various ages, Psychosom. Med. **27:**266, 1965.
Neugarten, B.L., and others: Women's attitudes toward the menopause. In Neugarten, B.L., editor: Middle age and aging—a reader in social psychology, Chicago, 1975, University of Chicago Press.
Notelovitz, M.: Gynecologic problems of menopausal women. I. Changes in genital tissue, Geriatrics, **33:**24, Aug. 1978.
Notelovitz, M.: Gynecologic problems of menopausal women. II. Treating estrogen deficiency, Geriatrics, **33:**35, Sept. 1978.
Notelovitz, M.: Gynecologic problems of menopausal women. III. Changes in extragenital tissues and sexuality, Geriatrics, **33:**51, Oct. 1978.
Novak, E.P., and others: Novak's textbook of gynecology, Baltimore, 1975, The Williams & Wilkins Co.
Overstreet, E.W.: Menopause and postmenopausal syndrome. In Benson, R.C.: Current obstetric and gynecologic diagnosis and treatment, Los Altos, Calif., 1976, Lange Medical Publications.
Peck, W.A., and others: Osteoporosis: exploring options and odds, Patient Care, Oct. 30, 1977, pp. 77-90.
Perlmutter, J.F.: A gynecological approach to menopause. In Notman, M.T., and Nadelson, C.C., editors: The woman patient—medical and psychological interfaces, vol. I, New York, 1978, Plenum Publishing Corp.
Rogers, J.: The menopause, N. Engl. J. Med. **254:**697, 1956.
Rogers, J.: Estrogens in the menopause and postmenopause, N. Engl. J. Med. **280:**364, 1969.
Rosenberg, L., and others: Myocardial infarction and estrogen therapy in post-menopausal women, N. Engl. J. Med. **294:**1256, 1976.
Rosenthal, S.H.: The involutional depressive syndrome, Am. J. Psychiatry, **124:**21, 1968.
Rutledge, F.N.: The female climacteric: current perspective in managing the menopausal patient, New York, 1977, Ayerst Laboratories.
Schindler, A., and others: Conversion of androstenedione to estrone by human fat tissue, J. Clin. Endocrinol. **35:**627, 1972.
Schneider, G.T.: Gynecologic malignancy in geriatric patients (65 years and over). In Greenblatt, R.B., and others, editors: The menopausal syndrome, New York, 1974, Medcom, Inc.
Segaloff, A.: The pros and cons of estrogen therapy, Postgrad. Med. **65:**106, 1979.
Seiler, J.C.: Estrogens for the menopause—maximizing benefits, minimizing risks, Postgrad. Med. **62:**73, 1977.
Smith, D.C., and others: Association of exogenous estrogen and endometrial carcinoma, N. Engl. J. Med. **293:**1164, 1975.
Stone, S.C.: Discontinuing contraception at menopause, Med. Asp. Hum. Sex. **10:**176, 1976.
Timiras, P.S., and Meisami, E.: Changes in gonadal function. In Timiras, P.S., editor: Developmental physiology and aging, New York, 1972, Macmillan, Inc.
Treloar, A.E.: Menarche, menopause, and intervening fecundability, Hum. Biol. **46:**89, 1974.
Tucker, S.J.: The menopause: how much soma and how much psyche? J.O.G.N. Nurs. **6:**40, Sept./Oct. 1977.

Utian, W.H.: The mental tonic effect of oestrogen administered to oopherectomized females, S. Afr. Med. J. **46:**1079, 1972.

Utian, W.H.: Scientific basis for postmenopausal estrogen therapy: the management of specific symptoms and rationale for long-term replacement. In Beard, R.J., editor: The menopause: a guide to current research and practice, Baltimore, 1976, University Park Press.

Utian, W.H.: Current status of menopause and postmenopausal estrogen therapy, Obstet. Gynecol. Surv. **32:** 193, 1977.

Wallach, S., and Henneman, P.H.: Prolonged estrogen therapy in postmenopausal women, J.A.M.A. **171:** 1637, 1959.

Willson, J.R., and Carrington, E.R.: Obstetrics and gynecology, ed. 6, St. Louis, 1979, The C.V. Mosby Co.

Wilson, R.A., and Wilson, T.A.: The fate of the non-treated postmenopausal woman: a plea for maintenance of adequate estrogen from puberty to grave, J. Am. Geriatr. Soc. **11:**347, 1963.

Winokur, G.: Depression in the menopause, Am. J. Psychiatry **130:**92, 1973.

Yen, S.S.C.: Estrogen and the menopause, Am. Fam. Phys. **16:**87, 1977.

Ziel, H.K., and Finkle, W.D.: Increased risk of endometrial carcinoma among users of conjugated estrogens, N. Engl. J. Med. **293:**1167, 1975.

Ziel, H.K., and Finkle, W.D.: Association of estrone with the development of endometrial carcinoma, Am. J. Obstet. Gynecol. **124:**735, 1976.

CHAPTER 8

Skin problems common to blacks: a nursing perspective

Betty L. Wilson

Literature that describes skin changes in heavily pigmented or black skin is largely unavailable. Therefore dermatological assessment of black clients may be difficult for some health care providers. If subtle skin changes go unrecognized, the provider may overlook underlying systemic disease. The focus of this chapter is to provide pertinent information that can assist the health care provider in the assessment and recognition of common changes and skin lesions frequently observed in black clients.

ANATOMY AND PHYSIOLOGY

The skin is composed of three major tissue layers: epidermis, dermis, and subcutaneous tissue (Fitzpatrick, 1971). The epidermis consists of two main cell types: melanocytes and keratinocytes. Melanocytes synthesize a pigment, melanin, which is responsible for the skin's brown hues. Racial pigmentation is not due to the number of melanocytes but is related to differences in the ability to produce melanin (Fitzpatrick).

The balance of red, brown, and yellow hues produces normal skin color. Oxyhemoglobin in superficial blood vessels produces red hues, melanin produces brown hues, and bile and carotene in collagen produce yellow hues (Judge and Zuidema, 1974). The key point in the assessment of skin problems is the ability to recognize where normal gradations of color occur on the body. Two areas where color variation occurs in the normal black client are the palms of the hands and soles of the feet. In addition, any change in the client's color since the previous observation is noteworthy.

ASSESSMENT
Emotional aspects of skin disorders

The approach that health care providers use with individuals who have skin disorders is of vital importance to the client's dignity. Individuals with severe skin problems are more likely to suffer from a distorted self-image. They may view skin alterations as unsightly or think they might have an incurable disease. Thus it is important to understand the meaning or value an individual attaches to a skin disorder. This assessment enables the practitioner to provide adequate support and reassurance to clients. The health care provider must be willing to discuss the client's feelings about a particular skin problem so that a unified plan of care can be developed.

The practitioner should remember that the cosmetic aspects of a skin disorder may seriously incapacitate an individual. Chronic skin problems may lead to rejection or to voluntary withdrawal from active life. The fear of rejection, either real or imagined, may be more incapacitating than the skin problem itself. Involvement of other members of the health team, such as social workers, psychologist, or physician, may be necessary.

The social significance of skin pigmentation is profound. People have tried throughout history to improve their social standing and sex appeal by modifying the color of their skin or hair. Consequently, much effort and money have been spent trying to straighten the hair and bleach the skin. This often led to hair loss and contact dermatitis, which created an increasing number of black clients who sought referrals to skin specialists. The emergence of new racial pride is beginning to reverse this trend.

History

Certain issues must be addressed by the health care provider during the initial contact with the client. The practitioner should assess the importance the client places on the skin conditions. Listening to a client's fears lends support and provides the framework for acceptance and trust between client and provider. If the initial assessment indicates further consultation or referral, the client should be prepared for this. If necessary, the limitations and scope of practice of the nurse practitioner should be explained. The initial assessment often provides the opportunity to prevent further skin problems and other health problems, since clients often seek prompt advice when the skin is affected.

Aspects of the history that are important in relation to diseases of the skin follow.

Chief complaint and history of present illness. The chief complaint of a client with a skin condition is often so vague or colloquial that it may be misleading. Symptoms such as pain, burning, and itching vary greatly and are subjective complaints. The following should be included in the history of present illness: (1) the type of skin lesions and their location and distribution; (2) the onset and duration of skin lesions; and (3) if chronic, the course of the disease, specifically remissions and exacerbations. It is essential to ask if any topical treatment has been tried. For example, use of steroids may reduce inflammation and change the appearance of the lesion.

Family history. The practitioner should inquire about a family history of diabetes, cardiovascular disease, tumors, or allergies. It is not sufficient to ask, "Is there allergy in your family?" Questions should refer specifically to hives, eczema, hay fever, or "sinus." Recent skin conditions or upper respiratory tract conditions in siblings, parents, and predecessors; current skin conditions occurring in family members; or hereditary problems such as sickle cell disease should be noted.

History of medication. All current prescribed and over-the-counter medications should be identified, including both topical and systemic drugs. The provider should remind the client to include regularly taken medications. Medicines such as aspirin, "cold tablets," "water pills," bacitracin, or antihistamines are so familiar that clients forget they are "medicine."

Environmental, occupational, and seasonal factors. Many lesions such as calluses or allergic reactions are due to excessive exposure to climatic elements or occupational irritants. Since the skin is subjected to numerous physical, chemical, and microbial attacks, such factors deserve consideration in almost every client with a disease affecting the skin. Certain diseases, such as impetigo, have seasonal peaks. Chronic skin disorders may be triggered by climatic factors. This may require prolonged questioning to elicit a seasonal association.

Physical examination

Examination of the client with a skin problem requires the health care provider to use the following modalities.

Observation and inspection. The first step is to view the client from a distance. After the entire skin surface is observed, the type and shape of individual lesions should be observed. Next, the distribution pattern of the lesions on the entire body surface should be assessed. The client should be completely disrobed to allow for inspection of the entire body. Poor lighting often prevents adequate observation of the individual. Subtle color changes in the absence of heavy pigmentation will be missed if there is poor illumination. The best light source is daylight. If that is infeasible, a standard 60-watt light bulb may be satisfactory (Williams, 1975). Flashlights are unsatisfactory light sources for identifying color changes in pigmented skin.

The position of the torso and the extremities influences the assessment of color change. The practitioner should carefully consider the relationship between color, position, and disease entity. For example, some vasomotor changes are influenced by position. An elevated or lowered extremity may alter circulation and produce temporary color change associated with some disease states.

Changes in color, contour, integrity, and cleanliness should be noted, as well as areas that have been scratched, chafed, picked, or rubbed. Color assessment of a deeply pigmented individual requires an awareness of shades of color. The practitioner should gauge the client's basic color by observing areas not exposed to sunlight; these are the palms, soles, torso, and medial aspects of the arms and legs. These should be compared with other areas of the body as well as with the site of specific lesions. One should remember that there may be more than one shade of black in the same person.

Palpation. The practitioner should evaluate the texture, temperature, and amount of secretions on the skin and hair and note areas of tenderness or warmth. Texture describes the feel of the skin; the provider should note soft, hard, or indurated areas. The temperature of the environment and the client's emotional state influence color changes and feeling of the skin. These influences should be noted if one is unable to alter them during the examination. When assessing the nail beds, the practitioner should note if the client recently smoked a cigarette because this may increase pallor or cyanosis.

Description of skin lesions

Skin disorders can occur in one location on the body (localized), on a larger portion of the body (regional), or over the entire skin surface (generalized).

Skin lesions are categorized by their size, shape, and color. They are macular, papular, papulosquamous, pustular, vesicular, nodular, urticarial, purpuric, petechial, or ulcerative. *Macules* are flat areas of altered skin pigmentation less than 1 cm in size. They cannot be felt on examination. Common examples of macules include rubella and petechiae.

Papules are palpable, solid, and raised. They are usually less than 1 cm in diameter.

Examples of these include acne and insect bites. Papules associated with plaque and scale formation are *papulosquamous* eruptions. Psoriasis, pityriasis rosea, and seborrheic dermatitis are examples. *Pustular eruptions* contain purulent material. A common example is folliculitis.

Vesicular eruptions contain fluid and arise from or below the epidermis. Examples are herpes zoster and contact dermatitis secondary to poison ivy. If the vesicles have a diameter over 0.5 cm, the eruption is called a bulla. Common examples include second-degree burns and bullous impetigo. Skin *nodules* are nonedematous swellings in the dermal or subcutaneous layers of the skin. They are greater than 1 cm in diameter. Examples include erythema nodosum and lymphoma cutis. *Urticarial eruptions* are erythematous and result from dermal edema. They are typically pruritic and migratory. Angioedema results from fluid accumulation in deeper skin layers. It is migratory but not necessarily pruritic or erythematous. Common causes are allergies to drugs, foods, and environmental agents, or parasitic infections.

Purpura refers to a purplish skin or mucous membrane discoloration due to subcutaneous collection of blood. The lesion is *petechial* if the diameter is less than 3 mm. Purpuric eruptions are commonly due to thrombocytopenia. Bleeding into the skin also occurs in a wide variety of vascular, connective tissue, or capillary permeability defects not associated with thrombocytopenia. *Ulcerations* are irregular-shaped lesions with central loss of dermis and epidermis. They leave a scar when healed. Common examples are stasis and decubitus ulcers.

Differences between pigmented and nonpigmented skin

Normal variations of pigment in blacks are often mistakenly labeled pathological. Some normal findings include prickling pigmentation of the mucosa of the mouth, lips, tongue, and the nail beds. The gums may appear uniformly blue or may have patchy areas of bluish pigmentation. The sclera may appear brown. Calloused extremities may appear opaque yellow (Galles, 1978).

Erythema may be difficult to detect in the black client. Occasionally it may appear purplish on heavily pigmented skin. To distinguish erythema from ecchymosis, pressure should be applied to the suspected erythematous area. If the area lightens, it is erythematous. One should not forget that reddened or inflamed skin does not always feel warm to the touch (Roach, 1977).

Pallor is difficult to assess on darkly pigmented skin. Pallor may be represented by a light gray color in a more lightly pigmented client. The ashen color is due to the absence of red hues arising from oxygenated hemoglobin. It is valuable to compare the skin with the client's skin on a previous visit. Pallor in brown-skinned clients will appear yellowish brown. An additional clue in assessment is to observe the mucous membranes and conjunctiva. The inner canthus appears normally more pale than the outer canthus. Both should be compared before final assessment. Applying pressure to nail beds or lips may determine the color and the extent of capillary refill. If necessary, the examiner's nail beds may be compared with the client's.

Occasionally edema may alter skin color so that the client appears pale. The visual error is due to the thickening of skin from accumulated fluid. The separation between the darkly pigmented layers and the vascular layers decreases the tone of red, thus lightening the overall hue.

Early *cyanosis* is difficult to assess in darkly pigmented clients. The lips and gums may be pigmented sufficiently to obscure beginning cyanosis. It is important to check all less-pigmented sites, including palms, soles, nail beds, and conjunctiva, before dismissing cyanosis. In addition, capillary refill is usually slower so that color returns slower to areas checked by pressure. Also, the character of refill is different. In cyanosis, the color returns from the periphery to the center. Normally peripheral and central refill should be simultaneous (Roach, 1974). Cigarette smoking and air conditioning may also alter capillary refill.

Jaundice may be difficult to assess in darkly pigmented individuals. The sclera of many clients normally may appear yellow to brown because of large amounts of carotene-containing subconjunctival fat. If the entire conjunctiva is yellow, the posterior hard palate should be observed in sunlight. Jaundice will appear in the suspected client if melanin pigmentation is not heavy. In addition, a thorough history might suggest other pertinent clinical data that should be collected (see Chapter 12).

Laboratory data

Common diagnostic aids used in a primary care setting are bacteriological culture, potassium hydroxide (KOH) preparation, Wood's lamp evaluation, and VDRL test. Bacteriological culture is helpful when infectious diseases are suspected. Material from the suspicious lesion is removed with a sterile cotton swab and inoculated onto the appropriate culture medium.

A KOH preparation may determine the presence of fungal elements. The lesion should be cleansed with alcohol. Epidermal scales, nail scrapings, or suspicious hairs should be removed for examination. The practitioner should place the material on a microscopic slide and add 1 or 2 drops of 10 to 20% KOH and a cover slip. The slide should be flamed slowly and observed under both low and high powers. Reduced light may help visualization. Fungal elements characteristic of the suspected problem will be identified.

A Wood's lamp evaluation will identify infected hairs or skin by demonstrating fluorescence of the lesion in some fungal infections. Tinea capitis is commonly identified in this way. The lamp must be used in a darkened room to ensure an adequate evaluation.

A VDRL test or other serological test for syphilis may aid in the evaluation of lesions that cannot easily be identified. Secondary syphilis appears as a variable rash. The provider should keep in mind that a false positive VDRL test may indicate another pathological condition or variation in a normal individual. A positive VDRL requires further testing and evaluation.

PLANNING AND EVALUATION OF SELECTED LESIONS

In assessing skin lesions, it is essential that the practitioner remember that a skin eruption may represent not only a dermatological condition but also a systemic one. If a rash appears suspicious or uncharacteristic, the provider should consider diseases that may affect multiple body systems. Such diseases include secondary syphilis, collagen diseases, and malignancies or chronic disease states. A high index of suspicion combined with a thorough evaluation may hasten diagnosis and possibly prevent further debilitation. It is not the focus of this chapter to discuss dermatological manifestations of systemic disease. Nor will problems that occur with equal frequency in all skin pigmentation be discussed.

Although black clients have a very high incidence of impetigo, the prevalence of pyodermas and parasitoses is often an index of the standard of living (Williams). Impetigo occurs commonly with poor hygiene and poor nutrition and is not influenced by pigmentation. The problem is similar for all skin types, and treatment is consistent for all clients.

Some skin diseases occur with lower frequency in black clients. Psoriasis, a papulosquamous dermatosis, occurs with relatively low frequency in the black American population (Fitzpatrick). Benign skin tumors occur with equal frequency in blacks and other racial groups. Skin cancers, including melanoma and precancerous skin lesions, rarely occur in heavily pigmented people.

The following selected problems represent skin conditions that either appear most often in darkly pigmented clients or appear differently in those clients.

Fungal infections: tinea versicolor

Hypopigmented scaly lesions noted on the upper trunk and neck typify tinea versicolor. However, a greater variation in color may appear in heavily pigmented skin. The offending organism is *Malassezia furfur*. Spores and hyphae ("spaghetti and meatballs" appearance) can be noted if the infected tissue is microscopically examined with KOH preparation. A Wood's lamp examination reveals a yellow or white fluorescence in suspected lesions. Other diagnoses to consider are other pigmentary disorders, such as vitiligo or seborrheic dermatitis (see Fig. 8-1).

Aside from a rare complaint of itching, most clients are chiefly concerned about their appearance. Occasionally lesions are so extensive that large patches of altered skin appear. During the summer, the lesions are more noticeable. Tinea versicolor is also more common in males.

A number of preparations are effective against the fungus if treatment lasts for several weeks. Common products are 2.5% selenium sulfide suspension (Selsun) or acrisorcin (Akrinol). Selsun should be applied to affected areas and left on for 5 to 10 minutes twice daily for 3 to 4 weeks. An alternative is Akrinol cream applied three times a day for 2 to 3 weeks. The provider should inform the client that scaling will resolve in a few days but complete treatment should be continued for the 3- or 4-week period. Pigmentation changes resolve more slowly; the practitioner should prepare the client for this gradual return to normal skin color. In addition, the provider should inform the client that thoroughly cleaning or steam-pressing clothing will prevent further reinfection.

Pigmentary disorders

The majority of changes in pigment involve benign medical conditions, although they may be extremely distressing to some clients. Hypopigmentation is more obvious on dark skin. In addition, evidence indicates that clients with pigmented skin are very cognizant of skin problems and are anxious to diminish them (Williams).

Albinism. Albinism is genetically acquired and results from failure of melanocytes to produce normal amounts of melanin (Fitzpatrick). Caucasian albinos appear pinkish white and negroid albinos appear tan or cream-colored with freckles on exposed skin surfaces (Williams). The hair of negroid clients is blonde to red to yellow brown. Negroid and Caucasian albinos have similar abnormalities of the eyes, including impaired vision, nystagmus, photophobia, rapid blinking, tearing, and central scotomas. The iris of the negroid albino appears pale blue to light brown, whereas the iris of the Caucasian albino is light gray changing to blue gray in adulthood.

The negroid albino probably suffers more social isolation because of the pigmentary difference between himself and peers and relatives. Psychological support is essential because the condition is permanent. In addition, protection of the eyes and referral for corrective lenses may improve the quality of sight. Although skin cancer is common in Caucasian albinos, it is rare in negroid albinos (Fitzpatrick). However, this does not exclude a thorough skin assessment at each visit. In addition, dry skin may be problematic. This can be improved by the use of a simple emollient.

Vitiligo. This problem affects about 3% of both blacks and whites. The macular depigmentation characteristic of this disorder is typically found on the face, axillae, neck, body openings, and extremities. In blacks, the border of the lesion is often transitional from dark brown to light tan to white. The border is also convex and smooth. The patches often appear suddenly and may increase in size. Upon exposure to sunlight, pruritus or sunburn may occur. Hairs growing in the affected area may become white. The color of the lesion is usually white but may appear gray blue because of melanin in a deeper dermal layer (Fitzpatrick). The cause of vitiligo is unknown, although inherited and autoimmune factors have been implicated. Half the cases develop before adulthood and before a familial history can be identified. The health care provider should consider other causes of hypopigmentation or depigmentation before arriving at the assessment of vitiligo. Other causes are Addison's disease, hyperthyroidism, and traumatic burns.

Cosmetic concerns are important to affected clients. The nurse practitioner can recommend covering the face (if affected) with makeup. In addition, protection of lesions from sunlight will prevent pain, since the hypopigmented skin is light-sensitive. If vitiligo is present on unexposed surfaces, the provider should stress the use of flattering garments. The treatment for vitiligo is evolving, although it is still experimental and costly. A third of cases spontaneously resolve; this may be important to stress for the client with marginal financial resources. The goal of therapy is to repigment visibly affected areas. A popular and somewhat successful therapy is the oral use of psoralen and subsequent sun exposure to the affected skin. Prior concern about systemic side effects of psoralen has decreased in the last decade, but management should still be conducted by a dermatologist familiar with the technique.

Mongolian spots (dermal melanosis). This lesion is flat, dark blue, and noted predominantly on the back and buttocks. The color is derived from pigment in melanocytes of the reticular layer of dermis. This pigment is usually congenital and may approach 10 cm in size, although this is uncommon. They are present in over 90% of black Americans, American Indians, and Orientals, while they exist in only 1% to 5% of Caucasian infants (Williams). The shape is variable without a definite border and may occur singly or in various numbers. They usually disappear in childhood and have never been associated with malignant degeneration. They should not be confused with bruises, which resolve more quickly and may undergo variation in color as the ecchymosis absorbs.

Dermatosis papulosa nigra. In the United States this skin condition is limited almost exclusively to blacks, with an incidence of 35% in that group. It occurs more often in women and appears in early to middle adulthood. The lesions may progress in size

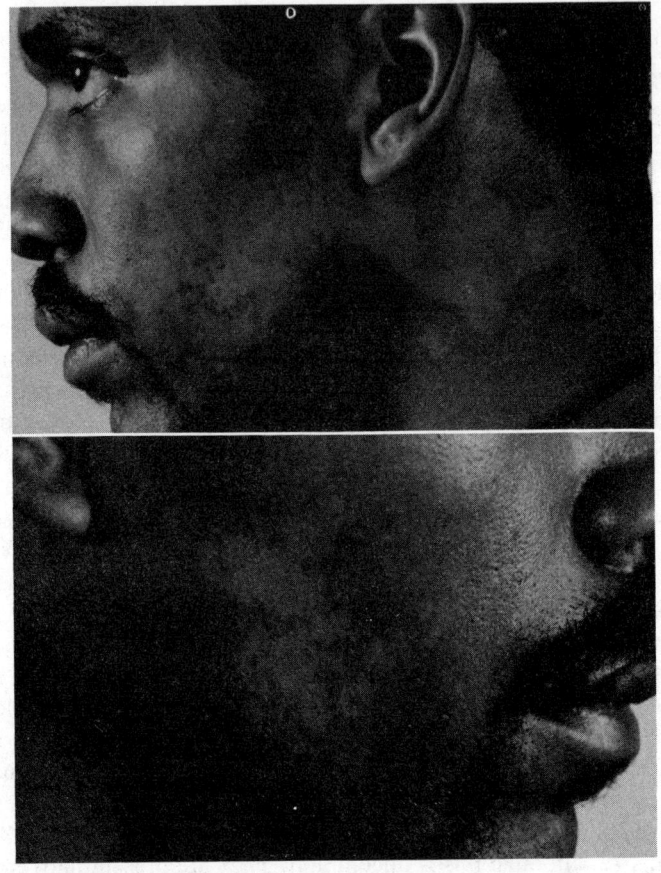

Fig. 8-1. Tinea versicolor seen as hypopigmented areas on cheek and neck. (Courtesy Lawrence J. Abramson, M.D., and Alfred D. Hernandez, M.D.)

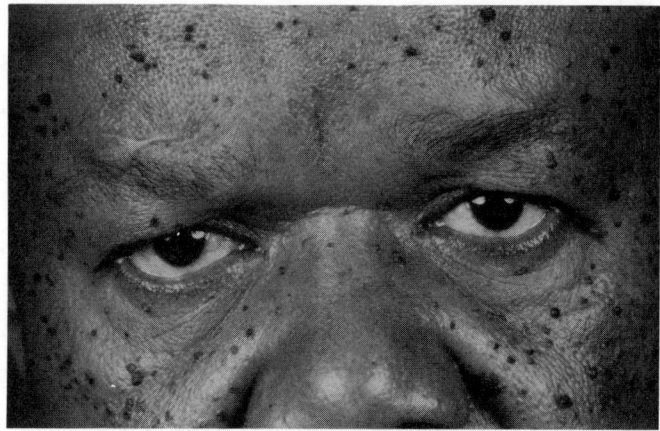

Fig. 8-2. Dermatosis papulosa nigra. (Courtesy Lawrence J. Abramson, M.D., and Alfred D. Hernandez, M.D.)

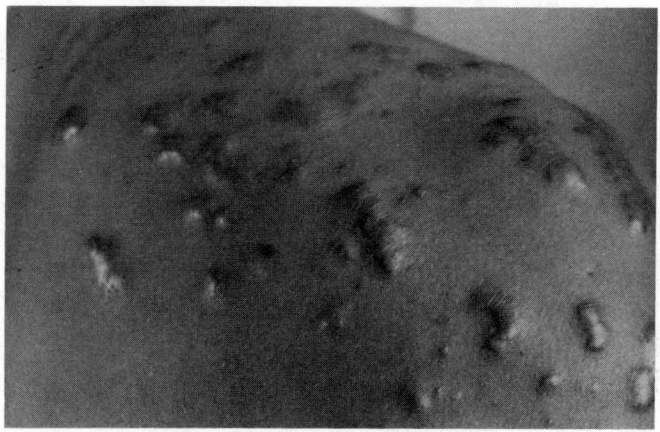

Fig. 8-3. Multiple keloids. (Courtesy Lawrence J. Abramson, M.D., and Alfred D. Hernandez, M.D.)

and number until the client is 50 to 60 years of age. They are well-demarcated papules. They occasionally may be pruritic but are not accompanied by redness, scaling, or telangiectasis. They occur most often on the cheekbones, although they may appear on the face, neck, and upper trunk. They are bilateral and may number in the hundreds. They are absent from the ears, lips, scalp, or bridge of the nose.

The major cause of concern for clients is a cosmetic one. Occasionally the lesions may be inflamed from shaving, picking, or other trauma. If the lesions are in a bothersome place, electrodesiccation will remove them. Otherwise, opaque makeup may cover the lesions. If removal is preferred, the client should be prepared for transient local skin color changes that will resolve in 4 to 5 months (see Fig. 8-2).

156 *Problems with family coping*

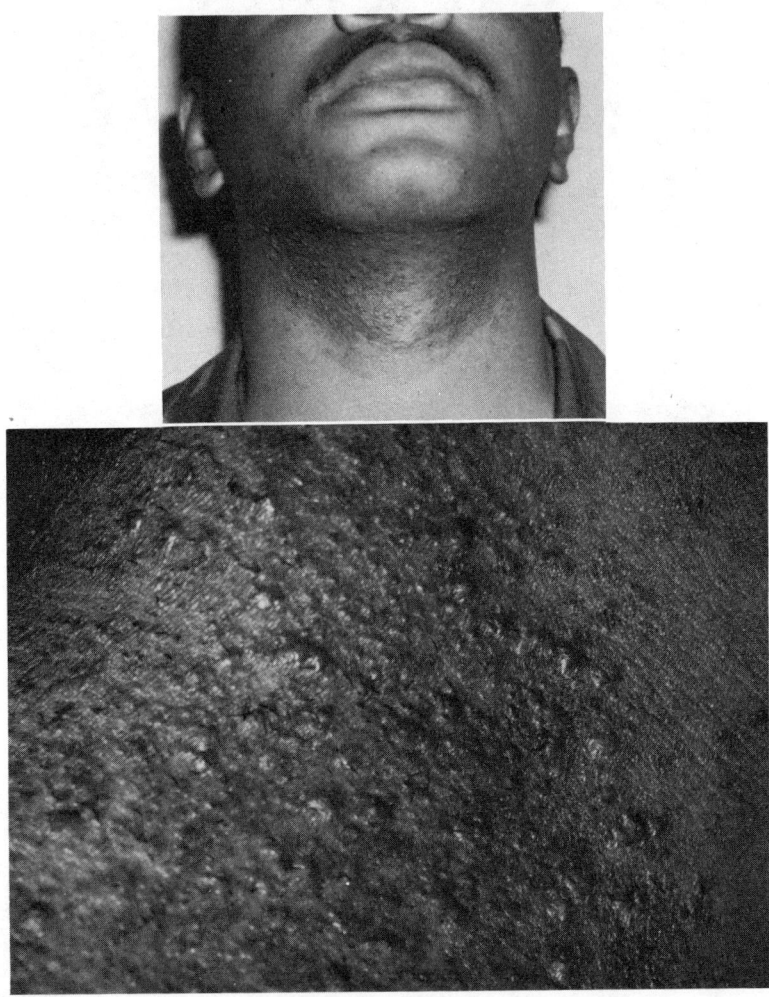

Fig. 8-4. Pseudofolliculitis barbae. (Courtesy Lawrence J. Abramson, M.D., and Alfred D. Hernandez, M.D.)

Problems of the hair

Pseudofolliculitis barbae. This problem, often called "ingrown hairs," is one of the most common dermatological conditions reported by blacks (Kennedy, 1977). This is due to the "kinkiness" of the hairshaft in blacks. When hair is cut, as in shaving, the pointed edge curls inward and penetrates the skin as the hair follicle grows. This causes inflammation, local skin infection, and occasional scarring. Inflamed papules, pustules, or keloids may be noted. The best remedy is to stop cutting or shaving the hair or beard. This may not always be feasible. An alternate treatment is use of a depilatory once or twice weekly as well as plucking out individual hairs. However, inflammation of the skin is common with depilatory products, and the treatment may have to stop. In addition, the use of hot compresses and an antibiotic cream may reduce pustular formations. If the condition is severe, systemic use of antibiotics may be necessary (see Fig. 8-4).

Alopecia. Loss of hair or baldness causes great concern to all clients. Hair loss in many men is hereditary, although total alopecia of the entire body occurs in 5% of clients who complain of losing hair. Common systemic causes of hair loss include fungal infection, discoid lupus erythematosus, secondary syphilis, and scars (Rorsman, 1976). However, the most common causes of hair loss in blacks are hair-grooming techniques (Williams). Such causes include the use of "hot combs," hair straighteners, and other hair products or styles.

A number of hair and skin products are marketed specifically for black consumers. In general, these products do not contain chemicals any different from those marketed for white consumers. One major difference is the marketing technique of adding oils and petroleum chemicals to grooming products for blacks. In addition, these products may be more expensive or difficult to obtain. It is not essential from a medical standpoint to recommend one brand over another. Many of the problems listed below occur in both whites and blacks. General education should focus on the discontinuation of the offending agents rather than switching to a different product to obtain a similar result.

Traction alopecia. As the name implies, hair is lost by pulling or tightly braiding the hair. A hair style known as "cornrowing," which consists of multiple tight braids, may leave balding at the parting of the hair. This occurs more often in teens and children; the sides and front of the scalp are most affected (Kennedy). Most balding is reversible if the hairstyle has not been continued over several months. If the client has this problem, a new hairstyle that does not include the use of curlers, hot combs, or chemicals should be encouraged. An "Afro" may be the best recommendation.

Hot comb alopecia. This type of hair loss results from the use of steam heat, pressing the hair with an iron, or the use of hot petroleum applications. Heat may cause inflammation and scarring of the scalp with subsequent hair loss. Hot petroleum may also initiate this process. Hot comb alopecia often occurs on the crown of the scalp. In some cases hair loss may be irreversible, but the majority of hair responds to discontinuation of the offending techniques.

Alopecia associated with hair straighteners. This form of alopecia occurs equally in black and white populations (Williams). Improper or excessive use of hair straighteners can be damaging to the keratin in the hair follicle, making it brittle and able to break off in pieces. This type of alopecia may be confused with trichotillomania or systemic causes of alopecia. Hair loss is reversible in this situation. Management should focus on discontinuation of the offending agent, recommendation of an alternate hairstyle, and avoidance of any other hair applications until normal hair growth resumes.

Alopecia associated with the Afro pick. "Afro picks" are forklike combs used to shape the Afro hair style worn by many black Americans. Using the comb breaks the individual hairshaft at the pilosebaceous apparatus just below the skin surface. In some cases, the comb may actually pull the hair out by the roots. The appearance is patches of uneven hair growth or hair loss. Hair loss is usually reversible. The solution is to wet the hair before "picking" because it is more manageable and less likely to break.

Sickle cell ulcer

Ulcerations of lower extremities develop in up to 75% of clients with sickle cell anemia (Williams). It may be the presenting symptom of the anemia and may be found in clients with sickle cell trait. Adults are most commonly affected, the plausible causes being stasis, ischemia, lodging of sickled cells in arterioles, and increased blood viscosity that leads to microthrombi. Sickle cell ulcer is clinically similar to a stasis ulcer. The elevated border is a well-defined circle or oval. The ulcer may be deep or shallow, single or multiple, and is usually found medially on the distal third of the legs. The lesion may be crusted, which may cause the disease to be confused with an infectious process. The diagnosis is verified by the presence of sickle cell anemia or sickle cell trait. Management includes decreased activity, treatment of the anemia, increased oxygen tension, and application of a clean dressing to the lesion.

Scars: keloid formations

A keloid is an abnormal scar that is a hard, smooth, and rounded mass of fibrotic tissue that occurs after injury to the skin, folliculitis, or infection. The size can vary immensely, and the shape may be irregular. Keloids are found more commonly in black skin, and they tend to be hereditary. Common sites for these scars include the ears, shoulders, upper chest, neck, back, and abdomen. If the scars are in prominent places or the client desires removal, referral to a dermatologist or plastic surgeon is necessary. Scar reduction procedures may be costly; the client should be informed of this. When adolescents with acne and keloids are counseled, it is essential that the practitioner discourage picking or pinching the skin. If acne is severe and keloid formation is present, referral to a dermatologist may prevent further disfigurement. Ear-piercing should also be discouraged in clients prone to keloids, because the procedure may initiate the development of large keloids (see Fig. 8-3).

REFERENCES

Allende, M.: The enigmas of pigmentation, J.A.M.A. **220**:1443, 1972.

Branch, M., and Paxton, P.: Providing safe nursing care for ethnic people of color, New York, 1976, Appleton-Century-Crofts.

Erkel, E.: The implications of cultural conflict for health care, Health Values **4**:51, March/April 1980.

Fitzpatrick, T.B., and others, editors: Dermatology in general medicine, New York, 1971, McGraw-Hill, Inc.

Galles, M.L.: Identifying dermatological conditions in blacks, J.E.N. **4**:56, Nov.-Dec. 1978.

Guyton, A.C.: Textbook of medical physiology, ed. 5, Philadelphia, 1976, W.B. Saunders Co.

Jeghers, H., and Edelstein, L.: Pigmentation of the skin. In MacBryde, C., and Blacklow, R., editors: Signs and symptoms, ed. 5, Philadelphia, 1970, J.B. Lippincott Co.

Judge, R.D., and Zuidema, G.D.: Methods of clinical examination: a physiologic approach, ed. 3, Boston, 1974, Little, Brown & Co.

Kennedy, J.A.: Dermatoses common in blacks, Postgrad. Med. **61:**122, June 1977.
Koshi, P., editor: Symposium on cultural and biological diversity and health care, Nurs. Clin. North Am. **12:**1, 1977.
Levene, G.M., and Calvan, C.D.: Color atlas of dermatology, Chicago, 1974, Year Book Medical Publishers, Inc.
Luckman, J., and Sorensen, J., editors: Medical-surgical nursing: a psychophysiologic approach, ed. 2, Philadelphia, 1980, W.B. Saunders Co.
Luckraft, D., editor: Black awareness: implications for black patient care, New York, 1976, The American Journal of Nursing Co.
McDonald, C.: Some thoughts on differences in black and white skin, Int. J. Dermatol. **15:**427, 1976.
Murray, R.B., and Zentner, J.F.: Nursing concepts for health promotion, Englewood Cliffs, N.J., 1979, Prentice-Hall, Inc.
Pegues, T.: Physical and psychological assessment of the black patient, Wash. State J. Nurs., 1979, p. 4-8.
Roach, L.B.: Assessing skin changes: the subtle and the obvious, Nursing (Jenkintown) **4:**64, March 1974.
Roach, L.B.: Color changes in dark skin, Nursing (Jenkintown) **7:**48, Jan. 1977.
Rorsman, H.: Dermatology, Chicago, 1976, Year Book Medical Publishers, Inc.
Rubin, B.A.: Black skin: here's how to adjust your assessment and care, R.N. **42:**31, March 1979.
Solomons, B.: Lecture notes on dermatology, ed. 3, Oxford, 1973, Blackwell Scientific Publications.
Szabo, G.: Racial differences in the fate of melanosomes in human epidermis, Nature, **222:**1081, 1969.
Thorne, N.: The problem of the black skin, Nurs. Times **65:**999, 1969.
Williams, R.A., editor: Textbook of black related diseases, New York, 1975, McGraw-Hill, Inc.

SECTION FOUR

Problems with nutritional alterations

CHAPTER 9

Assessment and guidance of nutrition during the first year of life

Stephanie McGhee

HISTORY AND TRENDS IN INFANT NUTRITION

Substituting proprietary formulas for human breast milk first occurred in the midnineteenth century. This was a radical dietary change. Considering that this change took place after some 1 million years of breast-feeding and involved vast numbers of infants, it may represent the world's largest uncontrolled in vivo experiment. Although for years some effects of the substitution were devastating, the practice remains. Among technological societies today, however, changing feeding practices show awareness of the benefits of the older methods of infant feedings.

Initially, the substitution of cow's milk for human milk resulted in the death of seven out of eight non-breast-fed infants (Fomon, 1974). The two main causes of these deaths were infectious gastrointestinal disease and cholera. These diseases often were transmitted through contaminated milk. The advent of technology in the late nineteenth and early twentieth centuries enabled scientists to determine the chemical composition and physiological action of human and cow's milk. Precise mathematical calculations were used to prescribe formulas in the hope of decreasing infant mortality (about 240/1000 in the United States) (Fried, 1977).

Two influential discoveries occurred in the latter part of the nineteenth century. Heinrick Finkelstein of Berlin, whose findings at first were ignored, believed a loving maternal-infant relationship was as necessary for healthy growth and development as was milk. Louis Pasteur's discoveries of 1876 were more readily accepted. It was his influence that led to strict sanitation codes in the preparation of milk in Europe in 1897. This ultimately led to the decrease in infant mortality (Fried). However, as late as the 1920s milk still became contaminated with tubercle bacilli from cattle and from lack of refrigeration.

With the processes of homogenization and pasteurization, bacterial counts in milk began to decrease; the heating also produced smaller milk curds, which facilitated digestion. Finally, infant mortality from enteric disease decreased dramatically. Cow's milk preparations became more precise and provided nutrients in proportion to human milk. In the 1940s ascorbic acid was added to formulas; over the next 30 years vitamin

B_6, iron, and zinc were added. Present formulas are an adequate substitute for human milk and meet an infant's nutritional needs.

From the time of its introduction, bottle-feeding escalated while the incidence of breast-feeding declined. By 1960 only 25% of American mothers breast-fed (Fomon). Modern technological advancement, commercial promotion, and lack of awareness among health professionals accounted for the decline in breast-feeding.

Developing societies, which traditionally used breast-feeding have also introduced bottle-feeding. As in Western society, its use grew rapidly. However, inadequate hygiene, funds, water, and education have led to diarrheal disease, marasmus, and malnutrition, which have increased infant mortality (Jelliffe and Jelliffe, 1978a). Although results in the United States are not as disastrous, infant disease and mortality have increased in the lower socioeconomic classes since the introduction of the bottle.

In addition to the advent of bottle-feeding, another significant change occurred when mothers altered solid food habits. Before 1920 the diets of infants under 1 year contained no solid food. In the 1930s pediatricians advocated semisolids at 6 months, and in the 1950s infants received semisolids in the first few days of life.

The 1970s saw a revolution in infant feeding. Forty-five percent of American mothers began breast-feeding and introducing semisolids at a later age; however, these trends predominated in more educated, higher socioeconomic classes (Frantz and others, 1978).

The goal of this chapter is to present guidelines for assessment and planning of nutrition during the first year of life. Recommendations focus on the healthy infant who is either breast- or bottle-fed. I emphasize breast-feeding because of its distinct nutritional advantages.

NUTRITIONAL REQUIREMENTS
Water

Water demands in proportion to body weight are greatest during infancy. This is due to the infant's relatively high metabolic rate, limited renal ability to conserve water, and increased sensible water losses from a relatively large body surface area. Requirements range from 120 ml/kg/day to 160 ml/kg/day. The largest amounts are necessary during the first 3 months. These are met by human milk and proprietary milk formulas, which supply 150 to 190 ml water per kg. Almroth (1978) demonstrated that well-breast-fed infants do not need additional water even in hot, tropical climates.

Renal and extrarenal water losses normally occur in healthy infants; however, these losses may be life threatening when coupled with illness. Additional extrarenal water losses occur with high environmental temperatures, fever, illnesses, and unusual diets. Diarrheal illnesses pose the greatest danger; water needs increase fivefold because of water lost in stools (Fomon).

Renal water losses depend on the renal solute load as determined by dietary intake of nitrogen, sodium, potassium, and chloride. Cow's milk presents a higher solute load, since it contains 4 times more sodium and 3 times more protein than human milk (Gamsu, 1975). Seventy five percent to 88% of bottle-fed infants have blood urea levels above normal limits (Davies and Saunders, 1973). Because of the uniquely low solute load of human milk, breast-fed infants need less water for excretion of excess solutes. This is compatible with the immature renal tubular function of the newborn and the limited ability to concentrate urine and conserve water for solute excretion. Because of this decreased ability to handle solute load, it is especially important that parents be taught proper formula preparation, since many mothers tend to overconcentrate feedings.

The intake of calorically concentrated formulas, such as cow's milk, skim milk, or 2% milk, causes increased solute loads and obligatory water losses. This is particularly dangerous when coupled with the additional water loss occurring in diarrheal illness. The infant tries to compensate for the loss by drinking more. Unfortunately, the only liquid available is calorically concentrated formula. This leads to a vicious cycle of dehydration. If uncorrected, hypernatremic dehydration may result and eventually produce permanent neurological damage, subdural effusion and hematomas, and death (Finberg, 1959).

Energy

Energy requirements are determined by body size and composition, physical activity, and rate of growth. Energy intake must equal energy output plus basal metabolic needs, which vary in every infant. The recommended daily requirement for infants up to 6 months is 117 kcal/kg. From 6 months to the end of the first year these requirements gradually decrease to 108 kcal/kg/day. These recommendations are based on a daily basal requirement of 55 kcal/kg, a growth requirement of about 35 kcal/kg, and an activity allowance of 10 to 25 kcal/kg (Alfin-Slater and Jelliffe, 1977).

Full-term infants have fat and water reserves at birth and do not need calories from feedings until 2 to 3 days of age. Carbohydrates should supply 35% to 65% of total daily calories, protein 7% to 16%, and fats 30% to 55% with 1% from linoleic acid (Fomon). Breast milk, and proprietary formulas and evaporated milk, if mixed properly, meet these requirements. During the first year of life, whole cow's milk, skim milk, or 2% milk may contribute to obesity, nutritional deficiencies, and dehydration.

Protein

Proteins are nitrogenous compounds essential for tissue growth. Their constituent amino acids are necessary for the formation of cell protoplasm. Nine of the amino acids must be supplied by the diet, since they cannot be synthesized in the body. The recommended daily intake of protein is 2.2 gm/kg for the first 6 months and 2.02 gm/kg for the second 6 months (Alfin-Slater and Jelliffe). Kwashiorkor and severe growth failure result from inadequate protein intake or utilization. In infancy an intake of protein that is greater than 20% of the caloric input is excessive and may result in hypernatremic dehydration due to a high solute load (Pipes, 1977).

There are major differences in the protein composition of human and cow's milk. In human milk, protein consists mainly of α-lactalbumin and lactoferrin with smaller amounts of lysozyme, serum albumin, IgA, IgC, and IgM. The antiinfective factors contribute bacteriostatic, antiviral, and antiallergic properties. The whey of cow's milk is predominantly β-lactoglobulin and bovine albumin, which are absent in human milk. The differences in protein composition have been implicated as causative factors in cow's milk allergy (Jelliffe and Jelliffe, 1978a).

The curd formation in human and cow's milk is not the same. This is because of differences in their amino acid content. Casein protein precipitates into curds in the low pH environment of the infant's stomach. This enables gastric enzymes to begin protein digestion (Hambraeus, 1977). The curd of the breast-fed baby is soft and flocculent, whereas the curd in the infant fed cow's milk is tough and rubbery and may cause bowel obstruction. Proprietary formulas produce less dense curds. However, if they are prepared with too little water, "milk bolus obstruction" may result, and the infant can develop an acute surgical abdomen. The human milk curd has never been observed to cause an obstruction (Graver and others, 1977).

The total level of amino acids is higher in cow's milk; however, human milk has more sulfur-containing amino acids, such as cystine and taurine. Some authorities consider these to be essential, rather than nonessential, amino acids in the neonatal period (Gauel and others, 1977). This is an important difference.

Carbohydrate

The body metabolizes carbohydrates to store and use for energy, reserving proteins for tissue synthesis. Too little carbohydrate intake results in the use of amino acids and fats as energy, with the risk of ketosis and fat breakdown. Excessive carbohydrate intake may cause diarrhea due to the increased osmotic load placed on the bowel (Christie, 1977).

Lactose is the carbohydrate present in human and cow's milk; formulas and commercial baby foods contain sucrose. Lactose levels are higher in human milk, which accounts for the loose, watery stool in the breast-fed infant. Lactose serves three essential functions: (1) lactose enhances calcium and magnesium absorption, which helps prevent rickets; (2) it is metabolized to galactose, which is necessary for development of the central nervous system; and (3) it contributes to the growth of intestinal lactobacilli, which contribute to a bacteriostatic effect against *Escherichia coli* (Jelliffe and Jelliffe, 1978a).

Fats

Fats provide energy, carry fat-soluble vitamins, and supply essential fatty acids. They are constituents of prostaglandins and sources of cholesterol. Vegetable sources supply polyunsaturated fatty acids, the most important being linoleic, linolenic, and arachidonic acids. When linoleic acid is only 1% of the total caloric intake, infants voluntarily ingest more than infants receiving the optimal 4% to 5% (Fomon). This may result in more rapid weight gain. However, deficiency signs do not occur, and rates of growth are as rapid as with higher levels. Deficient fat intake results in hunger; dry, thick, scaly, skin; hair loss; and failure to thrive (Crawford and others, 1978). Deficiencies result during infancy from the use of dilute formulas, skim milk, and 2% milk. These milks do not provide enough energy, calories, essential fatty acids, and vitamins; therefore, they are not recommended before 2 years of age. Excessive fat intake contributes to obesity and should be discouraged.

Infants digest and absorb fat from breast milk more efficiently than from cow's milk. Ninety five percent of fat from breast milk is absorbed as compared with 65% from cow's milk. The type of milk ingested is important because fat malabsorption may be high in the healthy preterm infant. Formulas that supply fats from medium-chain triglycerides of vegetable origin (corn, coconut, and soy oils) have absorption rates approaching 90%.

Cholesterol levels are higher in human milk than in cow's milk. Cholesterol is absent from proprietary formulas. Some authorities believe that cholesterol is necessary to develop enzyme systems and facilitate myelinization of the central nervous system postnataly (Tsang and Gluck, 1975). It may assist in the feedback mechanisms regulating the biosynthesis and catabolism of cholesterol (Fomon). Therefore during infancy the intake of cholesterol from human milk may decrease cholesterol levels later in life.

The fat content of human milk fluctuates diurnally, with higher levels occurring in the morning. It also varies during each feeding, with the fat content of the hind milk being greater than that at the beginning of breast-feeding. In addition, dietary fat intake of the mother directly affects the fat content of her milk.

Vitamins and minerals

Table 9-1 lists vitamins and minerals and states their functions and clinical implications. Differences between human and cow's milk are also included where applicable.

Undernutrition

Evaluation of feeding and nutrition is always an important part of every child's assessment. It should occur at each child's visit to the health care system and consist of both subjective and objective findings. This evaluation is never more important than in the first years of life, since proper nutrition in infancy is critical for normal growth and development. Brain growth is most rapid during the first year of life and almost complete by 2 years. Caloric deprivation during this phase of cellular hyperplasia may result in small cell size, decreased organ size, and depressed body growth. A 15-year follow-up study of malnourished infants indicated a higher incidence of visual motor perception disturbances, neurointegrative system defects, disturbed body concepts, organic brain dysfunction, abnormal electroencephalogram patterns, and irreversible intellectual impariment (Stoch and Smythe, 1976). Winick and Brasel (1977) found that dietary intervention and environmental change in a malnourished infant before the age of 5 can lead to improvements in intellectual capacity. Intervention before 2 years leads to almost complete recovery of intellectual functions.

Overnutrition

Excessive caloric intake may result in obesity, one of the most prevalent nutritional disorders of American society. The incidence of childhood obesity in the United States approaches 10% to 30%. The cause of obesity is the imbalance between energy intake and physical output; however, genetic factors are also thought to be important in interplay with the environment. The mother who forces the infant to empty the bottle, mixes an overconcentrated formula, begins solids too early, rewards the child with food, or misinterprets the child's every cry as hunger contributes to this energy imbalance.

The old adage that "a fat baby is a healthy baby" is grossly inaccurate. There are several complications associated with infantile obesity. Obese infants have an increased incidence of respiratory tract infections and have a more difficult time dealing with them because of the increased mechanical burden of breathing (Tracey and others, 1971). They have more skin diseases and infections that are difficult to treat because of increased moisture in large skinfolds. In addition, overfeeding may condition the child to do so throughout life.

Table 9-1. Vitamins and minerals: functions and clinical implications

	Functions	Clinical implications
Vitamins		
Fat-soluble		
A	Visual adaptation to changes in light, nerve activity, bone structure, lipid metabolism, protein synthesis, protection against infection	Human milk has higher levels than cow's milk Deficiency: failure to thrive, apathy, mental retardation, decreased resistance to infection, retarded bone and tooth growth Toxicity: anorexia, skin desquamation, vomiting, increased intracranial pressure
D	Maintenance of serum Ca and P and bone matrix	Deficiency: costochondral beading, cranial bossing, poor dental development, rickets Several cases of rickets reported in breast-fed infants without supplementation but were in areas of poor nutrition Other studies show that human milk may have enough vitamin D present as water-soluble conjugate of D
E	Antioxidant (protects A and C against oxidative destruction), provides erythrocyte resistance to hemolysis	Iron antagonistic to E and may lower E availability to infant; vitamin C may ↑ E requirements; as increased polyunsaturated fatty acids then increased need for E; E cannot be absorbed without fats, thus infants ingesting skim milk will not absorb E; supplements suggested for premature infants Deficiency: irritability, edema, hemolytic anemia
K	Biosynthesis of coagulation factors	Breast-fed infants require 0.5-1 mg IM at birth, since levels are lower in human milk and amount of consumption in first days is low Deficiency: neonatal hemorrhage, no RDA
Water-soluble		
B$_1$ (Thiamine)	Coenzyme in carbohydrate (CHO) metabolism	As increased CHO intake then increased need for thiamine
B$_2$ (Riboflavin)	Enzymes in metabolism of protein, lipids, and CHOs	Deficiency: seborrheic dermatitis, cheilosis, corneal vascularization
B$_6$ (Pyridoxine)	DNA synthesis, adrenocortical function, hemoglobin synthesis, coenzymes in protein, CHO, and lipid metabolism	As protein content of diet increases, increased need for B$_6$ and decreased niacin and pantothenic acid requirements Deficiency: failure to gain weight, anemia, convulsions
B$_{12}$ (Cyanocobalamin)	Coenzyme in protein lipid and CHO metabolism; red cell formation, DNA and nucleic acid synthesis	Deficiency: pernicious anemia, absent deep tendon reflexes, ataxia, paresthesias Since found only in animal sources must supplement if a strict vegetarian (no milk or eggs) or with breast milk from strict vegetarian mother

Nutrient	Function	Comments
C (Ascorbic acid)	Detoxification reactions; phagocytic control; coenzyme reducing and antioxidant in collagen formation, tissue repair, iron and folic acid metabolism, blood vessel integrity, hemoglobin formation and infection resistance	Human milk contains more than cow's milk; C in whole milk negligible. Deficiency: impaired wound healing, scurvy, anorexia, hemorrhages (gums, skin), irritability, weakness
Biotin	Nicotinic acid, pancreatic amylase synthesis; coenzyme in metabolism of CHO, lipids, and protein	Deficiency: hypotonia, anorexia, nausea, seborrheic dermatitis. No requirements known
Folic acid	Heme synthesis; coenzyme in synthesis of DNA, nucleic acids, and amino acid metabolism	Deficiency: megaloblastic anemia, growth and motor retardation, diarrhea
Niacin	Component of NAD and NADP	Deficiency: pellagra, skin lesions, nausea and vomiting
Panthothenic acid	Part of coenzyme A	No RDA
Minerals		
Calcium (Ca)	Skeleton and tooth formation; catalyst in reactions; blood coagulation, lactation	Vitamin D necessary for absorption; lactose increases absorption; phytic acid (husk of cereal grains) and oxalic acid (greens, spinach) form insoluble compounds with Ca and decrease absorption; Ca absorption poor in cow's milk. Low Ca-P ratio: restlessness, irritability, poor growth, soft tissue calcification. Deficiency: bone and tooth demineralization, tetany, failure to thrive
Chlorine (Cl)	Maintain acid-base balance, electrolytes, contractility of muscle tissue, nervous tissue irritability; maintains heart rhythm	Deficiency: alkalosis, dehydration
Chromium (Cr)	Necessary for insulin use in glucose metabolism	Deficiency may contribute to atherosclerosis and hypercholesterolemia. So far deficiency occurs only with impaired glucose tolerance
Cobalt (Co)	Part of B_{12}	No deficiency known
Copper (Cu)	90% as enzyme ceruloplasmin ferroxidase (converts ferrous to ferric iron); essential for erythropoiesis; normal bone growth, GI functions, cellular respiration	Deficiency: anemia, resistance to iron therapy, retarded growth, failure to thrive, cerebral degeneration. Phytates decrease absorption; mortality from coronary disease may be correlated with higher Zn-Cu ratio; Cu levels higher in human milk
Fluoride (Fl)	Reduces caries	Supplement according to content in H_2O supply. Toxicity: mottling of teeth occurs at intakes greater than 2 mg/day
Iodine (I)	Component of thyroid hormone; controls basal metabolic rate	Deficiency: goiter, cretinism. Toxicity: depressed thyroid. Colostrum very rich in iodine; I in human milk largely reflected by diet

Continued.

Table 9-1. Vitamins and minerals: functions and clinical implications—cont'd

	Functions	Clinical implications
Minerals—cont'd		
Iron (Fe)	Component of hemoglobin, myoglobin, cytochrome system; cofactor in enzyme systems	Vitamin C enhances absorption; eggs interfere with iron absorption from other sources ↑ availability of iron in human milk although levels are lower Deficiency: anemia
Magnesium (Mg)	Skeleton and tooth formation, protein synthesis, production and storage of energy, body temperature regulation; cofactor in metabolic systems	Fats and phytates decrease absorption; competes with Ca for absorption; if increased Ca in diet then must ↑ Mg; higher levels in human milk Deficiency: tetany, muscle weakness, behavioral disturbances
Manganese (Mn)	Mucopolysaccharide, cholesterol, and fatty acid synthesis	One of least toxic of trace elements; no RDA
Molybdenum (Mo)	Formation of uric acid, part of xanthine oxidase and aldehyde oxidase, may help release iron from ferritin	No deficiency known; no RDA; may prevent caries
Phosphorus (P)	Skeleton and tooth formation; forms ATP in citric acid cycle; component of phosphorylated compounds, nucleic acids, and nucleoproteins, maintains blood pH	Deficiency: poor bone and tooth structure, muscle weakness Vitamin D necessary for absorption
Potassium (K)	Maintains acid-base balance, electrolytes, contractility of muscle tissue, nervous tissue irritability; maintains heart rhythm	Deficiency: muscle weakness; slow, irregular heartbeat; anorexia Hyperkalemia: heart block
Selenium (Se)	Antioxidant at cellular level	Weight gains in infants with protein and caloric malnutrition when supplemented with Se; no deficiency known; no RDA
Sodium (Na)	Maintains acid-base balance, electrolytes, contractility of muscle tissue, nervous tissue irritability	Deficiency: dehydration, weakness, nausea, nervous irritability, tachycardia Increased sodium intakes in infancy may lead to high blood pressure as adults; lower Na levels in human milk
Zinc (Zn)	DNA synthesis; wound healing, enzyme systems	Cu competes with zinc for absorption; phytates decrease absorption Deficiency: growth retardation, anorexia, impaired wound healing, may cause pica and be responsible for congenital malformations; acrodermatitis enteropathica in the neonate may be caused by molecular defect related to Zn metabolism

Does infant obesity lead to obesity in adulthood with all the concomitant effects? The main theory of obesity, the "fat cell theory," states that during a critical period in infancy overfeeding will cause an increase in the number and size of adipocytes. After this critical phase there is an increase only in the size of adipocytes but not in the number. Once fat cells are present, the only way to lose body fat is to decrease cell size, which makes weight loss more difficult. The fat cell theory is debatable, and the explanation for obesity is complex (Taitz, Feb. 1977). It is the viewpoint of most authorities that food consumption during infancy should be regulated.

ASSESSMENT

Since early detection and intervention are vital, the nurse must obtain accurate nutritional assessments to detect malnourished infants and those at risk for nutritional problems such as obesity. An understanding of the nutritional requirements of the infant is necessary to evaluate feeding practices and types of feedings. Accurate measurements provide some of the best screening data for evaluating infant growth. Small errors may lead to inaccurate assessments and treatment. Fat-fold thickness and infant weight, length, and head circumference plotted on growth charts over a period of time show the rate and pattern of growth and provide a more reliable tool for diagnosis than do single measurements (Tanner and Whitehouse, 1967). This also provides a better view of familial influences on general body size. Excessively high (greater than 95th percentile) or low (less than 5th percentile) measurements as well as failure to demonstrate growth in any area should be investigated. Additionally, dental development, bone development, psychosocial development, and physical motor development assist in the assessment of nutritional status.

History

Accurate nutritional assessments to detect malnourished infants and those at risk for nutritional problems are essential for the nurse in a primary care setting. One of the most important aspects of the nutritional evaluation is the nutritional history. The boxed material on p. 172 provides guidelines for an appropriate infant feeding history. It can be expanded as needed for individual cases and is divided into the first and second 6 months of life, where some focuses differ.

Psychosocial problems. Psychosocial problems present within the family may influence feeding behaviors and problems. The psychosocial environment always needs exploring. For example, the practitioner should learn how much income is allotted to food. There are more nutritional disorders among families of low income (Owen and others, 1974). Water supply, sanitation, and food storage in the home are also important. Parenting styles may influence an infant's feeding. The parent may be unable to decipher the infant's cries and offer food each time the infant cries.

Past history. This includes perinatal history, birth weight and length, past illnesses, hospitalizations, surgeries, allergies, and immunizations. Allergies or past illnesses may be particularly helpful as clues to nutritional problems. Examples are chronic infection, heart disease, hepatitis, and asthma. Also, the best measure of iron endowment at birth is the birth weight because total body iron increases directly with weight. This is true for both term and low-birth-weight infants (Woodruff, 1977).

Family history. The practitioner should for conditions in the family history that may pose nutritional problems in the infant. Examples are anemias such as sickle cell, meta-

Feeding history during infancy

I. General
  A. Breast-feeding
     1. Duration of nursing session
     2. Interval between feedings
     3. Determination of need to feed (demand and schedule)
     4. Burping techniques
     5. Parental assessment of appetite
     6. Use of supplemental bottles
     7. Use of vitamin and mineral supplement
  B. Bottle-feeding
     1. Formula
        a. Type
        b. Preparation technique
        c. Sterilization techniques
        d. Frequency of opening new can of formula
     2. Feeding behavior
        a. Amount per feeding
        b. Number of feedings per 24 hours
        c. Burping techniques and frequency
        d. Type of nipple and bottle
        e. Parental assessment of appetite
        f. Use of other liquids
        g. Use of vitamin and mineral supplement
        h. Identity of primary food preparer and of feeder
II. Age-specific behaviors
  A. 0-6 months
     1. Introduction of semisolids
        a. Age of introduction
        b. Type
        c. Frequency
     2. Solids added to formula
     3. Bottle propping
  B. 6-12 months
     1. Introduction of semisolids
        a. Home-prepared
        b. Commercial
        c. Parental reaction to food refusal
     2. Self-feeding
        a. Introduction of spoon
        b. Types of finger foods
        c. Introduction of cup
        d. Bedtime or nap time bottle
     3. Meals
        a. Frequency
        b. Entire family present
        c. Safe high chair use
     4. Snacks
        a. Frequency
        b. Type

bolic conditions such as hyperlipidemias, diabetes or thyroid disorders, or milk intolerance. A positive family history for obesity should alert the practitioner that the infant is at risk for developing obesity (Taitz, Feb. 1977).

Diet history. The 24-hour dietary recall may be necessary for the practitioner to accurately assess an infant's diet. To be reliable the recall needs to be taken for a typical day. This excludes weekends, periods of erratic eating, periods of illness, or problems in the environment. If there are abnormal growth patterns, the nurse may wish to request a 3- to 7-day food diary. Another alternative is to determine how often key foods in major food groups are eaten; for example, if yellow vegetables are eaten more than once a day, only once a day, once a week, or seldom. Interpretation of food values can be complex. If the provider does not have an excellent understanding of nutritional requirements, it is best that a nutritionist's assistance be sought.

The practitioner should inquire about any areas of parental concern. Common problems parents identify are poor appetite, "picky" eating, and obesity. Exploration of the parents' concerns may both reveal misconceptions about "normal" behavior and the need for instruction. There may also be a problem that necessitates further investigation.

Physical examination

It is rare to see gross nutritional deficiencies in the United States; more likely are subclinical and subtle problems such as undernutrition, overnutrition, dental caries, and iron deficiency anemia (Ten-state nutrition survey, 1972). Growth patterns may be the prime indicators of nutritional deficiencies. The nurse has a responsibility to be aware of the leading nutritional problems of the population served. Pertinent examples include lack of fluoride in the water supply, pica, lead ingestion, and some culturally determined food patterns.

Physical examination begins with observation of the general appearance of the infant and the interaction with the parents. Some important questions include: Is the infant obese, edematous, or emaciated? Is the infant active and alert or apathetic, listless, and pale? Does the infant seem calm or irritable? Does the parent comfort and touch the infant or appear apathetic or hostile? The provider should observe the eyes, mouth, skin, hair, skeleton, mucous membranes, and nervous system for signs of vitamin or mineral deficiency (Table 9-1).

Growth standards. Growth charts allow both a recording of measurements over a period of time and a comparison with a growth standard. Measurements include stature-for-age, weight-for-age, and weight-for-stature. Charts prepared by the Center for Disease Control following recommendations by the National Academy of Sciences compare a range from the 5th to the 95th percentile. These charts reflect the standard of a larger sample and are thought to be more representative of the U.S. population than were the older Stuart-Merideth (Boston) charts. The Boston charts use the extremes of the 3rd and the 97th percentiles.

Isolated values on a growth chart may be of little vlaue. Velocities of growth over a period of time should be compared to detect growth patterns. For example, a child may be below the 5 percentile when compared with the standard for age, but the growth pattern over time shows a steadily increasing normal curve.

Head circumference. This measurement is most commonly used to screen for microcephaly and macrocephaly. Head circumference is a reliable indicator of brain growth during infancy. Measurements increase during the first 6 months and then reach a plateau. Infants with severe malnutrition have decreased total brain weight, protein, RNA, and DNA, with a proportional delay of head circumference growth. Familial size and general body size also influence head circumference.

Fat-fold thickness. The measurement of fat-fold thickness is probably the most valid tool for assessing obesity. Fifty percent of body fat is present in the subcutaneous tissue layers. Measurements with skinfold calipers reflect the relative fat deposition and correlate well with total body fat (Zerfas and Neumann, 1977). This measure is a better assessment of obesity than weight-for-age and weight-for-height, since those do not distinguish muscle and soft tissue bulk from fat. The routine use of skin calipers is important to prevent caloric restriction in the large but not obese child and false reassurance with the obese child of normal weight. This measurement is most commonly taken from the triceps

Table 9-2. Triceps fat-fold thickness: 90th to 97th percentile (boys and girls)

Age in months	Measurement in mm
0	10
3	11
6	12
9	13
12	14

Modified from Zerfas, A.J., and Neumann, C.G.: Office assessment of nutritional status, Pediatr. Clin. of North Am. **24:**253, Feb. 1977.

midway between the acromium and olecranon processes. Early in infancy this may be done while prone, but once the child can sit this is a more desirable position. Zerfas and Neumann indicate that values greater than the 90th to 97th percentile for triceps fat-fold thickness suggest obesity (Table 9-2).

Weight. The earliest sign of undernutrition is failure to gain weight despite relatively normal height. Also, serial weight measurements give an indication of excessive weight gain and likely obesity (Zerfas and Neumann). Obesity may be defined as weight-for-length greater than the 95th percentile.

Length. Length or height assesses linear skeletal growth, which reflects long-standing nutritional adequacy. This measurement correlates better with socioeconomic status than weight or other soft tissue measurements (Zerfas and Neumann).

Developmental patterns. Nutritional assessment includes ongoing examination of the infant's development, including gross and fine motor, social, and language development. A screening tool such as the Denver Developmental Screening Test may detect developmental delays. When administered periodically, it may be used to record the pattern of development in the same manner that other growth charts are used.

Laboratory data

Laboratory evaluations provide useful information in some clinical situations. Hemoglobin and hematocrit are the best screening tests to perform routinely. Evidence of anemia needs further testing, such as red cell indices, serum iron, total iron-binding capacity, and percent saturation. The presence of anemia or a family history of anemia may be an indication for a hemoglobin electrophoresis. Problems such as failure to thrive and endocrine or metabolic disease may require extensive evaluation; for example, radiographs for bone age and evaluations of serum or urine protein, vitamins, lipids, and minerals may be necessary. Suspision of such severe problems necessitates physician consultation.

PLAN
Breast-feeding

Human milk or proprietary formulas meet a healthy infant's needs for about the first 6 months of life. Although breast-feeding is not the most popular feeding choice, human milk meets the optimum requirements for growth and development of the human infant.

This section discusses the advantages of human milk, common concerns about breast-feeding, and problems in breast-feeding.

Benefits of breast-feeding. The antiinfective properties of human milk help the premature and full-term infant resist gastrointestinal and other diseases. These properties consist of humoral and cellular components. The major humoral components are the bifidus factor, lactoferrin, immunoglobulins, anitbodies, and lysozyme. Interferon and the lactoperoxidase system also are implicated. The bifidus factor, in combination with high lactose and low protein and phosphate levels in human milk, promotes the growth of *Lactobacillus bifidus* in the gastrointestinal tract. This contributes to the acidic pH of the gut, which helps inhibit pathogenic organisms, especially *E. coli* (Bullen and Willis, 1971). This is one way that breast-feeding protects against gastroenteritis (Mata and Urrutia, 1971). However, any supplemental milk increases intestinal pH and decreases resistance to *E. coli*. Thus this resistance lasts only during complete breast-feeding (Lavsen and Homer, 1978).

Immunoglobulins in human milk are IgA, IgC, IgG, IgD, IgM, and secretory IgA (sIgA). Secretory IgA is highest in colostrum (50 mg/ml) and drops to 1 mg/ml within a few days, but increased amounts of milk compensate for the drop. Unlike other immunoglobulins, sIgA is resistant to proteolytic gut enzymes and acts as an intestinal paint. Thus it protects the gut from invasion of bacteria and viruses. When inhaled by the infant during feeding, sIgA also coats the respiratory tract. Secretory IgA also binds to pathogens, retarding replication.

Secretory IgA helps decrease the risk of immunologically mediated allergic reactions. This is a result of the limited absorption of dietary antigens that is prevented by the intestinal coating action of IgA. About 100,000 yearly cases of milk allergy would be eliminated if all mothers breast-fed their infants (Jelliffe and Jelliffe, 1978a). Even with supplemental feedings, the sIgA from human milk would help decrease the antibody response to cow's milk protein (Hanson and others, 1977).

Specific antibodies (mainly sIgA) in human milk prevent the growth of bacteria such as *Clostridium tetani, Corynebacterium diptheriae, E. coli,* diplococci, salmonellae, shigellae, streptococci, and staphylococci. Human milk also contains antibodies against viruses, including Coxsackie virus, ECHO virus, alpha virus, influenza virus, parainfluenza virus, rotavirus, herpesvirus, poliovirus, and respiratory syncitial virus (Pittard, 1979). Mothers should refrain from breast-feeding 2 to 3 hours before and after a polio vaccination, since the human milk antibodies may inactivate the live polio vaccine virus. Antiinfective factors in the milk of poorly nourished mothers at different stages of lactation are comparable to those of well-nourished women (Reddy, 1977). This is significant in poor, crowded communities where infection rates are high. Mothers from these communities need encouragement to breast-feed and to give only breast milk to the infant for the first 6 months. After that time, the infant's own resistant factors become more mature and able to deal with invading organisms.

There are several disorders associated with formula-fed infants that are virtually unknown in breast-fed infants: obesity, iron deficiency anemia, hypernatremic dehydration, neonatal hypocalcemia, aminoacidemia, and acrodermatitis enteropathica (Jelliffe and Jelliffe, 1978a). Also, formula-fed infants have 8 times the incidence of otitis media as do breast-fed infants. Causes of this relate to the antiinfective, antiallergic properties of human milk and the positional phenomenon of bottle propping (Schaefer, 1971).

Human and artificial nipples require different sucking patterns. The tongue of the breast-fed infant moves posteriorly against the hard palate to squeeze milk from the nipple and areola. The lips purse downward with a jaw action. Sucking from an artificial nipple is easier. The tongue is thrust anteriorly to control milk inflow. An abnormal pattern of tongue thrusting occurs more often in bottle-fed infants and may be associated with dental malocclusion (Simpson and Cheung, 1976).

Maternal concerns. Economically, it is more expensive to bottle-feed than to breast-feed. Nurses should know the cost of different feeding practices, since parents who "economize" by diluting formulas or by other measures may seriously endanger a child's health.

In developing countries, complete breast-feeding provides more contraceptive protection than any current birth control program. Complete breast-feeding means that the infant feeds on demand without a bottle, pacifier, or early solid foods. This maintains high prolactin levels that are necessary to suppress menses and ovulation. Less than four feedings per day return prolactin levels to normal by 6 months. With greater than six feedings a day, prolactin levels will not decrease until a year (Delvoye, 1977). Kippley and Kippley (1977) found no pregnancies occurring during 12 months of complete nursing in 112 mothers. Mothers practicing scheduled feedings need other means of birth control, but the motivated mother should be informed that complete breast-feeding may provide adequate birth control for a year.

Some controversy exists about the caloric intake a lactating mother needs per day. Most authorities place the figure at 2,500 to 2,600 calories per day (Jelliffe, 1975; Thompson, 1970). These extra calories support milk output of 600 to 800 ml/day. The volume of daily milk production is a function of nutritional status and has little to do with fluid intake (Jelliffe and Jelliffe, 1978a). In a poorly nourished mother the volume of milk decreases, but the concentrations of protein, fat, and carbohydrate remain remarkably constant (Committee on Nutrition, 1960). Poor diet affects fatty acid and vitamin content predominantly. Supplementing malnourished mothers with protein increases milk volume and nutritional quality (Jelliffe and Jelliffe, 1978a). It is important to emphasize that caloric energy is necessary for milk production, not for increasing maternal fat stores. It is important that mothers do not diet during lactation.

Breast-milk jaundice occurs in 1% of breast-fed infants. A steroid found in breast milk interferes with the glucuronyl transferase system. This leads to accumulation of bile products (Guthrie, 1978). It appears about the second day of life and usually resolves in 7 days. Occasionally it may persist as long as 4 weeks (Chow and others, 1979). Bilirubin levels rarely exceed 15 to 20 mg/dl, whereas kernicterus usually occurs when levels reach 20 to 22 mg/dl. Other serious causes of jaundice should be excluded in the jaundiced breast-fed infant. Laboratory evaluation includes direct and indirect bilirubin, Coombs' test, and blood typing. If other laboratory values are normal, breast-feeding can be continued with close monitoring. Some physicians prefer to interrupt breast-feeding for 24 hours every other day. Concerns about continuing breast-feeding may arise at this time. To maintain milk supply, the mother must express milk with a manual or electric breast pump during the 24-hour absence of breast-feeding. Physician consultation is essential in the management of the infant with possible breast-milk jaundice.

Another concern of lactating mothers is the presence of environmental contaminants in breast milk. Levels of DDT and chlorinated hydrocarbons in human milk are almost always higher than the World Health Organization's limits set for cow's milk (Wilson and others, 1973). As of yet, however, there has been no evidence of damage to breast-fed infants from DDT. There is also much concern about drugs that are transmitted through breast milk and may be harmful to the infant. The mother should be instructed never to take any drug during lactation without seeking consultation from the health care provider. Physician consultation is warranted when the nurse anticipates the need for a drug. Certain foods that mothers consume may cause problems in their breast-fed infants. Chocolate, eggs, wheat, and peanuts may create an allergic response in susceptible infants. Although it is not a common occurrence, spicy and gas-producing foods eaten by mothers may cause abdominal discomfort and colic in the infant.

Problems in breast-feeding. Among those who breast-feed the failure rate is quite high. Sacks and associates (1976) found that within 2 weeks one third of the mothers in their study had stopped breast-feeding; at 1 month only one-half of those were still nursing. Some of the reasons for lack of initiation or continuation of breast-feeding include mother's work, fear of failure, ignorance of benefits, lack of familial or professional support, embarrassment, and commercial advertising. Many women feel that lack of milk supply or inhibition of the milk-ejection reflex explains their inability to breast-feed; however, improper feeding technique is probably the most common cause.

Feeding schedules may be a concern. Mothers may not allow the infant to nurse as frequently as necessary. Because of the easier digestibility of human milk, breast-feeding is almost a continuous process during the first few weeks of life. Most infants nurse every 2 to 3 hours. A few, especially premature infants, may even nurse hourly.

If nursing time is restricted, the letdown reflex is not adequately stimulated and too little milk is produced. Instructions to new mothers often restrict suckling time to 2 or 3 minutes, which is insufficient to trigger the letdown reflex. Infants should be allowed to terminate their own feedings. The use of both breasts at each feeding should be recommended. If this is not done, milk production decreases and milk pools in the unused breast. This increases the chance of engorgement and mastitis and further inhibits the letdown reflex.

Breast soreness may necessitate some limitation of the initial time at the breast. Studies provide conflicting information on whether or not "nipple preparation" prevents sore nipples. Generally, brunettes do not have the same degree of problems with soreness as do blondes and women with red hair. These women may have very sensitive skin; for the first few days, they may need to switch breasts after 5 minutes of nursing. The application of breast cream after nursing prevents the dryness that is often the cause of soreness. If soreness does occur, a heat lamp used for 2 to 3 minutes between feedings provides comfort and toughens nipples.

Proper positioning also helps prevent sore nipples. In addition, improper positioning while nursing may influence milk production. If the baby is not close enough, only the nipple rather than the entire areola may be grasped. As a result, the mother will have sore nipples as well as a poor letdown reflex.

Certain drugs reduce or stop lactation. Vitamin B_6 can block lactation by decreasing the release of prolactin from the pituitary. Caffeine in large amounts may inhibit lactation. Mothers should be aware that chocolate, in addition to coffee and tea, contains high levels of caffeine. Smoking should be decreased as well as alcohol intake. Although small amounts of alcohol (1 to 2 ounces) can stimulate the letdown reflex, larger amounts inhibit it.

Burping the breast-fed infant is very important and is often a difficult process. Persistence in burping the infant several times during a feeding may encourage the infant to take more milk.

The use of supplemental bottles, pacifiers and, early semisolid intake causes the breast-fed infant to go longer between feedings, thus decreasing nipple stimulation and milk production. Because it is easier to suck from an artificial nipple, the infant who is given the breast after a bottle may be unable to suck appropriately to elicit a letdown reflex. Nipple confusion may arise. However, there may be circumstances when supplemental bottles are necessary. When an infant demands to nurse constantly, a bottle may allow the mother time to rest and build up her milk supply. Mothers who go out or return to work must use supplemental bottles. In such instances, the Nuk nipple is recommended, since it simulates the human nipple; sucking action is also similar between the two. The problem with nipple confusion may also occur with the use of a nipple shield, which is often recommended when the mother's nipples become sore.

Mothers should evaluate the sucking patterns of their infants and compare these with any past experiences. The nurse should also observe and evaluate the sucking. Poor sucking patterns inhibit the letdown reflex. Negative-flutter sucking occurs when the infant does not draw the nipple into the mouth well, and the areolar area is not compressed. There is intermittant licking of the nipple, with a rapid gumming action. The "pauser" nurses well at the beginning, but then holds the nipple like a pacifier, barely sucking, but with occasional bursts of vigorous sucking. This is normal in premature infants who tire easily. Switching from side to side may help, since the infant sucks more efficiently during the first part of the feeding. Other infants are fussy and easily distracted when the letdown reflex does not occur quickly. The Lact-Aid Nursing Trainer is a device used to carry supplemental formula to the baby while he is sucking the mother's breast. The sucking may help build up a diminishing milk supply while the baby obtains milk. It is an excellent device for use with flutter-sucking, pauser, and premature infants (Frantz and others; Choi, 1978). Anxiety contributes to an inhibited, unstable letdown reflex. Mothers may not understand the reflex or may not be able to feel it and think they are not having one. Factors such as the infant's swallowing hard and leakage from the unsuckled breast indicate that a letdown reflex is occurring and should be pointed out to the mother who does not feel the letdown reflex. The practitioner should assess the maternal environment for stresses, since they interfere with the letdown reflex. Mothers may overexert themselves, may not get enough rest, or may have marital-family problems. Whether the mother has successfully breast-fed before also influences her anxiety level. Positive reinforcement from health care providers and family is mandatory.

Support is the most important factor in counseling the mother who is having problems with breast-feeding or a baby who is slowly gaining weight. Mothers need help in identifying and meeting their own needs and should not feel guilty for doing so. Most important, if the mother does not succeed at breast-feeding or decides to give it up, her decision should be respected and supported. The practitioner should remember that the ideal time to begin teaching about breast-feeding is the prenatal period, since the hospital routine may not foster learning and often there is no one to help. Early teaching may prevent later problems.

Formula feeding

Table 9-3 lists types of milk and proprietary formulas. It includes indications for use and the problems associated with each. More detailed information about these and other specialized formulas for low-birth-weight infants are available from nutritional statements made by the Academy of Pediatrics' Committee on Nutrition (1976, 1977).

Proprietary formulas are available in powdered, concentrated, and ready-to-use forms. Powdered formulas are seldom used in the United States because of the high incidence of error in their preparation. When mixed, formulas should provide 20 kcal/oz. Daily caloric needs are approximately 110 to 120 kcal/kg during the first 6 months and 90 to 100 kcal/kg during the second 6 months. The practitioner should determine the daily recommended amount of formula by dividing the infant's daily calorie need by 20. For example, a newborn weighing 8 pounds (3.6 kg) will need approximately 400 calories per day. Dividing this number by 20 (the number of calories per ounce of formula) determines that the infant needs 20 ounces a day. Milk intake should never be more than 32 ounces a day or less than 16 ounces a day. The American Academy of Pediatrics recommends that fortified formula (with iron, vitamins, and minerals) be given throughout the first year of life in the non-breast-fed infant. Mothers who do not comply with these recommendations (because of high cost) need to select appropriate alternative methods of feeding. Evaporated milk correctly prepared and supplemented with vitamins and minerals is the only milk other than formula that can provide adequate nutrition for growth and development during the first year of life.

Feeding schedule. Routines are not as rigid as they once were. With the focus on a positive mother-infant relationship, feeding infants on demand is the trend. Individual variabilities necessitate modification to meet both infants' and mothers' demands and needs. Night feedings are essential during the neonatal period to prevent hypoglycemia and may continue 6 to 12 weeks or longer. Because stomach capacity is so small at birth (2 ounces) and food is quickly digested, small frequent feedings are essential. No more than 4 hours should elapse between daytime feedings. Because of increases in stomach capacity at 6 and 12 weeks, hunger and intake may increase proportionally. Awareness of these needs is necessary to ensure adequate calories and nutrition. Similarly, appetite lags may occur during spurts of motor development during the first year.

Sterilization. Mothers frequently inquire about sterilization techniques. Hargrove and associates (1974) demonstrated no difference between the clean technique and terminal sterilization in relation to infant illness. The clean technique uses bottles and nipples washed well with hot sudsy water and rinsed with hot water. Milk is supplied from a sterile source and the desired amount poured only at the time of feeding. The remainder of the can is refrigerated, and hot tap water is added to the bottle.

Special formulas. Consultation with a physician is necessary when special formulas are used. Too often professionals blame an infant's formula for signs and symptoms of illnesses and change them needlessly. However, two of the most common problems that necessitate a special formula are cow's milk allergy and lactose intolerance.

Table 9-3. Composition, indications, and problems for major infant formulas

Formulas	Composition						Indications	Problems
	Protein (%)	Fat (%)	CHO (%)	Calories (oz)	Vitamins	Iron		
Milk								
Human	9	45	68	~20	+	+	Ideal for healthy full-term and premature infants	None in healthy infants May need vitamin D if not in sunlight, fluoride if not adequate in H_2O source
Whole	22	48	36	~20	−	−	After age 1	Milk allergy, lactose intolerance, increased protein content, supplement vitamins and iron
2% Lowfat	28	31	41	~17	−	−	After age 1 when caloric and/or fat restriction necessary	Same as whole milk
Skim	40	3	57	~12	−	−	After age 2 if caloric and 100% fat restriction necessary	Lack of calories, low fat content, very high protein content, same as above
Evaporated milk	19	50	31	20 (Prepared as indicated)	−	−	Can be used in healthy full-term and premature infants; mix: 13 oz evaporated milk 19 oz H_2O 1½ oz corn syrup	Lactose intolerance, milk allergy; must supplement vitamins and iron

Formula	Protein						Indications	Disadvantages
Enfamil, Similac, SMA	9-10 Protein: whey casein resembling human milk	48-50	41-43	20	+	+ or −	Healthy full-term and premature infants; Lower renal solute load and sodium content than other formulas	Milk allergy, lactose intolerance
Similac Advance	26	27	47	16	+	+	Obese infants older than 6 months, older infants	Milk allergy, lactose intolerance
Soy-based formulas								
Isomil, Prosobee, Nursoy, Soyalac	12-15 (soy protein)	45-48	39-40	20	+	+ or −	Cow's milk allergy, lactose intolerance, postdiarrheal	Soy allergy, sucrose intolerance
Special formulas								
Similac PM 60/40	9-10	48-50	41-43	20	+	+ or −	Lower renal solute load and low sodium for chronic renal and heart disease	
CHO-free	12 (soy)	48	39 (when added)	12 (depends on addition)	+	+	Disaccharide deficiency, milk allergy, glucose-galactose malabsorption, protein intolerance, short-term use only	Osmolality, cost, soy intolerance; if not supplemented with CHO, ketogenic diet results
Nutramigen	13 (hydrolyzed casein)	35	52	20	+	+	Milk allergy, lactose intolerance, severe diarrhea, protein intolerance, short bowel syndrome	Osmolality, cost, high acid load, powdered form only

Continued.

Table 9-3. Composition, indications, and problems for major infant formulas—cont'd

Formulas	Composition						Indications	Problems
	Protein (%)	Fat (%)	CHO (%)	Calories (oz)	Vitamins	Iron		
Special formulas—cont'd								
Pregestimil	13 (hydrolyzed casein)	36	51	20	+	+	Cystic fibrosis, sucrose intolerance, diarrhea, protein intolerance, liver disease	Same as Nutramigen
Portagen	14	42	44	20	+	+	Impaired fat absorption, pancreatic disease, liver disease, lactose-free	Cost, powdered form
Lofenalac	13	35	52	20	+	+	Phenylketonuria (phenylalanine removed)	Cost
Meat-based formulas	17 (made from beef heart)	38	45	20	+	+	Lactose intolerance, milk allergy	Cost
Ensure	14	31.5	54.5	30	−	−	High caloric density for infants with increased needs, lactose-free	Cost, osmolality, supplement D and calcium
Polycose			100	60			To provide extra calories	
Pedialyte	Oral electrolyte solution	−	−	6.2	−	−	Use with diet restricted in fat, protein, and electrolytes; rapid absorption without side effects	
Lytren	Same as Pedialyte	−	−	9	−	−	Mild to moderate diarrhea, replacement of body H_2O and minerals Same as above	

Cow's milk allergy. The most common allergy during infancy is cow's milk allergy. It occurs in 0.5% to 7% of the general pediatric population (Collins-Williams, 1956). Onset occurs between 2 days and 4 months and may disappear spontaneously between 2 and 3 years of age (Committee on Nutrition, 1979). Any milk protein or product of its digestion may induce an allergic response, but the main offender is thought to be β-lactoglobulin (May, 1974). These proteins (or antigenic substances) pass through the gut wall and into the circulation, where they stimulate a hypersensitivity response. Different levels of reactivity may occur. Allergic reactions mediated by IgE occur minutes to hours after ingestion and clear within 48 hours. Immediate systemic anaphylaxis is an example. Delayed reactions mediated by IgG and IGM occur hours to days after exposure to the antigen. Because it is difficult to determine causes of delayed reactions, challenge testing must be continued over a period of time (Goldman and others, 1963).

In addition, antigenic proteins from cow's milk may cause a direct toxic reaction in the mucosa of the intestine. This may also occur after prolonged diarrheal illness and may produce a secondary immunological response (May, 1974). The toxic reaction causes a protein-losing enteropathy and gastrointestinal bleeding, resulting in iron deficiency anemia. Intake of homogenized cow's milk greater than 1 liter per day results in protein and blood loss and is found in 50% of infants with iron deficiency anemia. Formulas and evaporated milk do not cause these reactions, since the antigenic protein has been removed during preparation (Wilson and others, 1974).

Gastrointestinal, dermal, and respiratory symptoms are most often encountered in cow's milk allergy. Of these symptoms, vomiting and diarrhea are the most common (Goldman and others). Vomiting may be effortless and unimpressive, continuing throughout the day, or it may be explosive and projectile. Very frequent watery stools that often contain blood and mucus are common. Weight loss may occur. The infant may be irritable and have decreased activity levels.

There is no laboratory test that diagnoses milk allergy. Immunoglobulin levels, skin testing, and rectal mucus evaluation for eosinophils and intestinal antibodies are inconsistent predictors. The most reliable method for diagnosis is to eliminate the cow's milk for at least a week, then give a test dose and observe for recurrent symptoms. Symptoms usually occur within 48 hours but respiratory symptoms may occur as late as 2 to 3 weeks after the challenge and be mistaken for a respiratory tract infection (Gerrard and others, 1974). The amount of milk used in challenge testing is variable. Often several feedings of cow's milk are used; but if there is a risk of a severe reaction or anaphylaxis, only a tablespoon at a time may be used. Physician consultation is necessary in those situations. Once the assessment of cow's milk allergy is made, all milk-containing substances are eliminated for the first year, and soy formula is given. Potentially allergenic foods such as eggs, wheat, chocolate, fish, and orange juice are eliminated for 9 to 12 months. Delayed introduction of semisolids is advised, with slow introduction of single foods.

When switching formula, the nurse should realize that any protein has allergenic potential. Frier (1973) found that 30% to 50% of milk-sensitive infants demonstrate adverse reactions to soy formulas. Whittington and Gibson (1977) state that mucosal damage from cow's milk may increase protein sensitivies (such as to soy protein) by increasing absorption of antigenic substances. Eastham (1978) cautions against soy protein formulas. Casein hydrolysate formulas, such as Nutramigen and Pregestimil, do not produce the same cross-reactivity as soy protein; however, they are expensive and have a bad taste and high osmolality. They should be used only in severe cases in which soy formulas produce sensitivity.

Lactose intolerance. This intolerance results from insufficient amounts of the enzyme lactase to metabolize lactose. The signs and symptoms of it relate to the osmotic load produced by the large amounts of undigested lactose traveling through the bowel. They may include abdominal distention and pain; watery, explosive, frothy diarrhea; flatus; vomiting; dehydration; failure to thrive; and steatorrhea (Christie). Occurrence is 1 to 4 hours after ingestion (Johnson and others, 1974). Lactose intolerance may be classified as congenital, primary, or secondary. Congenital absence of lactose is a rare life-threatening problem; the only treatment is the substitution of a lactose-free formula. The incidence of primary lactose intolerance in Greeks, Arabs, American blacks, Eskimos, American Indians, and Orientals exceeds 70% (Bayless, 1972). However, lactase levels are almost always adequate in all groups until after weaning occurs. These groups usually tolerate lactose as infants and do not show problems until after weaning (Kretchner, 1972).

Secondary lactose deficiency follows intestinal mucosal damage from surgery; chronic diseases, such as colitis, cystic fibrosis, and malnutrition; and severe gastroenteritis. Infants may have a lactose intolerance after severe diarrhea. This secondary lactase deficiency may continue for weeks or months (Speer, 1973).

When lactose intolerance is suspected, a screening test can be performed. Stool pH and stool-reducing substances are assessed with Clinitest tablets and Combistix; this is done after several feedings with a lactose formula. If reducing substances are greater than 0.25% or pH is less than 6, the diagnosis of lactose intolerance is a probability (Townley, 1966). With positive results, physician consultation is necessary and a lactose tolerance test may be ordered. Because of inconsistent results, some authorities rely on screening tests alone for a diagnosis or perform jejunal biopsy (Harrison and Walker-Smith, 1977). Management of acquired lactose intolerance is determined individually, since small amounts of lactose may be tolerated. Fermented products, such as yogurt, some cheeses, and buttermilk, may be tolerated. When lactose tolerance is a secondary problem, a soy isolate or casein hydrolysate formula is used until the mucosa heals. This may take a period of weeks or months (Garza and Scrimshaw, 1976).

Vitamin supplementation

Breast-fed infant. Jelliffe and Jelliffe (1978b) state that mothers who are well nourished during pregnancy and lactation do not need to supplement vitamins and minerals during the infant's first 6 months of life. However, a vitamin D supplement is recommended if there is inadequate sunlight exposure. Some studies suggest that a water-soluble conjugate of vitamin D appears in human milk; therefore, supplements may not be necessary as once thought (Lakdauala and Weddowson, 1977).

Supplementation with iron and possibly fluoride is necessary at some time during the first 6 months. Additional iron is needed at that time because iron levels in human milk decrease during the course of lactation; hemoglobin, serum ferritin, and transferrin saturation decline in the infant (Saarinen, 1978). Acceptable supplements are liquid iron or dietary sources such as dry infant cereal. Most authorities suggest iron supplementation at 4 to 6 months or when the birth weight doubles (Woodruff and others, 1977; Coulson and others, 1977). Iron is not given before that time, since it binds with lactaferrin, an iron-binding protein in breast milk that has bacteriostatic properties. Lactoferrin is thought to be largely responsible for the marked resistance of breast-fed infants to *E. coli* gastronteritis. Lactoferrin may also inhibit staphylococci and *Candida albicans*. In vitro, iron saturation of lactoferrin reverses its bateriostatic effect. Lactoferrin in formulas is ineffective because of destruction by heating.

The American Academy of Pediatrics Committee on Nutrition (1979) recommends fluoride supplementation for all infants and children if fluoride in the water supply is inadequate. The nurse should determine the level of fluoride in the infant's water supply. In the child from 2 weeks to 2 years of age, supplementation is unnecessary unless the water fluoride content is less than 0.3 ppm. In this case, 0.25 mg of fluoride should be given daily.

Breast-fed infants of poorly nourished mothers need a vitamin and mineral supplement. Water-soluble vitamins and vitamin A are particularly affected by maternal nutritional status. After the first 6 months, supplementation depends on the types of foods offered. With the intake of well-balanced meals, supplementation is unnecessary. However, those infants from poorer populations or those who are "picky eaters" need vitamin and iron supplements.

Formula-fed infant. Since most formulas contain vitamins and minerals, supplementation is unnecessary. However, only half of the formulas contain iron. Formulas without iron require supplementation after the first few months because of depleted infant stores and poor absorptive properties (Saarinen and Simes, 1977). Infants taking evaporated milk will need vitamin and mineral supplements, especially iron and vitamin C. The parent should supply iron during the second 6 months by giving fortified formulas, liquid iron, or iron-rich food.

Introduction of semisolids

The age for introducing semisolids has decreased during this century; today some infants under 1 month may eat semisolids. Some competitive mothers motivate the infant to achieve this developmental milestone. More often, mothers falsely interpret the child's physical or emotional needs as hunger and begin feedings earlier than necessary. Mothers who bottle-feed usually begin semisolids 8 weeks earlier than breast-feeding mothers (Averbach, 1978). Pediatricians develop permissive attitudes toward mother's wishes. Commercial industries promote early semisolids and have developed a syringelike device to force food into the neurologically immature infant.

Four main reasons support the delay in the introduction of semisolids: neuromuscular immaturity, allergy, obesity, and digestive immaturity. Before 16 to 24 weeks, the infant has poor head control, cannot sit without support, and may still have the Moro, rooting, and extrusor reflexes. Thus the infant is unable to participate in the feeding process. Once the primitive reflexes and postural responses disappear, the infant may begin semisolids.

The gut is permeable to proteins, and the introduction of foods may cause an allergic response. This is more likely to occur before 7 months when IgA levels begin to peak. In addition, an atopic family history predisposes a child to further risk of food allergy.

Some studies indicate that early feeding of semisolids (first 3 months) has no effect on weight gain in infancy (Davies, 1977). Others show that obesity in the first year of life does not necessarily continue into childhood (Poskitt, 1977). On the other hand, Eid (1970), among others, found that almost one half of obese infants became obese children. Most authorities conclude that excessive early food consumption during infancy can contribute to obesity and should be avoided (Fomon).

Pancreatic amylase, which is necessary for starch digestion, is insufficient early in life. Absorption of complex starches present in infant foods is inefficient during the first 6 months. Thus calories provided by these starches are lost in the stool (Lilibridge and Townes, 1973). If mothers drastically reduce their infants' milk intake in favor of semisolids, the diet may not provide adequate calories and nutrient intake.

Illingworth and Lister (1964) believe there is a critical or sensitive period in an infant's development during which the child begins to chew solid foods. If the mother withholds finger foods during this time, the child may refuse them at a later time, may not learn to chew well, or may develop later feeding problems. Developmental readiness occurs at about 6 months, but an active infant who grows rapidly and demands more nursing periods or formula (more than 1 quart daily) may begin solid foods a few weeks earlier. The quiet, placid baby may not demonstrate these signs and should begin semisolids around 6 months.

Feeding schedule. The following schedule should begin at 6 months and is suggested as a guideline. Rice cereal should be offered first because it is the least allergenic food. New foods should be given 2 tablespoons at a time and started every 3 to 7 days. This allows time for adverse reactions to occur. Dry infant cereals provide an excellent source of iron and B-complex vitamins. Cereal mixtures and ready-to-use products in jars should be avoided, since their nutrient value is lower than the dry product. During the seventh and eighth months, fruits and vegetables should be offered. Juices should be considered fruits when introduced; they are fortified with vitamin C and contain no sugar. Fresh-squeezed or adult juices should be diluted to 2:1, and then to 1:1.

Many commercial products contain sugar, tapioca, and cornstarch, which are empty calories and difficult to digest early in life. Vegetables are available as plain or as creamed, which contain milk solids and cornstarch. High nitrate–containing foods, such as beets, spinach, and greens, should be avoided until the end of the first year. When they are given before this time, methemoglobinemia may occur, which results in decreased oxygen to the tissues. Soups and dinners, which are highest in vegetable content, have less nutrient value than the individual servings of each constituent. Some vegetable-and-meat combinations have 6 times less protein than regular meats. Mothers should be discouraged from using these products.

At 9 months, meats and egg yolk should be introduced. Egg whites should not be given during the first year, since the risk of allergy is great. High protein dinners should be avoided, since they contain only one-half the protein of pure meats. Meats and egg yolks supply 20% of the infant's calories from protein, whereas other foods, including human milk, supply approximately 7%. In the breast-fed infant, a caloric intake of solids greater than 25% of total intake requires the addition of other protein sources. Protein requirements are met in the formula-fed infant as long as one third of total daily calories comes from formula (Anderson and Fomon, 1974). Milk intake should not be decreased too early, since it provides an excellent source of calories, vitamins, and minerals.

The infant who can sit and grasp objects is ready for finger foods, such as teething biscuits, meat, and cheese sticks. Drinking from a cup should be taught at 28 to 32 weeks; when the infant releases objects voluntarily (36 to 48 weeks), small bits of food should be offered to encourage self-feeding.

Home-prepared foods are an alternative to commercial infant foods. They are cheaper, have less sugar, and contain increased amounts of vitamins and minerals. They also have higher caloric densities; therefore, smaller amounts are necessary. Since sodium is high in canned foods, fresh or frozen foods are recommended.

Foods should be chosen to meet nutritional and developmental needs. Innovation is necessary to keep infants interested and to encourage positive feeding patterns. Food should be attractive and provide color, flavor, and texture. It should be cooked or ground well enough to prevent choking or aspiration. Dry foods mixed with moist ones and sharp flavors pared with mild ones encourage diverse intake. Food texture should include crunchy, chewy, and soft finger foods. Snacks should be nutritious. The use of sweets as a reinforcer only increases the desire for that food and may promote erratic nutrient intake.

Feeding environment. The environment should have few distractions and provide a pleasant atmosphere without turmoil and anxiety. The infant who is emotionally and physically healthy will have a good appetite. The infant who has not had a nap, has snacked all day, or is physically tired will not eat well. Age-appropriate dishes, utensils, tables, and chairs are necessary. Finishing a meal gives a child a sense of accomplishment and is impossible with too large a serving. The infant who finishes a meal should be allowed to play rather than made to sit through the rest of the meal. Parents should give verbal positive reinforcements of appropriate behaviors and ignore undesirable ones. Funny behaviors such as squirting out food should be ignored, since laughing reinforces inappropriate behavior. Parents must have patience and set limits to develop their child's food habits. They decide which habits to pass on and which to avoid. Since children eat what the parent buys, they usually develop the parent's food habits. For this reason, parents may have to change their own eating patterns (Pipes).

Food disinterest is a normal occurrence toward the end of the first year because of a decreased growth rate and concomitant need for fewer calories per body weight. As the infant becomes more independent and explorative, interest in food wanes. This may last for months or years. Food "jags" are common with the child, who may eat a few preferred foods over a period of time. Previously favorite foods may become hated ones. Infants may become ritualistic, demanding a specific plate or a specific food prepared only one way. A decrease in milk intake along with the decreased use of fortified cereals and disliked vegetables may lead to low values of vitamin A, calcium, phosphorus, and iron. A temporary vitamin and mineral supplement is necessary. It is important that mothers know that their child's food habits are transitory. What is eaten is more important than the amount. Brazelton states that 1 day's nutritional needs can be met with a pint of milk or its equivalent, an ounce of fruit juice or one piece of fruit, two ounces of iron-containing protein (one egg or meat), and a multivitamin preparation (Caplan, 1973). Lack of appetite may be a symptom of illness, and parents may become apprehensive. If the child is physically healthy and growth rates and development are normal, there is no need for concern. Nurses must provide reassurance and counseling on food preparation, eating environment, and normal development.

Food refusal may only mean a food dislike and may be temporary or long lasting. The child should not be forced to eat a refused food. Instead the food should be offered at other times or prepared another way. Substitution from the same food group is acceptable. For example, the addition of powdered milk may supply nutrients when milk is refused. The parents should set realistic goals, using positive reinforcement. Suggestions include letting the infant eat finger food, preparing food differently, avoiding fatigue, offering nutritious snacks, and letting a different person feed the child.

Picking at food and gorging are attention-seeking behaviors that signify independence-seeking or emotional problems. In assessing the problem, the practitioner should note onset, cause, and associated factors. Family attitudes, previous attempts to handle the problem, and interpersonal relationships should be explored. Continuous hunger is abnormal; pathological causes, such as malabsorption, hyperthyroidism, and diabetes, may need investigation. The child with inappropriate feeding behaviors may benefit from exercise. Limits should be set and appropriate behavior reinforced consistently. The infant should not be verbally or physically punished. Parents will need continual support and reassurance.

Changes in feeding habits are not immediate. Learning feeding behaviors is a complex task, which, like any other developmental milestone, progresses over a period of time. Failures and setbacks occur during this learning phase and should be expected.

EVALUATION

Feeding is a very important experience during infancy. During this time, infants learn to trust the mother and the environment if their needs are met appropriately, consistently, and without excessive waiting. This is also a time when good nutrition is essential to developing body structures. To ensure optimal nutrition during infancy, the nurse facilitates the following outcomes:

1. The choice of milk is appropriate for age and individual tolerance.
2. Mothers who choose to breast-feed are successful.
3. Formulas are prepared correctly.
4. The amount of food taken during each feeding is based on body weight and age.
5. Feeding techniques are based on safety, comfort, and developmental readiness.
6. Use of vitamin and mineral supplements is based on age, weight, and type of feeding.
7. Introduction of semisolids is based on age and developmental readiness.
8. Feeding practices promote social and motor development.
9. Feeding is a positive experience for the parents and infant.
10. Growth patterns are normal.

REFERENCES

Alfin-Slater, R.B., and Jelliffe, D.B.: Nutritional requirements with special reference to infancy, Pediatr. Clin. North Am. **24:**3, 1977.

Almroth, S.G.: Water requirements of breast-fed infants in a hot climate, Am. J. Clin. Nutr. **31:**1154, 1978.

Anderson, P.O.: Drugs and breastfeeding: a review, Drug Intel. Clin. Pharmacol. **2:**208, 1977.

Anderson, T.A., and Fomon, S.J.: Beikost. In Fomon, S.J.: Infant nutrition, ed. 2, Philadelphia, 1974, W.B. Saunders Co.

Averbach, K.G.: A study of timing of first solid foods: comparison of breast and bottlefeeding mothers, Birth Fam. J. **5:**27, 1978.

Baltimore, R.S., and others: Growth of *Esherichia coli* and concentration of iron in an infant-feeding formula, Pediatrics **62:**1072, 1978.

Barnes, R.H.: Points of concern with current interpretation of the effects of early malnutrition on mental development, Bibl. Nutr. Dieta **17:**1, 1972.

Bayless, T.M.: Milk intolerance: clinical developmental and epidemiological aspects. In Summary of the Conference on Lactose and Milk Intolerance, Washington, D.C., 1972, U.S. Department of Health, Education, and Welfare.

Bergmann, K.E., and others: Water and renal solute load. In Fomon, S.J.: Infant nutrition, ed. 2, Philadelphia, 1974, W.B. Saunders Co.

Brook, C.G.D.: Fat cells in childhood obesity, Lancet **1:**224, 1975.

Bullen, C.L., and Willis, A.T.: Resistance of the breastfed infant to gastroenteritis, Br. Med. J. **3:**338, 1971.

Caplan, F., editor: The first twelve months of life, New York, 1973, Grosset & Dunlap, Inc.

Choi, M.W.: Breast milk for infants who can't breastfeed, Am. J. Nurs. **78:**852, 1978.

Chow, M.P., and others, editors: Handbook of pediatric primary care, New York, 1979, John Wiley & Sons, Inc.

Christie, D.L.: GI symptoms related to feeding in the first two years of life. In Problems related to feeding in the first two years, Columbus, 1977, Ross Laboratories.

Collins-Williams, C.: The incidence of milk allergy in pediatric practice, J. Pediatr. **48:**39, 1956.

Committee on Nutrition, American Academy of Pediatrics: Composition of milks, Pediatrics **26:**1039, 1960.

Committee on Nutrition, American Academy of Pediatrics: Proposed standards for formulas for healthy infants, Pediatrics **57:**278, 1976,

Committee on Nutrition, American Academy of Pediatrics: Nutritional needs of low birth-weight infants, Pediatrics **60:**519, 1977.

Committee on Nutrition, American Academy of Pediatrics: Pediatric nutrition handbook, Evanston, Ill., 1979, The Academy.

Coulson, K.M., and others: Hematocrit levels in breastfed American babies: a preliminary study suggesting that nutritional anemias may not develop, Clin. Pediatr. **16:**649, 1977.

Crawford, M.A., and others: Fatty acid requirements in infancy, Am. J. Clin. Nutr. **31:**2181, 1978.

Davies, D.F., and Saunders, R.: Blood urea: normal values in early infancy to feeding practices, Arch. Dis. Child. **48:**563, 1973.

Davies, P.: Effects of solid foods on growth of bottlefed infants in the first three months of life, Br. Med. J. **2:**7, 1977.

Delvoye, P.: The influence of the frequency of nursing and of previous lactation experience on serum prolactin in lactating mothers, J. Biosoc. Sci. **9:**447, 1977.

Eastham, E.J.: Antigenicity of infant formulas: role of immature intestine on protein permeability, J. Pediatr. **93:**561, 1978.

Eid, E.E.: Followup study of physical growth of children who had excessive weight gain in the first six months of life, Br. Med. J. **2:**74, 1970.

Eiger, M.S., and Olds, S.W.: The complete book of breast feeding, New York, 1972, Workman Publishing Co., Inc.

Filer, L.S.: Salt in infant foods, Nutr. Rev. **29:**27, 1971.

Finberg, L.: Pathogenesis of lesions in the nervous system in hypernatremic states: clinical observation of infants, Pediatrics **23:**40, 1959.

Fomon, S.J.: Infant nutrition, ed. 2, Philadelphia, 1974, W.B. Saunders Co.

Food and Nutrition Board: Recommended dietary allowances, ed. 8, Washington, D.C., 1974, National Academy of Science, National Research Council.

Frantz, K.B., and others: Management of the slow gaining breastfed baby: keeping abreast, J. Hum. Nutr. **4:**287, 1978.

Fried, R.I.: One hundred years of infant feeding, Clin. Pediatr. **16:**215, 1977.

Frier, S.: Pediatric gastrointestinal allergy, Clinical Allergy **3**(suppl.):597, 1973.

Gamsu, H.R.: Medical evaluation of osmolar factors, J. Postgrad. Med. **3**(suppl. 51):31, 1975.

Garza, C., and Scrimshaw, N.S.: Relationship of lactose intolerance to milk intolerance in young children, Am. J. Clin. Nutr. **29:**192, 1976.

Gauel, G.E., and others: Milk protein quantity and quality in low birth weight infants: ill effects on sulphur amino acids in plasma and urine, J. Pediatr. **90:**348, 1977.

Gerrard, J.W., and others: Cow's milk allergy: prevalence and manifestations in an unselected series of newborns, Acta Paediatr. Scand. **14:**120, 1974.

Goldman, A.S., and others: Milk allergy. I. Oral challenge with milk and isolated milk protein in allergic children, Pediatrics **32:**425, 1963.

Good, J.C.: Does breast milk alone prevent iron deficiency amenia? Ohio State Med. J. **73:**562, 1977.

Graver, L., and others: Milk-curd bowel obstruction in the newborn infant, J.A.M.A. **238:**1050, 1977.

Greentree, L.B.: Dangers of vitamin B_6 in nursing mothers, N. Engl. J. Med. **300:**141, 1979.

Gunther, M.: The neonate's immunity gap: breastfeeding and cot death, Lancet **1:**441, 1975.

Guthrie, R.A.: Breast milk and jaundice, J. Hum. Nutr. **3:**49, 1978.

Hambraeus, L.: Proprietary milk versus human breast milk in infant feeding, Pediatr. Clin. North Am. **24:**17, 1977.

Hanson, L.A., and others: Secretory IgA antibody against cow's milk proteins in human milk and their possible effect in mixed feedings, Int. Arch. Allergy Appl. Immunol. **54:**457, 1977.

Hargrove, C.B., and others: Formula preparation and infant illness, Clin. Pediatr. **13:**1057, 1974.

Harrison, M., and Walker-Smith, J.A.: Reinvestigation of lactose intolerance in children: lack of correlation between continuing lactose intolerance and small intestine morphology: disaccharide activity and lactose tolerance tests, Gut **18:**48, 1977.

Hill, L.F.: Infant feeding: historical and current, Pediatr. Clin. North Am. **14:**255, 1967.

Illingworth, R.S., and Lister, J.: The critical or sensitive period with special reference to certain feeding problems in infants and children, J. Pediatr. **65:**839, 1964.

Jelliffe, D.B., and Jelliffe, E.F.P.: Human milk in the modern world, New York, 1978a, Oxford University Press, Inc.

Jelliffe, D.B., and Jelliffe, E.F.P.: The volume and composition of human milk in poorly nourished communities, Am. J. Clin. Nutr. **31:**492, 1978b.

Jelliffe, E.F.P.: Maternal nutrition and lactation. In Ciba Foundation Symposium: Breast feeding and the mother, Amsterdam, 1975, The Foundation.

Johnson, J.D., and others: Lactose malabsorption: its biology and history. In Schulman, I., editor: Advances in pediatrics, Chicago, 1974, Year Book Medical Publishers, Inc.

Joint FAO/WHO meeting: pesticide residues in food, WHO Technical Report Series, No. 474, Geneva, 1971, FAO/WHO.

Kippley, S.K., and Kippley, J.F.: The relation between breast feeding and amenorrhea: report of a survey, J. Trop. Pediatr. **23:**239, 1977.

Kretchner, N.: Lactose and lactase, Sci. Am. **227:**70, 1972.

Lakdauala, D.R., and Weddowson, E.M.: Vitamin D in human milk, Lancet **1:**167, 1977.

LaLeche League: The womanly art of breastfeeding, Franklin Park, Ill., 1963, The League.

Lavsen, S.A., and Homer, D.R.: Relation of breast versus bottle feeding to hospitalization for gastroenteritis in a middle-class U.S. population, J. Pediatr. **92:**417, 1978.

Lilibridge, C.B., and Townes, P.: Physiologic deficiency of pancreatic amylase in infancy: a factor in iatrogenic diarrhea, J. Pediatr. **82:**279, 1973.

Lowenberg, M.E.: The development of food patterns in young children. In Pipes, P.L.: Nutrition in infancy and childhood, St. Louis, 1977, The C.V. Mosby Co.

Mata, L.J., and Urrutia, J.J.: Intestinal colonization of breastfed children in a rural area of low socioeconomic level, Ann. N.Y. Acad. Sci. **176:**93, 1971.

May, C.D.: Food allergy. In Fomon, S.J.: Infant nutrition, ed. 2, Philadelphia, 1974, W.B. Saunders Co.

McMillan, J., and others: Iron sufficiency in breastfed infants and the availability of iron from milk, Pediatrics **58:**686, 1976.

O'Brien, T.E.: Excretions of drugs in human milk, Am. J. Hosp. Pharm. **31:**844, 1974.

Owen, G.M., and others: A study of nutritional status of preschool children in the United States, 1968-1970, Pediatrics **53:**597, 1974.

Pipes, P.L.: Nutrition in infancy and childhood, St. Louis, 1977, The C.V. Mosby Co.

Pittard, W.B.: Breast milk immunology, Am. J. Dis. Child. **133:**83, 1979.

Poivell, G.K.: Milk induced enterocolitis of infancy, J. Pediatr. **93:**553, 1978.

Poskitt, M.E.: Overfeeding and overnutrition in infancy and their relation to body size in early childhood, Nutr. Metab. **21**(suppl. 1):5, 1977.

Reddy, V.: Antimicrobial factors in human milk, Acta Paediatr. Scand. **66:**229, 1977.
Robinson, M.: Infant morbidity and mortality, Lancet **1:**788, 1951.
Saarinen, U.M.: Need for iron supplementation in infants on prolonged breast feeding, J. Pediatr. **93:**177, 1978.
Saarinen, U.M., and Simes, M.A.: Iron absorption from infant milk formula and the optimal level of iron supplementation, Acta Paediatr. Scand. **66:**719, 1977.
Sacks, S.H., and others: To breast feed or not to breast feed, Practitioner **216:**183, 1976.
Schaefer, O.: Otitis media and bottle feeding. Can. J. Pub. Health **62:**478, 1971.
Simpson, W.J., and Cheung, D.K.: Developing infant occlusion: related feeding methods and oral habits, J. Can. Diet. Assoc. **42:**124, 1976.
Speer, F.: Intolerance to foods. In Speer, F., and Dorkhoin, R.J., editors: Allergy and immunology in childhood, Springfield, Ill., 1973, Charles C Thomas, Publisher.
Stoch, M.B., and Smythe, P.M.: Fifteen-year developmental study on effects of severe undernutrition during infancy on subsequent physical growth and intellectual functioning, Arch. Dis. Child. **51:**327, 1976.
Taitz, L.S.: Obesity in pediatric practice: infantile obesity, Pediatr. Clin. North Am. Feb. **24:**107, 1977.
Taitz, L.S.: Sodium intake and health in infancy, J. Hum. Nutr. **31:**325, 1977.
Taitz, L., and Harris, F.: Accelerated height and weight gain in artificially fed babies, Acta Paediatr. Scand. **6:**499, 1972.
Tanner, J.M., and Whitehouse, R.N.: Standards for subcutaneous fat in British children: percentiles for thickness of skinfolds over triceps and below scapula, Br. Med. J. **1:**466, 1967.
Ten-state nutrition survey, 1968-1970, Pub. No. HSM 72-8132, Washington, D.C., 1972, U.S. Department of Health, Education, and Welfare.
Thompson, A.M.: The energy cost of human lactation, Br. J. Nutr. **24:**565, 1970.
Townley, R.R.W.: Disaccharide deficiency in infancy and childhood, Pediatrics **38:**127, 1966.
Tracey, U.V., and others: Obesity and respiratory infection in infants and young children, Br. Med. J. **1:**16, 1971.
Tsang, R.C., and Gluck, C.J.: Perinatal cholesterol metabolism, Clin. Perinatol. **2:**275, 1975.
Walker-Smith, J.: Cow's milk protein intolerance: transient food intolerance of infancy, Arch. Dis. Child. **50:**347, 1975.
Weil, W.B., Jr.: Current controversies in childhood obesity, J. Pediatr. **91:**176, 1977.
Whittington, P.F., and Gibson, R.: Soy protein intolerance: four patients with concomitant cow's milk intolerance, Pediatrics **59:**730, 1977.
Wilson, D.J., and others: DDT concentration in human milk, Am. J. Dis. Child. **125:**814, 1973.
Wilson, J.F., and others: Studies of iron metabolism versus further observation on cow's milk–induced bleeding in infants with iron deficiency anemia, J. Pediatr. **84:**335, 1974.
Winick, M., and Brasel, J.A.: Early malnutrition and subsequent brain development, Ann. N.Y. Acad. Sci. **300:**280, 1977.
Woodruff, C.W.; Iron deficiency in infancy and childhood, Pediatr. Clin. North Am. **24:**85, 1977.
Woodruff, C.W., and others: Iron nutrition in the breast-fed infant, J. Pediatr. **90:**36, 1977.
Zerfas, A.J., and Neumann, C.G.: Office assessment of nutritional status, Pediatr. Clin. North Am. **24:**253, 1977.

CHAPTER 10

Diverticular disease in the older adult

Winifred Still Hayes

The purpose of this chapter is to present an overview of diverticular disease and the management of those affected clients who appear in a primary care setting. The epidemiology, pathology, and etiology of diverticular disease include current and, at times, conflicting research findings. A discussion of assessment and plan (including prevention) is the major focus, with emphasis on primary care aspects relevant to the elderly. This chapter also covers indications for consultation and referral. A case study depicting the course of diverticular disease illuminates implementation and evaluation. The reference list at the end of the chapter should prove useful, if the reader desires further resources.

DEFINITIONS

The term "diverticula" means pouches or sacs in the wall of an organ or canal. Though diverticula may exist in various organs, such as the bladder and duodenum, diverticular disease refers to a wide range of disorders affecting the lower gastrointestinal tract. The most common characteristic of this problem is the presence of diverticula of the colon, primarily of the sigmoid and, to a lesser extent, of the descending colon. "True" diverticula are fairly uncommon and are congenital; they include all the layers of the wall from which they protrude. In contrast, the more common diverticula, or "false" diverticula, are acquired and are formed by rupture of the mucosa through the circular muscle layers of the bowel to the pericolic fat. This occurs at the point where the main colonic blood vessels pass through the circular muscle wall (Morson and Dawson, 1972).

EPIDEMIOLOGY

Diverticular disease, a relatively new problem of the twentieth century, is a disorder of the colon affecting approximately one third of our population over 60 years old and an increasing number of adults in their middle years. About 10% of those individuals diagnosed as having diverticular disease are symptomatic. Approximately 1% develop complications such as diverticulitis, hemorrhage, perforation, and obstruction (Painter, 1976; Waye, 1976; Painter and Burkitt, 1975).

Historical perspective

As recently as 1920 Sir John Bland-Sutton described diverticulitis as "a newly discovered bane of elders." Before the turn of the century diverticula were a medical rarity seldom resulting in clinical problems. Even though the clinicians of the nineteenth century rarely saw diverticular disease, their description of the problem and its etiological variables corresponds with current beliefs. In the early and middle 1800s various clinicians attributed diverticula to chronic constipation, high colonic pressures, excessive colonic muscle contraction, and eventual herniation of the mucous membrane through the muscle wall. In the midnineteenth century Cruveilhier pointed out the potential risk of diverticula as sites for infection.

By the 1920s authorities established diverticular disease as a significant clinical problem. The development of radiography and the use of contrast media documented the presence of diverticula. The medical profession's top priority was to prevent the complications of diverticulosis, such as inflamed, infected diverticula, a condition known as diverticulitis. In 1930 Mayo estimated the incidence of this former "curiosity" to be 5% in the over-40 age group.

The apparent change in incidence and prevalence of diverticular disease during the first quarter of the twentieth century may be the result of a number of factors. An inspection of global patterns of distribution, dietary habits, sex, race, age, bowel patterns, and stool characteristics is helpful. The examination of these data has generated recent advancements concerning the pathogenicity, etiology, assessment, and prevention of diverticular disease.

An understanding of research methodology is valuable to interpret epidemiological and clinical data. Studies attempting to determine the prevalence of diverticular disease in populations, especially among peoples of rural Africa and Asia, are predictions or, at best, estimates. The majority of data include barium enema and autopsy series obtained from individuals within the health care system. However, in underdeveloped countries, these data may not be representative of the population at large. Distinguishing between incidence and prevalence of the problem is difficult, because the disorder evolves over many years and many individuals remain asymptomatic or undiagnosed.

Most reports are ecological surveys, retrospective studies, or clinical trials. Study control groups, especially well-matched groups, frequently are missing. There is a lack of well-controlled, comprehensive, prospective studies that examine the relationship of hypothesized etiological factors, such as dietary fiber. Therefore, I avoid making firm conclusions about causal relationships and subsequent therapy. The clinician should maintain an awareness of additional data appearing in the literature in the future. Decisions regarding management should be based on the client's response and should reflect knowledge of advances in the subject.

Geographic distribution

Diverticular disease is infrequently found in underdeveloped areas of the world. The greatest differences exist between the Western world, including American blacks and Americans of Japanese extraction, and the peoples of rural Africa and Asia. Native Africans from Ethiopia, Kenya, Uganda, Ghana, Liberia, Nigeria, Sierra Leone, Zaire, Zimbabwe, and South Africa rarely develop diverticular disease. Painter and Burkitt's survey in Africa noted the absence of inflammatory diverticular disease and the existence of extremely rare cases of diverticulosis found on barium enema study and autopsy. Those diagnosed cases of diverticular disease occurred almost exclusively in the highest socioeconomic groups of Africans living in urban settings (Painter and Burkitt, Trowell and others, 1974).

Diverticular disease is also rare in India and the Middle East, where the problem occurs in urban regions, with clients from upper socioeconomic groups who report eating a Western diet. In rural areas diverticular disease is essentially unknown, although radiological studies have been largely unavailable. The same trend for diverticular disease occurs in Malaysia, Korea, and Thailand, with extremely rare or no cases identified by barium enema series and autopsies (Painter and Burkitt).

In countries with recent or partial industrialization, such as Japan, Finland, and Spain, the prevalence of diverticular disease is between that of the industrialized Western countries and that of underdeveloped countries. In contrast, the prevalence of diverticular disease in developed countries such as Great Britain, Sweden, the United States, France, and Australia is quite high. The estimates are 5% in populations over 40 years old, 30% to 35% in populations over 60 years old, and up to 66% in populations over 80 years old (Painter and Burkitt).

Age-specific morbidity and mortality studies for diverticular disease that compare underdeveloped and developed countries are unavailable. However, the difference in prevalence between underdeveloped and developed countries is so marked that extremes in rates may not be caused solely by differences in the age distribution of the populations in these countries. Even in the elderly of the underdeveloped countries, diverticular disease is extremely rare.

Dietary patterns

Accumulating evidence supports the hypothesis that removal of fiber from the diet and its replacement with refined carbohydrates are largely responsible for the development of diverticula of the colon. The diets of rural Asians and Africans are high in natural food fibers, including unrefined cereals, fruits, and vegetables. Refined carbohydrates, including sugar, constitute a very small percentage of their diets.

In contrast, since the 1870s the diets of residents of developed, industrialized countries have become devoid of fiber. Improved milling processes, which removed most of the fiber content of flour, occurred concurrently with the doubling of the intake of refined sugars, meat, and fats. The intake of cereal fibers dropped to one tenth its previous amount. A decrease in the consumption of bread also occurred, except during the two world wars. Given that diverticular disease evolves over a 40-year period, an increase in this disorder should have been expected in affected countries by the 1920s. Painter and Burkitt report that this in fact was true in Great Britain by 1920. Other developed countries also noted this pattern. Kocour (1937) and Cleave and associates (1969) documented similar dietary changes in black Americans, who subsequently have demonstrated increased prevalence of diverticular disease equal to that of white Americans.

Vegetable fiber reaches the colon in a relatively unchanged state and is largely responsible for determining the bulk, water content, and weight of the stool. Burkitt and others (1972) studied the stool transit times and stool weights of population groups from Great Britain, South Africa, South India, and Uganda, noting their dietary patterns as well. The rural African passes more than 400 g of soft stool daily in three bowel movements, with an average transit time of about 30 to 35 hours. Straining is never a problem.

The rural African's diet consists of unrefined foodstuffs. Urban Africans, Indians, and those whites in Great Britain who eat a mixed diet of both refined and unrefined foods pass about 200 g of stool daily, with an average transit time of 45 hours. In contrast, whites in South Africa and Great Britain who consume a refined diet pass less than 150 g of stool daily, with an average transit time of 80 hours. Their stools are viscous and often hard, with reports of straining to perform defecation.

Age, sex, and race

It is unlikely that race and sex are determinate factors in diverticular disease. Africans and Asians who live in industrialized countries and consume modern, westernized diets have prevalence rates equal to those of the whites of those countries. The female-to-male disease ratio increases gradually after the age of 40. However, the percentage of females as compared with males in the overall population also increases. When differences in sex distribution in the population are adjusted, sex is no longer a factor, although this matter remains somewhat controversial (Eastwood and others, 1976).

Increasing age positively correlates with increasing risk for diverticular disease. However, most studies refute the notion that diverticular disease results from degenerative changes caused by aging. Instead it seems that 40 years are necessary for high colonic pressures from fiber-deficient diets to produce diverticula. With markedly deficient fiber content in diets, individuals in their 30s are appearing with diverticular disease. (Eastwood and Mitchell, 1976; Almy, 1976).

Other possible variables

Other variables associated with the development of diverticular disease include obesity (Horner, 1958), genetic factors (Kohler, 1963), primary degeneration of the colonic muscle wall (Morson, 1963; Painter and Burkitt), arteriosclerosis and venous distention of colonic blood vessels (Cleave and others), psychosomatic factors or stressors (Lloyd-Davies, 1953). Current data do not support causal relationships for any of these factors. However, prospective and case-control studies are lacking. Differences in life-style excluding dietary patterns certainly exist between developed and underdeveloped countries. These factors deserve further exploration before they are eliminated as causal or contributing factors.

Other associated health problems

The epidemiology of diverticular disease is quite similar to that of other noninfectious gastrointestinal disorders, such as hiatus hernia, gallbladder disease, and cancer of the colon. Similarity also exists between diverticular disease and disorders associated with atherosclerosis, namely hypertension, coronary artery disease, and cerebral vascular accidents. Hemorrhoids and varicose veins also positively correlate with diverticula. One theory that links diverticular disease with these disorders is that of an association between the development of pathological conditions and Western dietary patterns, which are high in refined carbohydrates, saturated fats, and cholesterol and low in fiber. Food-content characteristics, delayed stool transit times, and small, hard stools typical of this dietary pattern promote increased gastrointestinal pressures and increased absorption of simple carbohydrates, fats, cholesterol, and bile salts. This may allow increased contact between the colon-rectal wall and postulated carcinogens found in stool. As outcomes of a Western diet, these factors may contribute to the disease entities discussed here (Burkitt, 1973; Burkitt and others, 1974; Trowell, 1973; Cleave and others).

Boles and Jordan (1958) estimate the association of diverticular disease, hiatus hernia, and gallstones (Saint's triad) to be as high as 6%. Burkitt, Painter and Burkitt, and Castleden and others (1978) report a positive association between the incidence of diverticular disease and gallstones as compared with the incidence of either disorder occurring alone. In contrast, Berardi and Siroospour (1976) found no common etiological factors between diverticular disease and the diseases postulated to be associated with it. The majority of available data seem to support causal or contributory relationships between a "refined" Western diet, diverticular disease, and associated disorders, although the specific pathways by which these disorders evolve are multifactorial.

PHYSIOLOGY AND PATHOPHYSIOLOGY

The colon has several primary functions. It completes the process of absorption, specifically the absorption of water, electrolytes, and bile acids. In this process, the colon secretes large quantities of mucus, variable amounts of potassium, and possibly bicarbonate. The colon also acts as a reservoir and transporter of stool. Voluntary control over this aspect permits defecation at socially acceptable times, with denial of the urge to defecate associated, in part, with constipation and possibly other disorders of the colon.

Neural and hormonal factors regulate colonic motility, an integral component of the transport, storage, and excretory functions of the left colon. Investigators have studied the left colon more intensively than the right. Available data reveal several forms of movements or waves. Slow waves are the simplest. They are segmental pressure changes that represent the basal electrical rhythm, or pacesetter potential, of the colon. Bursts of rapid electrical transients, or action spikes, accompany the slow waves, resulting in smooth-muscle contraction. Slow waves tend to occur less frequently and are more often singular in occurrence in the right colon as compared with the left colon. Transmission of slow waves occurs along longitudinal and transverse axes in a given colon segment independent of other segments. Segmentation occurs with the contraction of the smooth circular muscles of the colon while longitudinal muscle contractions form haustrations, an accordian-like effect (Fig. 10-1). Independently, segmental contractions do not contribute to the propulsion of stool through the colon. However, normal segmentation does promote stool movement back and forth between segments as a result of variations in pressure gradients, thus aiding the process of absorption. Clients who complain of constipation tend to have an increase in intrasegmental contractions with prolonged stool transit time (Connell, 1975). Although some studies are conflicting, most authorities agree that hypermotility and segmentation of the sigmoid colon will be found in clients with symptomatic diverticulosis.

A decrease of haustration and segmentation and the occurrence of high-pressure, progressive waves accompany the transport of a bolus of colonic wastes over a relatively long distance. This peristaltic movement is characteristic of defecation. Endogenous and exogenous factors stimulate its occurrence.

Endogenous factors include neural stimuli via the thoracolumbar and pelvic nerves

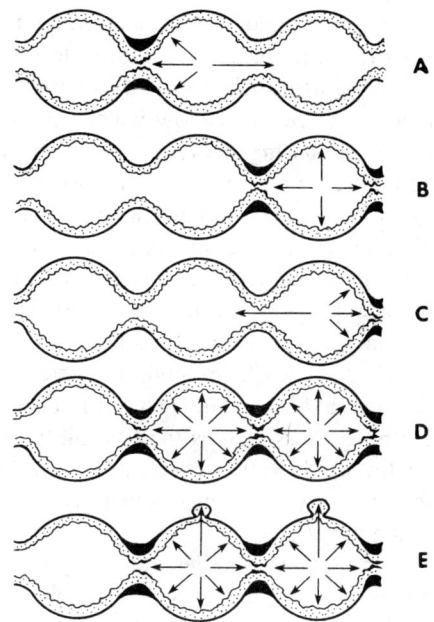

Fig. 10-1. Probable role of segmentation in the pathogenesis of diverticular disease. **A, B,** and **C,** Normal segmentation activity in the colon. With the contraction of the circular contraction rings, segments are formed, with a resulting intraluminal pressure increase. Fecal contents will be propelled from one segment to another as a result of contraction-ring relaxation and a difference in pressure gradient. Stool normally moves back and forth as well as halts within the colon before finally being expelled. **D,** Excessive segmentation seen with viscous stools as in chronic constipation. Increased intraluminal pressures are necessary to propel the fecal load through the contracted ring to the next segment. Fecal stasis also results. **E,** Chronic excessive segmentation with intermittent obstruction to the movement of stool. The colonic musculature has thickened at the contraction rings. With the high intraluminal pressure, herniation of the mucosa has resulted, forming diverticula. (Modified from Painter, N.S.: Geriatrics **31:**89, 1976.)

and the central nervous system. For example, lesions in the lumbosacral spinal cord disrupt colonic motility, resulting in increased segmenting contractions and intractable constipation. Emotional stimuli are more difficult to evaluate, since the effects of emotional state on colonic motility are variable (Connell).

Endogenous agents include gastrointestinal hormones such as cholecystokinin, secretin, and gastrin. Experimentally, endogenous cholecystokinin stimulates motor activity of the sigmoid, whereas secretin inhibits activity. Gastrin may be responsible for the postprandial stimulation of the terminal ileum that results in the emptying of ileal contents into the colon. Eating may be involved in this response. Prostaglandins may also mediate colonic motor function (Connell).

The quality and quantity of food and fluid intake are important exogenous determinants of colonic function and motility. Another exogenous factor, physical activity, can increase colonic motility, especially propulsive movements after meals. Posture too may influence colonic activity. Finally, drugs may promote or inhibit colonic motility. Laxatives, certain antacids and antibiotics, and other agents may contribute to changes in colonic movements or absorption, resulting in an increase in stool volume, propulsive force, or both. Morphine and codeine, along with cholinergic blocking agents, may disrupt normal motility patterns through hypersegmentation or paralysis of colonic musculature. Constipation may result (Goth, 1978).

The importance of food and fluid intake as a determinant of both normal and pathological colonic functioning appears to be integral to an understanding of diverticular disease. Food characteristics largely determine the volume, consistency, and transit time of stool, which in turn affect anatomical and physiological properties of the colon. Dietary fiber is a component of unprocessed, carbohydrate-rich foods such as whole grains, fruits, and vegetables. It determines the content and consistency of stool. Diets rich in fiber result in large, soft, bulky stools. In contrast, diets low in fiber and high in refined carbohydrates (refined sugar, sucrose, refined cereals, white flour) produce small, hard stools with relatively low water content.

In discussing fiber, the clinician needs to know the difference between crude fiber and dietary fiber; the terms are not synonymous. Dietary fiber consists of those remnants of the plant cell wall not hydrolyzed by man's alimentary enzymes. Celluloses, hemicelluloses, and lignin compose most dietary fiber (Trowell, 1972; Southgate, 1973; Southgate and Durnin, 1970). Cummings (1976) includes plant gums, mucilages, and storage polysaccharides in this definition because of their biochemical and physical property relationships to cell wall constituents. Most knowledge of fiber and its constituents comes from studies of grasses, woods, animal feeds, and ruminant nutrition. Studies involving human nutrition reflect the variability of dietary fiber content in different foods as well as the variability of effect of different fiber substances. For instance, pectin, a cell wall constituent, has cholesterol-lowering properties. It is unknown whether this property is retained when pectin is ingested as a component of the whole cell wall (Cummings).

Crude fiber, another frequently used term, is composed of a portion of the celluloses, traces of hemicelluloses, and lignin. Dietary fiber is the more comprehensive term, and I will refer only to this substance unless I specify otherwise. Dietary tables, however, frequently do not make this distinction, thus raising the possibility of altering dietary calculations (Cummings).

How does a lack of dietary fiber correlate with diverticular disease? The small, hard stools produced by a diet high in refined carbohydrates and low in fiber necessitate higher colonic pressures to expel. With the excessive circular-muscle contraction that results, the colon lumen narrows and hypersegmentation occurs, prolonging stool transit time. Food-residue transit time may be well over 36 to 48 hours. Individuals with chronic constipation, irritable colon syndrome, or diverticular disease demonstrate these colonic conditions. Over a period of 40 years, these conditions result in the propulsion herniation of the colon mucosa through the circular-muscle layer, especially in the area of the left colon where hypersegmentation is most marked. A thin layer of colonic longitudinal muscle and pericolic fat cover the pouch, or diverticulum, so formed. The herniation occurs through the circular-muscle layer at the points of entry of the main blood vessels that supply the colonic mucosa. Usually, two rows of diverticula are present, one on each side of the bowel wall between the mesenteric and antimesenteric teniae. Characteristically, there is thickening of the circular muscle, with a corrugated appearance evident on a barium enema study (Morson, 1975). Frequently, considerable fat surrounds the sigmoid colon in people with diverticulosis. Lymphoid tissue in the affected region may increase as a result of fecal stasis.

Diverticulitis, a complication of diverticulosis, involves inflammation of diverticula. This usually involves one or at the most three or four diverticula and is secondary to fecal stasis at the neck of the diverticulum. A chronic inflammatory response, including mucosal and lymphoid hyperplasia, results in inflammation of the diverticulum and surrounding fat. Additionally, a local peritonitis often occurs. Perforation of the sac and generalized peritonitis may occur, although this is much less common. Adhesions of the colon and surrounding structures (such as the bladder), with subsequent fistula formation, is possible though rare. Erosion of blood vessels at the point of mucosal herniation can cause hemorrhage, at times necessitating surgery. Abcess formation is an additional complication (Morson, 1975; Hughes, 1975; Waye; Painter).

ASSESSMENT
Assessing risk factors

A Western diet high in refined carbohydrates and low in dietary fiber is the major predisposing factor in the development of diverticular disease. Americans of all ages eat large quantities of refined sugars and starches in the form of candies, snack foods, soft drinks, refined cereals and breads, and other "quick" foods. In addition, the consumption of complex carbohydrates rich in dietary fiber is often lacking or absent. Generally, complex-carbohydrate sources such as fresh fruit and vegetables, whole-grain breads, and unprocessed rice and cereals are more expensive, less readily available, have shorter storage lives, or take longer to prepare than do refined, simple-carbohydrate foods. These factors are particularly significant for the older adult, the individual most prone to diverticular disease.

Because the older adult is frequently on a fixed, limited income, food costs are of great concern. Problems with food purchasing, preparation, and storage also contribute to a life-style incorporating a refined carbohydrate diet. With dentition problems common in the elderly, refined-carbohydrate foods may be easier to chew and ingest than high-fiber sources such as fresh fruits. Furthermore, food patterns established over a lifetime are likely to persist.

Another risk factor predisposing individuals to diverticular disease is increasing age, although this correlates with a history of 40 or more years' ingestion of a Western diet rather than with degenerative changes characteristic of aging. Obesity, commonly seen in clients with diverticular disease, probably is not a causal factor in the development of diverticula. Rather, obesity frequently is caused by excessive refined-carbohydrate intake.

Chronic constipation results largely from a lack of dietary fiber. The percentage of individuals with chronic constipation who later develop diverticular disease is unknown. However, a high percentage of clients with diverticular disease report histories of chronic constipation. Available data indicate that chronic constipation predisposes individuals to the formation of diverticula. Further studies may confirm or refute this association.

Research data that associate activity patterns with the development of diverticular disease are unavailable. However, an increase in daily exercise is accompanied by improved bowel motility with more frequent emptying of contents. For this reason, an increase in activity may prove beneficial in preventing and treating diverticular disease.

The degree to which emotional state is a risk factor in the development of diverticular disease is unknown. Anxiety, depression, and other psychological disorders may affect appetite, hormone secretion, nervous system function, and secondarily, colon function. The effects are variable and the improtance of these factors remains undetermined.

Irritable colon syndrome

The relationship of the irritable colon syndrome to diverticular disease, specifically as a prodromal state, is unclear. Clients with irritable bowel syndrome are frequently in their late 20s to mid-40s. Many clients with documented diverticula have a long history of abdominal discomfort characteristic of irritable or spastic colon. However, many clients with diverticula may be asymptomatic, without pain or colonic dysfunction, at the time of or just before the diagnosis of diverticular disease. There is also an unknown percentage of clients having histories compatible with less severe manifestations of irritable colon syndrome (such as constipation, intermittent cramping, intermittent diarrhea, flatus, straining with defecation, and occasional mucus excretion).

Asymptomatic and symptomatic diverticulosis

History. Approximately half of those clients diagnosed as having diverticulosis have no antecedent history of lower abdominal pain or irritable colon. They may report chronic constipation and straining with defecation. Research indicates that slow-wave motility and intralumen pressure patterns of individuals with asymptomatic diverticular disease are different from those of individuals who are symptomatic. This may indicate that other mechanical events could produce herniation besides an excess of slow-wave activity. In these situations, a workup for another problem usually identifies diverticula (Almy and Howell, 1980).

The symptoms of diverticulosis include constipation, flatulence, anorexia, left lower quadrant tenderness, cramping, vague dyspepsia, nausea, straining with defecation, distention, a heavy sensation in the lower abdomen, and a feeling of "never completely emptying the rectum." At times pain and colicky cramping in the left lower quadrant or the central abdomen can become intense, frequently in the absence of complications such as diverticulitis. The client's diet history is characteristic of a low-fiber, high–refined-carbohydrate diet. Bowel habits are irregular, with hard, small, at times pellet-like stools reported. Occasionally the client complains of intermittent diarrhea, especially in the presence of laxative use. Clients' activity patterns, especially with increasing age, are sedentary. Therefore, life-style is a valuable clue in the assessment of and planning for the client with diverticular disease.

Symptoms of diverticulosis are quite similar to those of other bowel disorders characteristic of the older population. These disorders include irritable bowel syndrome, cancer of the colon, Crohn's disease, biliary disease, hiatus hernia, peptic ulcer, intestinal obstruction, and other colonic disorders. Hemorrhoids frequently occur concomitantly with diverticula as well. Along with mimicking diverticular disease, these disorders may coexist with it, thus complicating the diagnostic process.

Physical examination. In addition to the historical findings described above, changes may be evident on physical examination. At times the examination may be completely normal. In the absence of complications of diverticulosis, tenderness in the left lower quadrant in the area of the sigmoid and descending colon is a frequent finding. Rebound tenderness should be absent. A mass may be palpable in this area and is usually sausage shaped. Its presence is the result of thickening of the colon's muscle wall, the presence of adipose tissue, and an accumulation of feces within the bowel lumen and diverticula. Pain or masses elsewhere in the abdomen are not characterisitc of diverticular disease.

Rectal examination may be normal, or the examiner may palpate clusters of small masses through the anterior wall if diverticula are extensive. Palpation does not exclude carcinoma. Hemorrhoids or fissures may be present. Systemic manifestations or inflammation and infection may or may not be present. The masking of early signs of infection is characteristic of the older adult, and this may complicate diagnosis. In the older adult who has left lower quadrant pain, an elevated white cell count, and possibly rebound tenderness, a diagnosis of diverticulitis is a strong consideration.

Diagnostic studies. Additional investigatory steps are appropriate to arrive at a diagnosis of diverticular disease. For diverticulosis, the stool guaiac test should be negative for occult bleeding unless complications or other disorders, such as cancer of the colon, are present. Although its use is not a routine procedure, an abdominal flat-plate x-ray film may reveal excessive stool and gas in the colon. Referral for sigmoidoscopy may be appropriate, although this procedure will not generally aid in the diagnosis of diverticula. However, sigmoidoscopy will facilitate the confirmation or exclusion of a carcinoma in the rectal-sigmoid area.

The barium enema study is the most revealing investigatory procedure. The provider should use this to confirm the diagnosis of diverticular disease. Occasionally the radiologist may identify irritable bowel syndrome by the appearance of edema with thickening of the folds of the sigmoid, or a "picket-fence" (serrated) colon pattern. In the presence of symptoms characteristic of irritable bowel syndrome, some providers may diagnose irritable bowel syndrome or spastic colon in spite of an absence of radiological abnormalities. Radiologists may label a barium enema study "normal" when in fact there are subtle changes indicative of a prediverticular state.

On barium enema study diverticula have a characteristic appearance. The barium-filled diverticula are saclike projections from the lumen of the colon. The diverticula may take on a sawtooth appearance because of muscular contractions or partial filling by residual stool. This sawtooth effect occurs with diverticulitis as well, but it does not necessarily indicate the presence of inflammation.

Preparation for a barium enema study, especially in an older individual with long-standing constipation and laxative abuse, may be somewhat trying for both the clinician and the client. Specific, written step-by-step instructions are helpful. At times a home nursing referral to assist with colon preparation is useful. Thorough cleansing of the colon is important and usually involves both low– and high–soap suds and saline enemas and colonic stimulators such as dulcolax tablets. The client should be instructed to abstain from food or fluids (except water) after the evening meal on the night before the scheduled barium enema study. The elderly may need more vigorous measures, but such clients should not be made overtired. Excessive colonic irrigation may also disrupt their electrolyte balance. Radiology departments generally have guidelines for barium enema preparation that specify agents and the timing involved.

Colonoscopy is not a standard procedure for the client suspected of having diverticular disease. A history of bleeding or abnormalities identified on the barium enema study are indications for this procedure. Because of muscle contraction and thickening, with subsequent narrowing of the bowel lumen, colonoscopy is a difficult procedure for both the client and the colonoscopist. However, the procedure is useful to exclude other disease processes, specifically cancer, telangiectasia, and Crohn's disease (Waye).

PLAN
Diet

Prevention of diverticular disease is of prime importance. A high-fiber diet that is low in refined carbohydrates is the principal preventive measure. Because this kind of diet involves a permanent life-style change, it may, for many individuals, be a difficult pat-

Table 10-1. Fruit and vegetable fiber and water-holding capacity

Food source	Fiber (percent of foodstuff)	Water-holding capacity (g water/g fiber)	Capacity of fiber in 100 g foodstuff to absorb water (g water)
Apple	14.6	12.1	177
Banana	22.7	2.9	68
Bran	89.3	3.0	447
Brussel sprouts	7.5	17.3	129
Carrot	8.9	23.4	208
Cauliflower	11.6	5.9	68
Celery	6.0	16.2	97
Corn	86.1	1.5	129
Cucumber	3.7	20.9	77
Green bean	12.4	8.1	100
Lettuce	4.2	23.7	99
Mango	15.3	20.4	312
Orange	9.9	12.4	122
Pea	21.6	4.6	99
Pear	15.3	7.4	113
Potato	19.5	2.0	41
Rhubarb	4.2	14.4	60
Tomato	6.6	10.8	71

Modified from Eastwood, M.A., and Mitchell, W.D.: Physical properties of fiber. In Spiller, G.H., and Amen, R.J., editors: Fiber in human nutrition, New York, 1976, Plenum Publishing Corp.

tern to establish. Adolescents, young adults, and the elderly may have particular problems in changing their eating patterns, although these difficulties may arise for different reasons. Individuals may find compliance with a high-fiber diet achievable by adding bran to food or by taking bran tablets daily. Foods high in fiber content and potent in water-holding capacity are numerous and include whole-grain breads, whole-grain cereals (though many "natural" cereals have sugar added), whole-grain rice (versus "instant" or "quick" rice), and fresh fruits and vegetables. A food's ability to hold water is a manifestation of its fiber content, a property that contributes to the stool characteristics of consistency and volume. Table 10-1 summarizes the water-holding characteristics of many common fruits and vegetables. Water-holding capacity may vary with the age and variety of a given fruit or vegetable. Generally speaking, raw fruits and vegetables are more beneficial than those that are cooked, though both add fiber to the diet.

By weight, bran is one of the most potent water-holding substances (Eastwood and Mitchell). Although its fiber has only moderate water-holding ability, bran's fiber content is extremely high (nearly 90%). Because of bran's capacity to produce a large, soft stool and thus alleviate symptoms of constipation, straining, and cramping, it is one of the treatments of choice in managing constipation, irritable colon, and diverticular disease. A decrease in intraluminal pressure and more effortless, frequent emptying of the colon decrease the degree of abdominal discomfort reported by the client. Studies document that a reduction in pressure is measurable in clients who eat a high-fiber diet. Over time, increased stool bulk resulting from the water-retention properties of a high-fiber diet results in a normalization of bowel habits.

In recommending dietary changes to clients at risk for or suffering from documented diverticular disease, the clinician needs to reinforce the goals of therapy. Consultation with a dietician and at times referral of the client to the dietician are beneficial practices in all phases of management. Alleviating symptoms and reestablishing healthy bowel habits certainly are of major importance. Achieving a balanced nutritional intake is also a priority. For this reason, I recommend a variety of high-fiber foods rather than total reliance on bran. This variety also should ensure the intake of all needed vitamins and minerals. In the presence of additional life-style or gastrointestinal problems such as vitamin deficiencies or lactose intolerance, vitamin and mineral supplementation is necessary. In addition, bran may not be palatable for all clients, and the option of alternate high-fiber foodstuffs should be available. Since little is known about the need for different types of fiber, reliance on bran alone is undesirable. Future study of fiber properties and their specific effect on bile salt reabsorption, cholesterol levels, motility, and other functions may indicate recommending certain foods high in a desired fiber constituent.

The introduction of bran into the diet is often accompanied initially by distention, excessive flatulence, and even diarrhea for the first 2 to 6 weeks of therapy. The clinician must make individual adjustments in the amount of bran consumed either as an additive to cereals, juices, and salads or as chewable tablets. The clinician should plan increases in bran and other high-fiber foods every 2 or 3 days. The client should begin with 2 tablets or 1 tablespoon of bran once or twice a day and increase the amount regularly (up to 25 g per day or until the desired results are obtained: bulky, soft stools defecated effortlessly once or twice daily [Almy and Howell]). An alternate source of bran is five slices (150 g) of unrefined whole wheat bread per day. Vegetable fiber also contains valuable water-absorptive properties. Recommended are carrots, apples, oranges, and salad greens.

Drugs

If the client is having difficulty tolerating or adhering to a high-fiber diet or if the client's symptoms are particularly severe, other agents may be useful. Psyllium (Metamucil) or methylcellulose preparations are convenient hydrophilic colloids refined from vegetable fibers. Metamucil, 1 or 2 tablespoons daily, is useful in producing bulky, soft stools. Although not all authorities agree, anticholinergic drugs may help reduce the hypermotility of the sigmoid in the initial treatment of diverticular disease. The practitioner should use caution with these drugs because the elderly client may have problems (such as glaucoma, urinary retention, or hiatus hernia) that contraindicate their use. I find propantheline bromide (Pro-Banthine), 95 mg three times daily, a useful drug for this purpose. Anticholinergics are not satisfactory alone, and the practitioner should recommend them in conjunction with high-fiber additions to the diet. Their need should last no longer than 1 or 2 months of therapy. Stool softeners, such as dioctyl sodium sulfosuccinate (Colace), may also be helpful. The practitioner should discourage the regular use of laxatives and enemas, because these actually contribute to poor bowel habits (Waye; Almy and Howell).

Life-style

Other therapeutic measures should include increased fluid intake, specifically six or more 8-ounce glasses of fluid daily. The practitioner should encourage the client to change from a sedentary to a more physically active life-style. Chronic disorders such as arthritis and cardiopulmonary problems need special consideration when planning for exercise programs. An improved activity pattern may also benefit the older adult's mental outlook. Improved appetite and bowel function should result. The practitioner should help the client establish a regular unhurried time for daily bowel movements and should ensure that the client's dentures fit properly to ease the chewing of high-fiber foods. Gum and bone changes with aging and weight loss make poorly fitting dentures or loss of teeth common problems in the older adult. Referral for dental care is important for these individuals.

Social and economic problems contribute to poor nutritional patterns. These may require the practitioner's working with the client and family to modify food purchases and preparation. If such actions are necessary, the practitioner should help the client obtain food stamps, enroll the client in a "Meals on Wheels" program, help the client obtain additional financial assistance, and attempt to involve the client in social groups, such as a senior citizens' club. With the life-style changes needed for effective prevention or management of diverticular disease, the client and the client's family must help determine appropriate goals and interventions.

Health education

For the elderly client, dietary interventions may be a total reversal of the dietary regimen he or she has followed for years. The "traditional" low-residue diet was the hallmark of therapy for the irritable bowel syndrome and diverticular disease until the late 1960s and early 1970s. Authorities now consider this approach physiologically unsound. There is no evidence supporting the notion that seeds or other materials found in a high-fiber diet will get caught in or perforate diverticula (Waye). However, with the drastic change in therapy, clients may be confused or skeptical of the new diet. Sharing with the client the rationale for the high-fiber, low–refined-carbohydrate diet and its relation to bowel function and diverticular disease will usually improve the client's understanding and compliance. Jointly prepared menus and written schedules for bran, fluid, and drug therapy are useful as well.

A written contract clarifies even further a mutually acceptable plan of care and makes compliance more likely. It should include the health goals, management plans, time frame for implementation and evaluation, responsibilities of the practitioner and client, and their signatures. The contract should be open to revision as the need arises and should consider other health problems that may coexist (Hayes and Davis, 1980).

EVALUATION
Expected outcomes

If additional health problems do not surface, therapy should prevent the occurrence of diverticular disease. If the disorder is present, therapy will alleviate the symptoms. Whether the addition of fiber to the diet can prevent diverticulitis and reverse the physiological and anatomical changes that occur has not been demonstrated (Painter and others, 1972).

Additional gains with therapy may include prevention or improvement of other disorders linked to diets high in refined carbohydrates and fat and low in fiber. These are gallbladder disease, hiatus hernia, arteriosclerotic cardiovascular diseases, and diabetes mellitus. An increase in physical activities is beneficial for these disorders as well.

Complications and indications for referral

Certain signs and symptoms herald the onset of complications of diverticular disease. Inflammation of one or more diverticula, diverticulitis, is the most common complication. Waye estimates that nearly one third of clients with symptomatic diverticulosis develop diverticulitis at some point in their life. This figure may change in the future, because more people are adhering to a high-fiber diet. However, the number of people at risk for diverticulitis remains high, with some evidence supporting an increased chance of occurrence the longer an individual has diverticular disease (Waye).

Diverticulitis may localize to a single diverticulum and its peridiverticulum structure, or it may involve multiple diverticula. The only symptoms may be an acute onset of pain in the left lower quadrant and tenderness with palpation. Leukocytosis, fever, and rebound tenderness are absent in earlier stages. A sudden change in the bowel pattern is uncharacteristic except for some increase in constipation and discomfort with defecation. In some clients the lesion may heal spontaneously (Waye; Almy and Howell).

The inflammatory process may progress with systemic manifestations (such as fever and leukocytosis) occurring. Rebound tenderness in the left lower quadrant or over a greater area of the abdomen indicates peritoneal inflammation. With clients in the seventh and eighth decades of life, signs and symptoms indicative of infection may be obscure. Physician consultation or referral is essential. Interventions might include a well-absorbed antibiotic, such as ampicillin or tetracycline. Because there may be edema at the neck of the diverticulum, poorly absorbed drugs such as sulfonamides and neomycin do not reach the site of infection. Blood cultures for a specific organism are usually not helpful. A liquid diet or gastric suction may decrease colonic contents, depending on the severity of the symptoms. Analgesics may be necessary. In some situations, hospitalization may be necessary (Almy and Howell).

Perforation, obstruction (partial or complete), or an aberrant presentation of appendicitis, Crohn's disease, or carcinoma should be excluded. An abdominal flat-plate x-ray film may clear the clinical picture. If needed, a barium enema study may be obtained, preferably 2 weeks after the inflammatory episode. In severe situations, where the client has marked pyrexia or profound signs of toxicity, surgery may be necessary.

Hemorrhage associated with diverticular disease usually results from erosion of a blood vessel by hardened retained stool at the site of a noninflamed diverticulum. With acute inflammation, the blood vessel supplying the diverticulum frequently seals off (Waye). The "bleeder", usually an arterial source, produces bright red blood from the rectum. The colonic bleeding episode may be the client's initial presentation of diverticular disease. The client may also report the urge to defecate every 10 to 15 minutes, though only blood is passed. Syncope may also be present, but evidence of clinical shock is unusual. Immediate consultation and referral are essential to identify the site of and the reason for the bleeding. These studies may include abdominal angiography, sigmoidoscopy, barium enema study, and last, colonoscopy, if the other tests fail to reveal the problem.

CASE STUDY
Subjective

A 63-year-old housewife comes to the neighborhood primary care clinic for her annual checkup. From the client's records, the clinician is aware that she has a long-standing history of chronic constipation and laxative abuse, specifically abuse of Correctol and Ex-Lax. She reports "bouts" of lower abdominal cramping three or four times weekly, for which she "doses [herself] with a laxative." Bowel movements are irregular, with stools described as pelletlike, except after laxative use, when bowel movements become watery. The client's appetite is not particularly good, though she denies weight loss in the last year. Excessive belching and flatus are also problems, especially after dinner.

The client lives with her husband, a 67-year-old retired carpenter. They live on his Social Security check and a small pension fund established by his labor union. The client describes their eating preferences as "meat and potatoes," though she does admit to a "sweet tooth." The client does not take vitamin and mineral supplements. Her activity pattern is sedentary.

Objective

General. Ht, 5 ft 3 in; wt, 154 lb; BP, 138/80; T, 98.2°; P, 78; R, 22. The client does not appear to be in acute distress.

HEENT. Test results are normal.

Cardiovascular. Normal S_1 and S_2 sounds are heard, without murmurs or gallop rhythm.

Abdomen. Palpatory tenderness is present over both lower quadrants, though more marked in the left. There is no rebound tenderness. A firm, sausage-shaped mass is palpable in the left lower quadrant.

Pelvic exam. The findings are normal.

Rectal exam. No tenderness or masses are present.

Laboratory data. The complete blood count is normal. The stool guaiac test is negative. Fasting triglyceride and cholesterol levels are within normal limits.

Problems

1. Alteration in comfort—abdominal pain
2. Alteration in elimination—chronic constipation
3. Nutritional alteration—fiber-deficient diet and excessive caloric intake
4. Limited income

Plan

This situation describes a typical presentation of diverticulosis. A concomitant problem is obesity, a disorder frequently seen in clients with diverticular disease. The client is approximately 20% overweight; her ideal body weight is between 115 and 125 lb. Dietary and activity patterns contribute to her health problems. Underlying socioeconomic factors, such as a low, fixed income, and her food preferences are complicating factors.

Diagnostic studies. Refer the client for barium enema study and sigmoidoscopy to confirm diverticulosis and exclude other causes, such as cancer of the colon, Crohn's disease, and irritable bowel syndrome. Prepare the client for radiography with appropriate medications, enemas, and diet and fluid requirements. Obtain a stool guaiac test for occult blood three times in the next 2 weeks (Chapter 4). No diagnostic studies are necessary for obesity at this time.

Diet. Recommend a high-fiber, low–refined-carbohydrate diet. Teach diet and meal planning with the aid of a dietician, if appropriate. Limit the caloric intake to 1,500 calories for weight reduction, and stress the importance of a low-fat diet. Encourage the client to join a weight-reduction group such as Weight Watchers, if she appears motivated. Recommend six to eight 8-ounce glasses of fluid daily to help alleviate the problem of constipation. Most important, start the client on 1 tablespoon of bran twice daily with meals. Increase this amount to 2 or 3 tablespoons twice or three times daily, depending on the client's stool characteristics. Also encourage the intake of carrots, oranges, and salad greens as substitutes for snack foods.

Medication. Discontinue all self-prescribed over-the-counter laxatives and enemas. Recommend Metamucil, 1 tablespoon twice daily in a full glass of fluid, if the client is unable to take bran. After 2 to 3 months of use discontinue the drug. Possibly give an anticholinergic agent of choice (such as Pro-Banthine, 15 mg three times daily for 1 or 2 months). Use this only if the client has marked discomfort. A stool softener of choice (such as Colace, 100 mg twice daily, by mouth) may be necessary for 1 to 2 months. These drugs should be given only with a clear explanation of their expected results, as these may be different from those of harsh laxatives.

Activity. Encourage brisk walking for 30 to 40 minutes twice daily as tolerated. The husband may want to participate. This may improve bowel function and reduce the frequency of abdominal complaints.

Counseling. Incorporate mutual health goals and plan of care. Teach the client about the association between a fiber-deficient diet and constipation. Encourage the client to participate in group education sessions with older adults having similar problems. Consult with the social worker and dietician, if they are available, to plan strategies for affording a high-fiber diet on a limited income. Substitution of specific snack foods for high-fiber foods may improve the client's nutritional status. Explain to the client that diverticulosis is a possible diagnosis, and give a brief explanation of this disease. Request the client to return in 2 weeks, after completion of diagnostic studies.

Evaluation

At the return visit, the client reported abdominal pain only once in the previous 2 weeks. She felt that the pills she was taking (Pro-Banthine and Colace) were so helpful that she did not need a laxative. She reported daily bowel movements that were formed and soft after the first week. She also was taking bran with meals and voiced no dislike for this additive. She started eating salads at lunch and an occasional piece of fruit. She has not lost any weight, but she promised that she would start Weight Watchers the next week. She complained of difficulty sticking to the 1,500 calorie diet. Her activity pattern had not changed measurably. The barium enema study revealed multiple diverticula in the left descending colon. The provider shared this information with the client and reinforced the teaching about diverticular disease discussed previously. The client would return in 2 weeks for a "weigh in." The practitioner reinforced the temporary nature of the medications and prepared the client not to fear further constipation if the low–refined-carbohydrate, high-fiber diet was followed.

SUMMARY

Diverticular disease consists of a continuum of disorders. It encompasses prediverticular states, such as chronic constipation and possibly irritable colon syndrome. These may progress to diverticulosis, with both asymptomatic and symptomatic manifestations, and may include complications such as diverticulitis and hemorrhage. The preponderance of research findings implicates a diet low in fiber and high in refined carbohydrates as the probable causal factor in the development of diverticular disease. Over approximately a 40-year period, anatomical and physiological changes in the colon occur. These include shortening of the longitudinal smooth muscles, excessive haustration and segmentation, increased intraluminal pressure, smooth-muscle thickening, and eventually colon mucosa herniation through the circular-muscle layer.

The older adult is most frequently affected by diverticular disease. Primary prevention through early institution of a high-fiber diet is of major importance. With clients having established diverticulosis the goals of therapy are to relieve symptoms, reestablish a normal bowel pattern, and prevent complications. The first two outcomes are achievable through adherence to a high-fiber, low–refined-carbohydrate diet. Additional wheat bran is a useful adjunct to a high-fiber diet. Other life-style changes, such as increased physical activity and alternative coping strategies, may also be helpful. Problems of the elderly may complicate the achievement of therapeutic goals.

Many unanswered questions deserve further exploration in the attempt to prevent and manage diverticular disease, a highly prevalent disorder of Western man. A great deal of progress has been made in this direction. However, our continued effort is certainly indicated if continued progress is to be made.

REFERENCES

Almy, T.P.: The role of fiber in the diet. In Winick, M., editor: Nutrition and aging, New York, 1976, John Wiley & Sons, Inc.

Almy, T.P., and Howell, P.A.: Medical progress: diverticular disease of the colon, N. Engl. J. Med. **302:**324, 1980.

Becker, M.H., and Maiman, L.A.: Sociobehavioral determinants of compliance with health and medical care recommendations, Med. Care **13:**10, 1975.

Berardi, R.S., and Siroospour, D.: Diverticular disorders of the colon and associated pathology, Am. J. Proctol. **27:**45, 1976.

Berman, P.M., and others: Guide to the diagnosis of problems of the aging gut, Hosp. Med., May, 1975, pp. 112, 115-116, 118, 122-123.

Bland-Sutton, J. Cited in A discussion of diverticulitis at the Royal Society of Medicine, Proc. R. Soc. Med. **13:**64, 1920.

Boles, R.S., Jr., and Jordan, S.M.: The clinical significance of diverticulosis, Gastroenterology **35:**579, 1958.

Burkitt, D.P.: Some diseases characteristic of modern Western civilization, Br. Med. J. **1:**274, 1973.

Burkitt, D.P., and others: Effect of dietary fibre on stools and the transit-times, and its role in the causation of disease, Lancet **2:**1408, 1972.

Burkitt, D.P., and others: Dietary fiber and disease, J.A.M.A. **229:**1068, 1974.

Castleden, W.M., and others: Gallstones, carcinoma of the colon and diverticular disease, Clin. Oncol. **4:**139, 1978.

Cleave, T.L., and others: Diabetes, coronary thrombosis and the saccharine disease, ed. 2, Bristol, England, 1969, John Wright & Sons, Ltd.

Connell, A.M.: Applied physiology of the colon: factors relevant to diverticular disease, Clin. Gastroenterol. **4:**23, 1975.

Cummings, J.H.: Dietary fiber, Gut **14:**69, 1973.

Cummings, J.H.: What is fiber? In Spiller, G.A., and Amen, R.J., editors: Fiber in human nutrition, New York, 1976, Plenum Publishing Corp.

Diekelmann, N.: Primary health care of the well adult, New York, 1977, McGraw-Hill, Inc.

Eastwood, M.A., and Mitchell, W.D.: Physical properties of fiber, In Spiller, G.A., and Amen, R.J., editors: Fiber in human nutrition, New York, 1976, Plenum Publishing Corp.

Eastwood, M.A., and others: Epidemiology of bowel disease. In Spiller, G.A., and Amen, R.J., editors: Fiber in human nutrition, New York, 1976, Plenum Publishing Corp.

Flynn, K.T.: Iron deficiency anemia among the elderly, Nurse Pract. **3:**20, Nov.-Dec. 1978.

Goth, A.: Medical pharmacology, ed. 9, St. Louis, 1978, The C.V. Mosby Co.

Hayes, W.S., and Davis, L.L.: What is a health care contract? Health Val. **4:**82, 1980.

Haynes, R.B., and others, editors: Compliance in health care, Baltimore, 1979, The Johns Hopkins University Press.

Horner, J.L.: Natural history of diverticulosis of the colon, Am. J. Dig. Dis. **3:**343, 1958.

Hughes, L.E.: Complications of diverticular disease: inflammation, obstruction and bleeding, Clin. Gastroenterol. **4:**147, 1975.
Hymovich, D., and Underwood, M., editors: Family health care, vol. I, ed. 2, New York, 1979, McGraw-Hill, Inc.
Kocour, E.J.: Diverticulosis of the colon, Am. J. Surg. **37:**430, 1937.
Kohler, R.: The incidence of colonic diverticulosis in Finland and Sweden, Acta Chir. Scand. **126:**148, 1963.
Lloyd-Davies, O.V.: Diverticulitis, Proc. R. Soc. Med. **46:**407, 1953.
Mayo, W.J.: Diverticula of the sigmoid, Ann. Surg. **92:**739, 1930.
Morson, B.C.: The muscle abnormality in diverticular disease of the sigmoid colon, Br. J. Radiol. **36:**385, 1963.
Morson, B.C.: Pathology of diverticular disease of the colon, Clin. Gastroenterol. **4:**37, 1975.
Morson, B.C., and Dawson, I.M.P.: Gastrointestinal pathology, Oxford, 1972, Blackwell Scientific Publications.
Painter, N.S.: Diverticular disease of the colon: a bane of the elderly, Geriatrics **31:**89, 1976.
Painter, N.S., and Burkitt, D.P.: Diverticular disease of the colon: a 20th century problem, Clin. Gastroenterol. **4:**3, 1975.
Painter, N.S., and others: Unprocessed bran in treatment of diverticular disease of the colon, Br. Med. J. **2:**137, 1972.
Palmer, E.D.: Gastrointestinal problems in the elderly, Hosp. Med., Dec., 1978, pp. 32, 34-39.
Plein, J.B.: Drug dosing for geriatric patients, Nurse Pract. **4:**30, Mar.-Apr. 1979.
Shields, E.M.: Introduction to drug therapy for older adults, J. Gerontol. Nurs. **1:**8, Mar.-Apr. 1975.
Southgate, D.A.T.: Plant foods for man, **1:**475, 1973.
Southgate, D.A.T., and Durnin, J.V.G.A.: Caloric conversion factors: an experimental reassessment of the factors used in the calculation of the energy value of human diets, Br. J. Nutr. **24:**517, 1970.
Tarpila, S., and others: Effects of bran on serum cholesterol, faecal mass, fat, bile acids and neutral sterols, and biliary lipids in patients with diverticular disease of the colon, Gut **19:**137, 1978.
Tilkian, S., and others: Clinical implications of laboratory tests, ed. 2, St. Louis, 1979, The C.V. Mosby Co.
Trowell, H.C.: Ischemic heart disease and dietary fiber, Am. J. Clin. Nutr. **25:**926, 1972.
Trowell, H.C.: Dietary fiber, ischemic heart disease and diabetes mellitus, Proc. Nutr. Soc. **32:**151, 1973.
Trowell, H.C., and others: Aspects of the epidemiology of diverticular disease and ischemic heart disease, Am. J. Dig. Dis. **19:**864, 1974.
Walker, A.R.P.: Gastrointestinal diseases and fiber intake with special reference to South African populations. In Spiller, G.A., and Amens, R.J., editors: Fiber in human nutrition, New York, 1976, Plenum Publishing Corp.
Waye, J.D.: Diverticular disease, Prim. Care **3:**91, 1976.
Williams, S.R.: Nutrition and diet therapy, ed. 3, St. Louis, 1977, The C.V. Mosby Co.

SECTION FIVE

Problems with infectious diseases

CHAPTER 11

Acute salpingitis

Ann M. Biderman and Richard L. Sweet

Acute salpingitis is a common gynecological problem that affects approximately 600,000 women a year in the United States (Eschenbach, 1976). Furthermore, salpingitis rates are rising on a curve parallel to the increasing incidence of gonorrhea (Dans, 1975). Ten percent to 17% of women with untreated endocervical gonorrhea will develop salpingitis (Rees, 1969).

The woman with salpingitis suffers more than the physiological pain related to tubal inflammation. She may also feel embarrassed about having a sexually transmitted disease. In addition, the client may be left with serious sequelae, such as infertility, chronic pelvic pain, or recurrent salpingitis. The nurse practitioner who treats the woman with salpingitis combines nursing process skills with medical protocol to create an effective plan of care. Such a plan addresses the client's psychosocial as well as her physiological needs. The aim of this chapter is to provide a guide that presents a comprehensive approach to the management of acute salpingitis in an ambulatory setting. The goal of this management is to facilitate the client's return to a state of wellness and to prevent psychosocial problems and chronic residua of inflammation.

Acute salpingitis, an acute inflammation of the fallopian tubes, is commonly referred to as pelvic inflammatory disease, or PID. However, increasing numbers of practitioners favor the term "salpingitis," which is more accurate and produces far less social stigma than the nonspecific term "PID." In addition, much of the general public mistakenly thinks that PID is always a result of gonorrhea. There are two forms of acute salpingitis: gonococcal and nongonococcal. Differentiation is made on the basis of positive or negative *Neisseria gonorrhoeae* culture of the endocervix at the time of the initial evaluation. Tubercular and parasitic salpingitis is rare in industrialized countries.

EPIDEMIOLOGY
Etiology

There are many unanswered questions about the cause of acute salpingitis. Numerous studies show that 33% to 80% of salpingitis cases will be associated with cervical gonorrhea (Sweet, 1977). Chow and associates (1975) found that *N. gonorrhoeae* was the only difference in cervical flora between gonococcal and nongonococcal salpingitis groups. It has been shown that cervices of healthy women reveal a great variety of aerobic and anaerobic microorganisms. (Chow and others; Thadepalli and others, 1973). Even when a pathogenic organism is isolated from the cervix, it may not be the cause of an upper tract infection. Investigators have used laparoscopy, laparotomy, and culdocentesis to obtain intraabdominal specimens of peritoneal or tubal fluid for culture. A poor correlation was found between organisms from the intraabdominal cultures and those from the cervical cultures of the same client (Chow and others; Eschenbach and Holmes, 1975; Jacobson, 1964; Lip and Burgoyne, 1966; Sunden, 1959).

There are several theories for the low recovery rate of *N. gonorrhoeae* in intraabdominal specimens. One theory, originally presented by Curtis in 1921 and recently supported by Chow, is that the gonococcus initiates the infection and paves the way for other cervical and vaginal pathogens. The gonococci are present only for a short time at the start of the disease process. A second theory that Eschenbach (1976) proposes is that *N. gonorrhoeae* is extremely difficult to recover from pus and demands meticulous culturing techniques. A third explanation may be related to the gonococci's ability to attack epithelial cells. Perhaps the organism is in the tissue rather than in the purulent discharge. Studdiford and associates (1938) were able to recover *N. gonorrhoeae* from tubal tissue in 67% of patients with gonococcal salpingitis. They were unable to isolate the organism from the purulent exudate discharged from the tubes in these same women. While the precise role of the gonococcus in the cause of salpingitis remains unclear, many authorities consider this disease to be the result of a mixed aerobic and anaerobic infection (Sweet, 1977; Swenson and others, 1973).

Mycoplasma and *Chlamydia trachomatis* are two other microorganisms that have been implicated in the cause of salpingitis. Studies of mycoplasma revealed that it is not a major pathogen, but it may play a role in a few cases of acute salpingitis (Eschenbach and Holmes; Mardh and Westrom, 1970). In Sweden *C. trachomatis* has been implicated as a significant pathogen in salpingitis; however, in the United States its role needs further investigation.

Pathogenesis

There is little doubt that sexual intercourse is a factor in the pathogenesis of gonococcal salpingitis. However, what part, if any, intercourse has in the epidemiology of nongonococcal salpingitis remains unclear. In gonococcal salpingitis the infection spreads from the endocervix through the endometrial cavity to the lumen of the fallopian tubes. The exact mechanism by which *N. gonorrhoeae* accomplishes this is unknown. It is also unknown why only 10% to 17% of women with endocervical gonorrhea (untreated) will develop upper tract infection, while the majority of these women will manifest only a localized disease.

Carney and Taylor-Robinson (1973), using fallopian tube organ cultures, have described what happens when the gonococci reach the endosalpinx. After the organisms attach to the epithelial cells of the tubal mucosa, they invade the cells by phagocytosis and destroy them. Ciliary motility of the tubal lumen is lost in 2 to 7 days. A purulent exudate, which results from the destruction of the endosalpinx, oozes out of the fimbriated end of the tube into the abdominal cavity, causing peritonitis. This peritonitis may affect adjacent structures such as the omentum, bowel, and ovary.

Another example of peritoneal involvement occurs in Fitz-Hugh–Curtis syndrome,

Table 11-1. Gonococcal and nongonococcal salpingitis

Gonococcal salpingitis	Nongonococcal salpingitis
Onset usually at end of or after menstrual period	Onset distributed throughout menstrual cycle
Fever more common	Fever less common
Abnormal vaginal discharge more common	Discharge uncommon
Presence of liver tenderness	Liver tenderness rare
Rapid response to treatment	Slower response to treatment

From Sweet, R.L.: Diagnosis and treatment of acute salpingitis, J. Reprod. Med. **19**:21, 1977.

in which gonococcal salpingitis is associated with perihepatitis. Presumably, the purulent exudate deposited into the peritoneal cavity from the tube travels upward to inflame the liver capsule. Although this syndrome was once thought to be a relatively rare occurrence (1% to 10%) in salpingitis cases, Eschenbach and Holmes reported that 31% of clients with gonococcal salpingitis had liver tenderness; they presumed this was due to gonococcal perihepatitis.

In the later stages of salpingitis, the fimbriated ends of the tubes become occluded. The continuing accumulation of pus is then trapped, causing the tubes to enlarge and form pyosalpinges. Abscess formation is not uncommon in a case of unchecked salpingitis and may appear as a tuboovarian abscess or pelvic abscess in the cul-de-sac.

Much less is known about the pathogenesis of nongonococcal infection. An intrauterine device (IUD) or previous gonococcal infection predisposes a woman to subsequent nongonococcal infection (Eschenbach and Holmes). In addition, a nongonococcal salpingitis may result as a complication of tubal ligation, pregnancy termination, parturition, or other uterine instrumentation. In all of these situations the assumption is made that the salpingitis results from an infectious continuum that begins with an endometritis. The endometritis progresses to myometritis, then to parametritis, and finally to salpingitis. Investigations are currently in progress to further delineate the pathogenesis of nongonococcal salpingitis (Sweet and others, 1979). The clinical differences between gonococcal and nongonococcal salpingitis are summarized in Table 11-1. The practitioner should recognize that nongonococcal salpingitis does not demonstrate a well-defined clinical picture.

ASSESSMENT

The nurse practitioner uses a combination of nursing process and medical management skills to assess the woman with acute salpingitis. The practitioner uses problem-solving theory to solve the dilemma of the disease process of acute salpingitis. In addition, the needs of the woman affected by salpingitis are determined through the nursing process.

If the nurse practitioner assesses the salpingitis client using the medical model alone, almost total emphasis is placed on physiological needs. By using the nursing process model of assessment, the practitioner assigns top priority to physiological problems but will subsequently address other important client needs.

Risk factors

A number of factors increase the likelihood of acquiring salpingitis. These factors should be noted during the history because they may precipitate events that lead to clinical disease.

Menstruation. It is recognized that menstruation plays a significant role in salpingitis. Sixty-six percent to 75% of women with gonococcal salpingitis develop symptoms during or within 7 days of menses. It is theorized that menstruation is involved in the breakdown of local host defense mechanisms that usually prevent vaginal and cervical flora from ascending into the endometrium (Falk and Krook, 1967). The cervical mucous plug dissipates during menses and may allow bacterial access to the endometrium. Menstrual blood may act as a transport system for gonococci when it refluxes into the tube and carries the organisms with it. In addition, menstrual blood is an excellent culture medium for bacteriological growth. Most authorities believe that hormonal changes during the menstrual cycle do not affect growth of gonococcus.

Previous history of gonorrhea. A past history of gonorrhea increases the incidence of either gonococcal or nongonococcal salpingitis. Of the 10% to 17% of women with cervical gonorrhea who develop salpingitis, most will develop it during the first one or two menstrual cycles after acquisition of gonorrhea (Eschenbach, 1976). In addition, gonorrhea may increase the risk of upper tract infection from other bacteria by mucosal damage to the endosalpinx.

It is also important to note a history of gonorrhea and subsequent treatment in the male sexual contact. Most recurrences of gonococcal salpingitis are due to reinfection. In addition, the general public believes that all gonorrhea in males is symptomatic; thus men informed of venereal contact are not likely to seek treatment if they are asymptomatic. However, asymptomatic gonorrhea may occur in 40% of a selected male population (Handsfield and others, 1974).

Method of contraception. Much controversy exists over the role of the IUD and the development of acute salpingitis. Initially, salpingitis occurring more than 2 months after IUD insertion was considered unrelated to the device (Mishell and Moyer, 1969). More recently Ishihama and associates (1970) noted a constant rate of positive endometrial cultures of 4% to 5.5% up to 5 years after insertion. Eschenbach (1976) postulates that bacteria do not persist but are reintroduced in the endometrium during menses or coitus. The IUD may alter the normal local host defense mechanisms in some manner and lead to pelvic infection. IUD users have a significantly increased risk of salpingitis (Wright and Laemmle, 1968; Targum and Wright, 1974). The risk of acute salpingitis for any woman using an IUD increases eightfold as compared with nonusers; for nulliparas the risk is even greater (Westrom and others, 1976). The frequency of cervical gonorrhea is unrelated to IUD use. There is also no difference related to type of IUD, whether plastic or copper containing. In Westrom's study, 25% of salpingitis occurred within 4 weeks of insertion, and 58% occurred longer than 2 months after insertion. The frequency of sexual intercourse, the length of contraception, and the number of sexual partners do not appear to influence the rate of salpingitis in IUD users (Faulkner and Ory, 1976).

Eschenbach (1976) has noted that IUD users with salpingitis have a clinical picture different from that of non-IUD users with salpingitis. In both gonococcal and nongonococcal salpingitis, temperatures greater than 100.8° F were less common in IUD users than in non-IUD users. Adnexal masses were more common in nongonococcal salpingitis clients with IUDs than in non-IUD users. The isolation of *N. gonorrhoeae* from the peritoneal fluid was similar in both groups, but there was an increased rate of isolation of nongonococcal bacteria from the peritoneal fluid of IUD users with salpingitis as compared with that of non-IUD users. No particular type of IUD has been associated with an increased risk of pelvic infections in nonpregnant women, although the Dalkon Shield has been implicated in septic abortion (Christian, 1974). The above findings have far-reaching implications in the recommendation of IUDs for nulliparas or women with prior history of salpingitis. Oral contraceptives have been associated with a lower rate of salpingitis than normally expected for women who use contraception (Hager and Wiesner, 1977).

Number of sexual partners. Targum and Wright revealed no difference between salpingitis and control groups in the number of sex partners in the previous 4 months. The frequency of sexual intercourse was the same for the two groups. Flesh and associates (1979) found the number of sex partners in the previous 12 months in an indigent population to be a significant risk factor. The investigators do not know if the same risk factors would emerge among salpingitis clients in a high socioeconomic group. This discrepancy requires further investigation.

Race, blood group, health-seeking behavior. Black women have a higher incidence of salpingitis than nonblack women (Hager and Wiesner). A number of factors may explain this phenomenon. The average time between onset of symptoms and treatment may be greater for blacks than for whites. Many studies use lower socioeconomic populations; thus these results do not generalize to all women. Poor women in general have limited access to medical care and may seek treatment only when a problem is severe. ABO blood type gene frequencies may contribute to the acquisition of gonorrhea. The prevalence of gonorrhea was significant for blood type B in one study of black indigent women (Hager and Wiesner). Further study in these areas is needed to identify specific risk factors in the development of salpingitis.

History

Chief complaint. Evaluation of the chief complaint of acute abdominal pain should include its location, duration, intensity, radiation, onset, and relieving or exacerbating factors. Any symptoms that accompany the pain, including vaginal discharge, diarrhea, constipation, dysuria, nausea, vomiting, fever, or anorexia should be noted.

Review of systems. The client should be questioned about any urinary symptoms such as frequency, urgency, dysuria, hematuria, nocturia, or flank pain. The practitioner should ask about a history of kidney stones. Dark or brown urine may be a helpful clue. Questions relevant to gastrointestinal system relate to color of stools (black, tarry, clay colored), presence of melena, rectal bleeding, diarrhea, or constipation. The practitioner should ask about nausea, vomiting, anorexia, indigestion, or pain related to food intake and note if the client reports the onset of jaundice.

The gynecological review should include gravidity, parity, and date of the last menstrual period. Menstrual symptoms of importance are amenorrhea, intermenstrual vaginal bleeding, and presence of cramps before or throughout menses. The presence, duration, color, and amount of vaginal discharge are important. The practitioner should record the type of contraception and whether it is routinely used. The client should be asked if she thinks she may be pregnant or if she has ever had an abortion and when. Any gynecological conditions such as endometriosis, prior salpingitis, or history of gonorrhea should be noted. The practitioner should question the client about treatment for gonorrhea and determine if the sexual partner was also treated for venereal disease (VD). The client should also be questioned about surgeries, particularly appendectomy or tubal surgery.

Life-style. The social history should include a sexual history. The practitioner should note the frequency of intercourse, its recency, type of contraception used, number of partners, and new sexual partners within the last year. The client should be questioned about the presence of VD or penile discharge in a male partner. The variability of sexual expression, including vaginal, rectal, and oral penetration, should be noted. Painful vaginal intercourse is also an important finding. Marital status, number of children, and working status are important in the planning of the client's care.

Past history. The practitioner should question the client about any serious illnesses, particularly pyelonephritis, duodenal ulcer, pancreatitis, gallbladder disease, Crohn's disease, or diverticulitis. Any surgeries, especially abdominal ones, should be noted. The practitioner should note any allergies and the names of medications or treatments tried recently.

Physical examination

Assessment of acute abdominal pain challenges the skills of even the most advanced practitioners. Before abdominal assessment, the skin, lymph nodes, chest, heart, head, and neck should be examined. A thorough assessment of the female client requires pelvic examination.

During inspection of the abdomen, contour, scars, dilated veins, color changes, peristalsis, pulsatile movements, and masses should be noted. Auscultation may detect a murmur in an abdominal blood vessel or increased peristalsis. The absence of bowel sounds is abnormal and should be noted only if the examiner listens for at least 5 minutes. Percussion should note any areas of tympany or dullness. Palpation should locate areas of light or deep abdominal tenderness as well as rebound tenderness. The femoral pulses should be palpable. The location, size, shape, consistency, mobility, pulsatility, and tenderness of any masses should be noted.

Pelvic examination notes the presence of discharge and whether it is vaginal or originates from the upper tract (uterus, tubes, ovaries). The practitioner should note the appearance of the cervix and determine its color, the presence of blood or tissue at the os, and the presence of any lesions. The practitioner should note if tenderness is present with speculum insertion; this can be assessed only in a relaxed and cooperative client. All necessary laboratory data should be obtained. Bimanual examination may reveal local heat in the pelvic region, cervical motion tenderness, adnexal tenderness, enlarged uterus or ovaries, or thickened tubes or masses. A full bladder may be mistaken for an abnormal mass.

Rectal examination and rectovaginal examination may confirm findings with the vaginal bimanual examination. The practitioner should also note any rectal masses, tenderness, and the presence of any stool or hemorrhoids. Table 11-2 notes pertinent physical findings in the female with acute abdominal pain and the likely associated pathological conditions.

Table 11-2. Possible physical findings and the likely associated pathological conditions in females with acute abdominal pain

Findings	Pathological conditions
General	
Fever	Salpingitis
	Pyelonephritis
	Appendicitis (if fever low grade)
	Septic abortion
Orthostatic change in blood pressure, pulse	Ruptured ectopic pregnancy
	Ruptured appendix
	Hemorrhagic ovarian cyst
Abdominal examination	
Abdominal distention	Ovarian cyst
	Pregnancy
	Feces
	Hepatomegaly
	Splenomegaly
Bluish umbilicus	Blood in peritoneum
Abdominal murmur	Possible aortic aneurysm
Absent bowel sounds	Peritonitis (multiple causes)
	Advanced bowel obstruction
Abdominal tenderness	
Acute epigastric	Early appendicitis
	Perforated peptic ulcer
	Pancreatitis
	Dissecting aneurysm
Right upper quadrant (RUQ)	Cholecystitis
	Cholelithiasis
	Hepatitis
	Right-sided pleurisy
	Right ureteral colic
	Pyelonephritis
RUQ radiating to right scapula	Cholecystitis
Left upper quadrant	Ureteral colic
	Pyelonephritis
Right lower quadrant	Appendicitis
	Meckel's diverticulum
	Crohn's disease
	Perforated duodenal ulcer
	Ectopic pregnancy
	Ovarian cyst
	Mittelschmerz
	Unilateral salpingitis
Left lower quadrant	Diverticulitis
	Ectopic pregnancy
	Ovarian cyst
	Mittelschmerz
	Unilateral salpingitis

Continued.

Table 11-2. Possible physical findings and the likely associated pathological conditions in females with acute abdominal pain—cont'd

Findings	Pathological conditions
Abdominal tenderness —cont'd	
Bilateral lower quadrant	Salpingitis
	Torsion of ovarian cyst
RUQ and bilateral lower quadrant	Gonococcal salpingitis (perihepatitis)
Costovertebral angle (right or left)	Pyelonephritis
Four quadrant with rebound	Peritonitis: multiple causes
Pelvic and rectal examination	
Bleeding and/or tissue present at os	Threatened inevitable or incomplete abortion
Purulent exudate from os	Salpingitis
	Endometritis
	Septic abortion
Cervical softening or cyanosis	Pregnancy
	Fibroid tumors
	Uterine neoplasm
Uterine tenderness	Endometritis
Bilateral adnexal tenderness	Salpingitis
Unilateral lower quadrant tenderness	Salpingitis
	Ectopic pregnancy
	Ovarian cyst
	Torsion of ovarian cyst
	Acute inflammatory bowel disease
Adnexal mass	Ectopic pregnancy
	Ovarian cyst
	Tuboovarian cyst
	Neoplasm
	Endometriosis
	Oophoritis
	Tuboovarian abscess
Pelvic mass	Endometriosis
	Neoplasm
	Ectopic pregnancy
	Feces
Vaginal discharge	Salpingitis
	Septic abortion
	Coincidental vaginitis
	Normal leukorrhea of pregnancy

Table 11-3. Laboratory data and associated pathological conditions in the woman with acute pelvic pain

Test	Findings	Pathological conditions
WBC	15,000-30,000/cu mm	Salpingitis
	10,000-18,000/cu mm	Appendicitis
	6,000-15,000/cu mm	Ectopic pregnancy
	6,000-20,000/cu mm	Septic abortion
ESR	Markedly elevated	Salpingitis
	Mildly elevated	Ectopic pregnancy
	Mildly elevated	Appendicitis
Hct	Falling serial measurements	Ectopic pregnancy (ruptured)
		Hemorrhagic ovarian cyst
Serum pregnancy (qualitative)	+	Ectopic pregnancy
		Threatened abortion
Urine pregnancy	−	Does not exclude ectopic pregnancy
	+	Ectopic pregnancy, threatened abortion
GC culture	+	Gonococcal salpingitis
Gram stain of urine (clean catch or catheterized)	Bacteria	Urinary tract infection
Endocervical Gram stain	Gram-negative intracellular diplococci	Gonococcal salpingitis
Wet mount of vaginal secretions	Bacteria	Vaginitis existing with other pathological conditions
	Yeast	
	White blood cells	
	Trichomonads	

Laboratory data

Clinical laboratory tests that are helpful in the assessment of acute pelvic pain include a complete blood count with differential, sedimentation rate, VDRL, urinalysis, urine pregnancy test, and possibly a serum pregnancy test. A wet mount evaluation of the vaginal discharge also is suggested. A Gram stain of endocervical exudate may not be reliable. When used by experienced personnel, the identification of gram-negative intracellular diplococci may be helpful to distinguish between gonococcal and nongonococcal salpingitis. A negative smear does not exclude gonorrhea, and false positive smears can occur in women. Thus final results in most instances must rely on gonorrhea culture. Historical and physical findings may help differentiate between gonococcal and nongonococcal salpingitis. Table 11-3 summarizes laboratory data and associated pathological conditions in the client with abdominal pain. It is pointless to obtain aerobic and anaerobic cultures from the endocervix to distinguish organisms other than gonorrhea. However, a specimen should be obtained for culture of *N. gonorrhoeae*. This is plated directly onto a solid medium, such as Thayer-Martin agar. These cultures can have 10% false negative rate. The use of two consecutive swabs in the endocervix for each Thayer-Martin plate may improve recovery of cervical gonococcus. Throat and rectal cultures may also be appropriate, depending on the client's sexual history or the institution's protocol.

Culdocentesis is useful in diagnosis especially when intraabdominal bleeding is suspected. A needle is introduced into the cul-de-sac and the contents are tested. A culdocentesis that returns nonclotting blood is diagnostic of intraabdominal hemorrhage and may suggest a ruptured ectopic pregnancy or a ruptured hemorrhagic cyst. These situations necessitate immediate surgical intervention. A return of purulent aspirate indicates an infection. A negative culdocentesis is one in which clear peritoneal fluid is obtained. A culdocentesis that does not yield any return is nondiagnostic. There is some controversy as to the accuracy of bacteriological data obtained by culdocentesis (Sweet and others).

Laparoscopy is a method used to obtain material from the fallopian tubes. In addition to microbiological specificity, laparoscopic examination allows the establishment of a definite diagnosis. Because of the serious prognostic implications for the woman with acute salpingitis and the difficulty in establishing an accurate diagnosis, laparoscopy may become more widely used.

Sonography (pelvic ultrasound) is not helpful in the assessment of acute salpingitis unless abscesses are present. However, it is useful to confirm the presence of adnexal masses, especially in women who have not responded favorably to adequate antibiotic therapy. Serial sonography is also helpful to evaluate the resolution of tuboovarian abscesses that have been treated with medical management.

Differential diagnosis

The classic description of acute salpingitis includes pelvic pain, abnormal vaginal discharge, cervical motion tenderness, adnexal tenderness, fever, leukocytosis, and increased erythrocyte sedimentation rate. However, objective clinical data to substantiate these signs and symptoms are without confirmation (Sweet, 1977). Many believe that acute salpingitis demonstrates a variety of symptoms (Eschenbach and Holmes). Laparoscopic confirmation shows that diagnosis of acute salpingitis based on commonly accepted clinical criteria may be inaccurate. Jacobson and Westrom (1969) found that 65% of subjects diagnosed initially with salpingitis actually had salpingitis on laparoscopic examination. Twenty-three percent of symptomatic women had normal pelvic anatomy, and 12% revealed other lower abdominal conditions. In addition, only 20% of documented salpingitis cases demonstrated the classic symptoms of acute salpingitis. The practitioner should keep in mind that reliance on the presence of all symptoms before diagnosis will lead to inaccurate assessment and poor planning (Eschenbach and Holmes). Table 11-4 lists common diseases in the differential diagnosis of acute salpingitis.

Acute salpingitis. Lower abdominal pain, typically bilateral, and adnexal tenderness are the most reliable findings in acute salpingitis (Eschenbach and Holmes). Unilateral salpingitis occurs less often but has been documented laparoscopically (Falk, 1965). Cervical motion tenderness is usually present, but not always; diagnosis of salpingitis cannot be excluded based on the absence of this finding. Likewise, cervical motion tenderness may be present in other conditions, such as ectopic pregnancy. No adnexal masses are palpable unless pyosalpinx is present. A purulent vaginal discharge exuding from the os, not merely in the vaginal pool, also suggests upper tract infection. Liver tenderness and onset of pain after menses are more common with gonococcal salpingitis. In nongonococcal salpingitis, fever, menstrual association, and liver tenderness are less common (Table 11-1). A history of IUD use is often associated with salpingitis. An

Table 11-4. Comparative signs and symptoms in differential diagnosis of acute pelvic pain

	Salpingitis	Appendicitis	Ruptured ovarian cyst	Ectopic pregnancy	Urinary tract infection	Inflammatory bowel disease	Endometritis
Fever	40%+*	Low grade, <101° F	—	—	+ or −	+ or −	—
Location	Bilateral adnexal or RUQ	Periumbilical to RLQ with + rebound	Unilateral adnexal, Resolves in few hours	Unilateral adnexal	Suprapubic, flank pain	Variable cramping	Lower abdomen
Radiation	—	—	To shoulder with hemorrhage	To shoulder with rupture	To vulva with pyelonephritis	—	—
Relationship to menses	Menstrual changes; GC: onset during or within 7 days of menses	—	May be late, may not	Amenorrhea possibly, 90% late spotting common	—	—	Most severe before menses and during maximal flow
GI symptoms	Nausea, vomiting late in disease; infrequent	Anorexia, nausea, vomiting	Rare	Nausea or vomiting of pregnancy Vomiting after rupture	Nausea, vomiting, variable	Diarrhea, nausea, constipation, vomiting	+ with extensive disease
GU symptoms	Dysuria with GC	—	—	—	+	—	+ with extensive disease
Sexual activity	GC: new or multiple partners	Unrelated	Dyspareunia	History of unprotected intercourse or poor contraception	—	Possible dyspareunia	Dyspareunia
Cervical motion tenderness	Exam +; also dyspareunia	—	—	+	—	—	+ or −
Adnexal tenderness	+	—	+	+	—	—	+ or −
Other findings	Possible mass, IUD user	Possible rectal tenderness	Faintness at onset of pain with rupture	Mass unilateral or in cul-de-sac, prior tubal surgery or salpingitis, IUD user	—	—	—

*+ Positive, − negative.

endocervical Gram stain may reveal gram-negative intracellular diplococci in gonococcal salpingitis. An elevated white blood count with relatively more polymorphonucleated cells (left shift) may be present. Sedimentation rate may be markedly elevated, and urinalysis should be normal. If infection has progressed significantly, the peritoneum will be inflamed; this is indicated by generalized abdominal tenderness, distention, rebound tenderness, and hypotonic bowel sounds. Nausea, vomiting, and fever are likely. The practitioner should keep in mind that peritoneal signs are nonspecific and that all other causes of peritonitis need consideration.

Appendicitis. The history is helpful to exclude an inflamed appendix. When the appendix is typically placed, the sequence of events is initial epigastric pain, followed by nausea and vomiting. Next the pain shifts to the right lower quadrant and is expressed by tenderness there. Fever then appears and finally leukocytosis. When right lower quadrant tenderness is present, the temperature is usually between 101° and 103° F. If the appendix ruptures, fever, pain, and leukocytosis increase with the formation of a tender abscess or the appearance of peritoneal signs. Atypical presentations of appendicitis do occur occasionally. When one is in doubt about the assessment, close observation, consultation, and hospitalization may be necessary to prevent a ruptured appendix.

Ruptured or hemorrhagic ovarian cyst. Follicle and corpus leuteum cysts are normal structures that represent accumulation of fluid from an incompletely developed follicle. A follicle cyst usually disappears with ovulation. It may continue to grow and become a palpable mass at the surface of the ovaries. Before rupture, it can cause local lower abdominal pain, dyspareunia, and occasionally abnormal uterine bleeding. The corresponding ovary-adnexal area may be tender on examination. The pain may appear as severe as that in salpingitis or appendicitis, but after rupture it usually resolves within several hours. The pain may also radiate to the ipsilateral shoulder and may be accompanied by nausea or vomiting. Rarely during the normal course of rupture (before ovulation) a blood vessel on the surface of the ovary may tear and bleed. If it is a large vessel, intraperitoneal bleeding may be extensive, producing tachycardia, hypotension, falling hematocrit levels, and syncope. Vaginal bleeding is usually absent. History reveals a normal prior menstrual period. The serum pregnancy test is negative. With extensive bleeding, surgery may be required. Fever, leukocytosis, and dysuria are absent. A corpus luteum cyst may fail to involute and may continue to grow and secrete progesterone, delaying menses. The ovary may approach 4 to 6 cm in size. A persistent cyst may cause severe and sudden adnexal pain and tenderness. A mass is palpable, and it too may rupture and bleed, causing blood to collect in the peritoneum. A prior history of ammenorrhea or delayed menstruation followed by brisk bleeding before the expected date of menses are helpful clues. Hemorrhagic ovarian cysts may be confused with ectopic pregnancy and require consultation and referral. Leukocytosis is absent, and serum pregnancy test is negative. Most ovarian cysts resolve in 60 days and are asymptomatic.

Mittelschmerz. Cyclic intermenstrual pain is associated with ovulation and is common in young women. The pain may range from mild to severe, with acute abdominal pain lasting less than 1 day. It is noncramping and nonradiating, and unaccompanied by fever, nausea, vomiting, or vaginal discharge. The appearance of midcycle pain is highly suggestive, and the client should have a normal prior menstrual history.

Ovarian torsion. A corpus luteum cyst or teratoma may cause the ovary to twist, resulting in severe, sudden adnexal pain or suprapubic pain accompanied by vomiting, obstipation, and adnexal mass. The pain is unrelated to menses, the pregnancy test is negative, and leukocytosis occurs later in the disease process. Consultation and referral are essential.

Ectopic pregnancy. Extrauterine pregnancy may cause unilateral adnexal pain and cramps before rupture. Almost half of ectopic pregnancies occur in the right tube; afflicted clients may give a history of prior salpingitis or may be using an IUD. History includes vaginal bleeding within 1 to 8 weeks after a missed period. The pain is usually severe and may radiate to the shoulder. The client may have pregnancy symptoms, but the pregnancy test may be negative. On examination an adnexal mass is palpable, and cervical motion tenderness is present. Intraabdominal bleeding may be present with bulging of the cul-de-sac. Leukocytosis, low hematocrit values, fever, and slightly increased sedimentation rate may be observed. Consultation and referral are essential.

Threatened abortion. When the client complains of severe lower abdominal cramping, a "missed period," nausea, vomiting, and vaginal bleeding, the possibility of threatened abortion should be suspected. A negative pregnancy test will not exclude this consideration. Rebound tenderness, adnexal tenderness, and cervical motion tenderness should be absent. White blood count, urinalysis, and sedimentation rate should be normal. Threatened abortion may also appear as painless vaginal bleeding. Consultation may be necessary.

Infected septic abortion. Occasionally a client will have a therapeutic abortion performed with subsequent infection due to instrumentation. The client will have a tender uterus, cervix, and possibly adnexa. Vaginal bleeding, discharge, fever, nausea and vomiting, and rebound phenomena may be present. With a clumsy attempt, the cervix or upper vagina may be injured. If this situation is suspected referral is essential.

Urinary tract infections. The client may have cystitis with accompanying fever, dysuria, and suprapubic pain. The pain is usually not severe or sudden and may be worsened during micturition. The pelvic examination should be normal; urinalysis may reveal bacteria or pyuria. Many women with cystitis complain of concomitant vaginal discharge. In pyelonephritis, costovertebral angle tenderness may be present, along with fever, nausea, vomiting, and abnormal urinalysis. With renal colic, flank pain radiating to the vulva may be excruciating and sudden. Urinalysis may show pyuria and blood; the client may complain of hematuria, nausea, vomiting, or a prior history of kidney stones. Pelvic examination should be normal.

Inflammatory bowel disease. Gastroenteritis, ulcerative colitis, regional enteritis, and diverticulitis may be confused with salpingitis. With gastroenteritis, abdominal pain may be sudden and generalized, and accompanied by nausea, vomiting, and diarrhea. With severe diarrhea or vomiting, dehydration may be present. The symptoms are unrelated to menses, and the pelvic examination is normal. Generalized tenderness may be present over the abdomen, and bowel sounds may be hyperactive. With diverticulitis, the pain may be localized to the left lower quadrant. A sausage-shaped mass in the left lower quadrant may be palpable on abdominal examination. The client is usually over 40 and gives a history of chronic constipation. If diverticulae rupture, fever and peritonitis may occur. A prior history of intermittent left lower quadrant pain and a negative menstrual history are common. During pelvic examination, cervical-adnexal tenderness and mass are absent. With ulcerative colitis, diarrhea with mucus or blood accompanies generalized abdominal pain. Fever may be present; weight loss is present with excessive diarrhea. Defecation may cause severe abdominal cramping. The pelvic examination is normal. With regional enteritis (Crohn's disease) right lower quadrant pain occurs with diarrhea, which is usually chronic and may lead to weight loss. Abdominal pain may be similar to that of appendicitis.

Endometriosis. Abdominal pain is constant and most severe before menses. The history includes deep-thrust dyspareunia. Dysmenorrhea occurs before menses, with the most pain during maximal flow. In the early stages of the disease, only tenderness of involved structures is present. No abnormal vaginal discharge is noted. As disease progresses, implants or tender pelvic masses are palpable. The uterus may be fixed and painful on manipulation. The ovaries may be enlarged. Infertility is a common complaint; fever and leukocytosis are absent. Consultation and referral for laparoscopic verification are necessary. Occasionally an endometrioma may rupture, accompanied by sudden severe abdominal pain requiring surgical attention.

PLAN

The literature documents the difficulties in accurately diagnosing acute salpingitis. Usually this refers to problems differentiating salpingitis from other serious pathological conditions. An equally troubling situation is management of the woman with fewer and milder signs and symptoms. The practitioner must decide if there is sufficient evidence to commit the client to a course of therapy or to simply observe the client without beginning therapy. It is not uncommon for a woman to complain of low abdominal pain after the onset of menses, have a minimally tender exam, and be sent home with a diagnosis of dysmenorrhea only to return a few days later with a classic and severe picture of acute salpingitis. Although no one wants to needlessly treat a woman with antibiotics, many physicians prefer to overtreat than to undertreat by withholding therapy.

In the assessment of acute salpingitis without laparoscopic visualization, decisions are based on probabilities and not on absolutes. After assessing the situation in which a woman has acute pelvic pain, the practitioner must decide whether a diagnosis can be made and a treatment plan initiated, or whether consultation with a physician is appropriate. There are also times when referral to another health care facility may be necessary. The goal of management of acute salpingitis is to prevent infertility and chronic residua of tubal infection, such as adhesions, chronic pain, hydropyosalpinx and tubo-ovarian abscess, which often require surgical intervention.

Medication

In order for antibiotic therapy to be effective to prevent the sequelae of salpingitis, it must be instituted early in the disease process. The antibiotic regimen should also cover the polymicrobial cause of acute salpingitis. Controversy has arisen over the issue of outpatient treatment with oral antibiotics versus inpatient treatment with parenteral antibiotics in clients with acute salpingitis. No prospective investigation has been done to evaluate which is more appropriate and effective. We believe that in-hospital therapy with high-dose parenteral antibiotics will result in the best prognosis for these women. However, this is often infeasible or uneconomical; the majority of clients with acute salpingitis are treated in ambulatory care settings.

Table 11-5 presents outpatient treatment of acute salpingitis. Cuningham and asso-

Table 11-5. CDC-recommended schedule for outpatient treatment of acute salpingitis, 1979

Drug	Dosage	Nursing implications
Tetracycline hydrochloride	500 mg p.o. q.i.d. × 10 days	Do not use in pregnant women
		Take ½ h a.c. or 2 h p.c.
		Do not take with milk or antacids
		May eliminate coexisting chlamydial infection
	or	
Procaine penicillin G	4.8 million units IM	Divide dose to give at two sites
plus probenecid	1 g p.o.	Give at time of injection
followed by amoxicillin or ampicillin*	500 mg p.o. q.i.d. × 10 days	Determine allergic history with all drugs
	or	
Ampicillin	3.5 g p.o. in one dose	Take simultaneously
plus probenecid	1 g p.o.	
followed by amoxicillin or ampicillin*	500 mg p.o. q.i.d. × 10 days	
	or	
Amoxacillin*	3.0 g p.o. in one dose	Take simultaneously
plus probenecid	1 g p.o.	
followed by amoxicillin or ampicillin*	500 mg p.o. q.i.d. × 10 days	

*Amoxicillin achieves higher blood levels than ampicillin, and may cause less diarrhea. Either may be taken with food.

ciates (1977) compared tetracycline with penicillin-ampicillin salpingitis treatments and reported excellent results with both regimens. However, preliminary evaluation of a Centers for Disease Control (CDC)–sponsored, multicenter investigation revealed both regimens to be associated with a significantly higher failure rate for treatment of both gonococcal and nongonococcal disease (Thompson, 1979). Changes in the currently recommended antibiotic regimens for the treatment of outpatient salpingitis must await future investigation and confirmation of these preliminary findings.

Activity

The practitioner should encourage bed rest and reduced activity level for at least 2 or 3 days. If nausea is present, small frequent feedings may be helpful. Although many clinicians recommend semi-Fowler's position to promote pelvic drainage, there is little documentation of its effectiveness (Wright, 1976).

Pain relief

Abdominal discomfort can be reduced by the use of analgesics. Aspirin or Phenaphen with codeine may be necessary, depending on the severity of pain. Aspirin, 10 grains every 4 hours as needed, is useful in most ambulatory care settings because masking pain may prevent assessment of resistance to antibiotics or clinical deterioration. Pelvic heat is also comforting, although of unproven therapeutic value. Sitz baths 2 or 3 times daily may reduce pain. Restricting garments, such as belts, tight pants, or girdles, should be discouraged.

Psychosocial support

For some clients gonococcal salpingitis can initiate a marital or relationship crisis. Anticipatory guidance may give the client an opportunity to discuss methods of presenting and working through the moment of disclosure. The client should be reminded that the practitioner is available for further counseling and, if necessary, can arrange referral to a professional counselor. Personal embarrassment may also accompany the diagnosis of gonococcal salpingitis; the practitioner should allow the client to verbalize feelings.

Sexual contact

Sexual activity should be discouraged for approximately 2 weeks. Vaginal or rectal intercourse may increase discomfort as well as reinfect the client. When the assessment is gonococcal salpingitis, the practitioner should stress the importance of having the partner treated. Specific instructions regarding sexual contact need to be shared with the client. This may also serve as an opportunity for the client to receive contraceptive information.

Health education

The practitioner should discuss situations that require an early return visit. Localized or increasing abdominal pain, persistent vomiting, pain on inspiration, decreased urination, or prostration require immediate return for evaluation. Otherwise the client should be informed that abdominal pain and fever should decrease markedly within 48 hours.

A lack of understanding and appreciation of the scope of acute salpingitis and its consequences has specific adverse effects on the woman with this disease. A client is much less likely to comply with a treatment schedule when she does not clearly understand the goals of that treatment and also the potential hazards of ignoring the recommendation. Lack of compliance in taking the medication may appear as a treatment failure. Taking a tablet 4 times a day for 10 days is much more difficult than it seems. The client must be highly motivated in order to be compliant. It is hoped that motivation can be fostered through health education. It is important to get the message across to the client that she effects the cure and that the providers serve as advocates and consultants. The client is ultimately responsible for her own health care status.

The practitioner is usually not in a position to carry the burden of being a total resource person and should be aware of community agencies that offer appropriate services. Most cities now have efficient, confidential clinics for sexually transmitted disease that can be useful for partner referral. In addition, the city health departments have outreach workers who are experienced in dealing with the often awkward aspects of notifying and treating consorts. The CDC offers a telephone hot line (VD national hot line) to handle inquiries on sexually related diseases. The number is 1-800-227-8922.

EVALUATION
Expected outcomes

The client's subjective pain is generally the first criterion used to evaluate treatment effectiveness. If the client complies with the antibiotic regimen and maintains pelvic rest, abdominal pain should decrease significantly within 48 to 72 hours after antibiotic therapy is initiated. The endocervical gonorrhea culture results are ready at this time as well, and they may be shared with the client.

The next evaluation is 1 week after starting therapy. At the 1-week follow-up repeat endocervical, rectal, and throat cultures should be obtained to ensure eradication of *N. gonorrhoeae* in those clients who had positive cultures. The practitioner should ask if the partner has been treated. Abdominal tenderness should be decreased by client report, since a bimanual pelvic examination is deferred at this time.

After completion of the 10-day course of antibiotics, the 2-week follow-up visit should find the client essentially pain free and without other associated signs or symptoms. Not uncommonly, a woman will return for follow-up with *Candida* vaginitis superinfection. Some practitioners will treat this prophylactically with an antifungal agent at the initiation of therapy. This may be preferable for women with recurrent candidiasis, those taking oral contraceptives, or those with diabetes. We prefer to advise the client of the possibility of a *Candida* vaginitis infection, discuss the options of prophylactic or symptomatic treatment, and let the client decide which plan she prefers.

The physical examination at the 14-day follow-up visit should be essentially normal. Any tests that previously had abnormal results are repeated. A common and difficult problem occurs when there is some residual adnexal tenderness. It may be appropriate to prolong therapy or try an alternative antibiotic regimen. Because the inflammatory process involved in salpingitis can produce adhesions, a woman may persist to have a minimally tender examination for years after the infectious episode. It is difficult, if not impossible, to differentiate between an acute low-grade resolving salpingitis and chronic residua of inflammation on the basis of pelvic examination. An increased sedimentation rate may indicate infection as opposed to adhesions. The practitioner must evaluate each case individually and seek consultation.

Guidelines for referral

The logistics of nurse practitioner–physician collaboration are determined by the individuals involved and by specific work settings. Obviously the consultation needs and practices of the practitioner in a remote, rural setting will differ from those of a practitioner in a large university medical center.

What follows are some general guidelines and specific criteria to identify the high-risk salpingitis client. This client will warrant, when feasible, physician consultation and perhaps hospitalization. The practitioner should consider the woman with an unclear diagnosis as high risk. Unless the practitioner can exclude with reasonable certainty the potentially serious problems of ectopic pregnancy, appendicitis, and ruptured hemorrhagic cyst, physician consultation is needed. Also considered high risk is the woman who has more than mild, uncomplicated salpingitis. Women in this latter category are those salpingitis clients with one or more of the following findings:

1. Possible or actual adnexal mass
2. IUD
3. Temperature greater than 100.4° F
4. Upper abdominal peritoneal signs
5. Pregnancy
6. Unable to take oral medications

7. Failure to respond to outpatient therapy
8. Adolescents with their first episode
9. Serious concomitant illness, such as pyelonephritis or diabetes

Infertility

Before the use of antibiotics, many cases of acute salpingitis spontaneously resolved without sequelae (Curtis, 1921, 1933). It has been claimed that the advent of antibiotics has improved the prognosis for acute salpingitis: mortality has been eliminated; the frequency of ruptured pelvic abscesses and persistent masses requiring surgery has decreased; and the subsequent fertility rate has improved (Hedberg and Anberg, 1965). Westrom (1975) has shown that reinfection is the factor with the strongest effect on fertility rates. Compared with a 3% rate of involuntary infertility among controls, a single episode of salpingitis resulted in a 13% incidence of infertility. A second episode was associated with a 33.5% infertility rate. With three episodes of salpingitis, the infertility rate rose to 75%. In this study, one quarter of the clients had more than one episode of acute salpingitis. Eschenbach (1975) has found a high incidence of early gonorrhea recurrence among women with gonococcal salpingitis. Within 10 weeks of obtaining a posttreatment negative endocervical culture of *N. gonorrhoeae,* 25% of women had a recurrence of endocervical gonorrhea. This high recurrence rate is felt to be a result of reinfection acquired from untreated asymptomatic male carriers. These data emphasize how important it is for the practitioner to adequately inform the client about salpingitis and sexually transmitted diseases and to be involved in the referral process or in the evaluation and treatment of male contacts. Negligence in these areas may be the major cause of recurrent salpingitis and its associated poor prognosis for fertility.

CASE STUDY
Subjective

A 17-year-old black, gravida 1, para 1, girl has come to the outpatient department with an 18-hour history of lower abdominal pain. Her menstrual period started 3 days previously. The client was well until the day before seeking care, when she noted gradual onset of continuous lower quadrant pain. The pain increased in intensity, with the right lower quadrant pain greater than the left. The pain is described as sharp and aching and radiated to the back. She denies fever, chills, nausea, vomiting, and urinary symptoms. Her last bowel movement was on the day before the visit and was normal. The client denies any pregnancy symptoms and says that her appetite has been fair. She has been sexually active with a new partner for the past 2 weeks. She has not used any form of birth control since the normal, spontaneous vaginal delivery of a healthy boy 2 years previously. She reports her menstrual periods as regular, every 28 to 30 days, with 4 days of flow and with minimal cramping.

Past medical history. There is no prior history of salpingitis, gonorrhea, or other problems. There are no known allergies, chronic illnesses, surgeries, or routinely taken medications. She denies alcohol and tobacco use.

Family history. This is noncontributory.

Social history. The client lives with her 23-month-old son and is not working or attending school. She receives financial assistance from the state and reports a close relationship with and support from an older sister who lives nearby.

Review of systems. This is noncontributory.

Objective

General. Ht, 5 ft 2 in; wt, 100 lb; BP, 84/64; T, 99; P, 92; R, 20. The client is a well-developed, well-nourished female in mild distress, yet very cooperative. The entire physical examination is normal except for the following.

Abdomen. The abdomen is soft and flat; bowel sounds are present. There are no masses. There is moderate bilateral, lower quadrant palpatory tenderness without rebound.

Pelvic and rectal exam. Examination reveals purulent discharge in the vagina and from the cervical os, cervical motion tenderness, mild uterine tenderness, and bilateral adnexal tenderness without masses. The rectovaginal exam is confirmatory.

Laboratory data. Hct, 37.3%; Hb, 12.8; WBC, 11.9, with a normal differential; ESR, mildly elevated. Urine is contaminated by many epithelial cells. Urine pregnancy test is negative. Wet mount of vaginal discharge reveals many WBCs. Endocervical culture for GC is positive after 48 hours. Cervical Gram stain shows gram-negative intracellular diplococci.

Problems

1. Acute gonococcal salpingitis
2. Alteration in comfort due to infection
3. Impaired home management due to illness
4. Disturbance in self-concept
5. Potential need for contraception

Plan

In making the assessment of the case just described, the practitioner had many indications that this might be acute gonococcal salpingitis: recent onset of bilateral abdominal pain and yellow discharge around time of menses, absence of nausea and vomiting, and a new sexual partner. The most worrisome factor was a history of unprotected coitus. Fortunately, there was no evidence of pregnancy. The diagnosis in this client was fairly straightforward. Acute salpingitis was certainly the most likely cause of her illness.

Many factors pointed toward the treatment of this young woman as an outpatient. She had negligible elevations of temperature, white blood count, and sedimentation rate; she had no evidence of peritonitis or adnexal masses. By most standards she was well within the criteria to receive oral antibiotic therapy; yet the practitioner considered admission because of the client's age. This line of thinking was a result of the bias, albeit unproven, that parenteral antibiotic treatment will afford the salpingitis client with the best prognosis. Yet hospitalization is often not practical.

An important issue in the decision-making process was the client's 23-month-old child. Certainly it would be traumatic for the child to be separated from his mother because of hospitalization. On the other hand, it is unrealistic to expect the client to rest if she had to care for her son. The practitioner discussed her concerns with this client and explored various solutions. This particular young woman had a strong sense of responsibility and was quite eager to cooperate and participate in her health care planning. She arranged to stay at her sister's house to recuperate while her sister cared for her son.

The client started a 10-day course of tetracycline, 500 mg orally 4 times a day, and pelvic rest (minimal activity and no intercourse) and was advised to call or return if she was not substantially better in 48 hours.

Evaluation

At her first follow-up visit, the client reported that her symptoms had decreased dramatically after 36 hours of antibiotic therapy. She was feeling generally well and having only occasional abdominal pains. Results of the physical exam done at the second-week follow-up visit were essentially normal, with only minimal adnexal tenderness. The client was informed that she should return promptly if any similar signs or symptoms recurred. Recurrent pelvic infections can lead to infertility if they are not treated quickly and adequately.

Cultures from this visit were negative for *N. gonorrhoeae*. However, the client arrived at this visit looking obviously distraught and on the verge of tears. She described a violent argument she had had with her boyfriend (her alleged gonococcus contact) centering around the origin of the gonorrhea infection. He refused to be treated because he was without symptoms and had accused the client of being promiscuous. The practitioner let the client ventilate some of her frustration and hurt. They discussed the possibility of having a health department worker assist her in having the partner receive treatment and, it was hoped, to give him some correct information. The partner did ultimately receive medication, but their relationship seemed to have been permanently marred by the chain of events.

The practitioner also offered to discuss contraception if the client was interested; a handout of contraceptive methods and commonly asked questions was made available. The client appeared interested in the reading material but was not anxious to seek contraceptive counseling at this visit.

This particular case presents a good example of some of the most common problems a practitioner must address with acute salpingitis. Not only is there the challenge of establishing a diagnosis based on physiological criteria, but there is also the need to consider the client's social and biological situation when determining the most beneficial plan of care. There is also the important aspect of helping the client cope with the ramifications of having a sexually transmitted disease.

SUMMARY

Acute salpingitis is one of the most common acute gynecological diseases in the United States. Use of laparoscopy to confirm the diagnosis of acute salpingitis has shown that the signs and symptoms classically ascribed to this disease are not specific to it. Fever, leukocytosis, elevated ESR, and adnexal masses or swelling is not necessary to make a diagnosis of acute salpingitis. Lower abdominal pain and adnexal tenderness are the most consistent findings.

Microbiological data obtained by laparoscopy and culdocentesis have raised questions about the role of *N. gonorrhoeae* in salpingitis. The data have demonstrated that both gonococcal and nongonococcal acute salpingitis are associated with mixed aerobic-anaerobic bacterial flora.

Good results in the treatment of acute salpingitis depend on (1) early diagnosis, (2) bed rest, (3) the use of antibiotic therapy that accounts for the polymicrobial cause of acute salpingitis, and (4) prevention of recurrent episodes of salpingitis through health education and identification of sexual contacts. The future reproductive potential of a young woman must be weighed against both client and practitioner convenience and cost. Finally, the practitioner should be prepared to address the significant psychosocial components of acute salpingitis.

Further investigative efforts are essential to determine the role of IUDs in pelvic infections, to discover the true microbiological cause of salpingitis, and to establish appropriate antimicrobial treatment as determined by prospective, microbiologically controlled investigations.

REFERENCES

Carney, F.E., and Taylor-Robinson, D.: Growth and effect on *Neisseria gonorrhoeae* in organism cultures, Br. J. Vener. Dis. **49:**435, 1973.
Chow, A.W., and others: The bacteriology of acute pelvic inflammatory disease, Am. J. Obstet. Gynecol. **122:** 876, 1975.
Christian, C.D.: Maternal deaths associated with an intrauterine device, Am. J. Obstet. Gynecol. **11:**441, 1974.
Cuningham, F.G., and others: Evaluation of tetracycline or penicillin and ampicillin for treatment of acute pelvic inflammatory disease, N. Engl. J. Med. **296:**1380, 1977.
Curtis, A.H.: Bacteriology and pathology of fallopian tubes removed at operation, Surg. Gynecol. Obstet. **33:**621, 1921.
Curtis, A.H.: Obstetrics and gynecology, vol. XI, Philadelphia, 1933, W.B. Saunders Co.
Dans, P.O.E.: Gonococcal anogenital tract infection, Clin. Obstet. Gynecol. **18:**103, 1975.
Eschenbach, D.A.: Pelvic inflammatory disease. Presented at the Fifteenth Interscience Conference on Antimicrobial Agents and Chemotherapy, Washington, D.C., Sept. 24-26, 1975.
Eschenbach, D.A.: Acute pelvic inflammatory disease: etiology, risk factors and pathogenesis, Clin. Obstet. Gynecol. **19:**147, 1976.
Eschenbach, D.A., and Holmes, K.K.: Acute pelvic inflammatory disease: current concepts of pathogenesis, etiology, and management, Clin. Obstet. Gynecol. **18:**35, 1975.
Falk, V.: Treatment of acute non-tuberculous salpingitis with antibiotics alone and in combination with glucocorticoids, Acta Obstet. Gynecol. Scand. **44**(suppl. 16):65, 1965.
Falk, V., and Krook, G.: Do results of culture for gonococci vary with sampling phase of menstrual cycle? Acta Derm. Venereol. (Stockh.) **47:**190, 1967.
Faulkner, W.L., and Ory, H.W.: Intrauterine devices and acute PID, J.A.M.A. **235:**1851, 1976.
Flesh, G., and others: The intrauterine contraceptive device and acute salpingitis: a multifactor analysis, Am. J. Obstet. Gynecol. **135:**404, 1979.
Hager, W.D., and Wiesner, P.J.: Selected epidemiological aspects of acute salpingitis: a review, J. Reprod. Med. **19:**47, 1977.
Handsfield, H.H.: Disseminated gonococcal infection. Presented at the Thirteenth Interscience Conference on Antimicrobial Agents and Chemotherapy, Washington, D.C., Sept. 9-12, 1973.
Handsfield, H.H., and others: Asymptomatic gonorrhea in men, N. Engl. J. Med. **290:**117, 1974.
Hedberg, E., and Anberg, A.: Gonorrheal salpingitis: views on treatment and prognosis, Fertil. Steril. **16:**125, 1965.
Hedberg, E., and Septz, S.O.: Acute salpingitis: views on prognosis and treatment, Acta Obstet. Gynecol. Scand. **37:**131, 1958.
Ishihama, A., and others: Bacteriological study on the users of intrauterine contraceptive devices, Acta Obstet. Gynecol. Jap. **17:**77, 1970.
Jacobson, L.: Laparoscopy in the diagnosis of acute salpingitis, Acta Obstet. Gynecol. Scand. **43:**160, 1964.
Jacobson, L., and Westrom, L.: Objectivized diagnosis of acute pelvic inflammatory disease, Am. J. Obstet. Gynecol. **105:**1088, 1969.
Lip, J., and Burgoyne, X.: Cervical and peritoneal bacterial flora associated with salpingitis, Obstet. Gynecol. **23:**561, 1966.
Lukasik, J.: A comparative evaluation of the bacteriological flora of the uterine cervix and fallopian tubes in cases of salpingitis, Am. J. Obstet. Gynecol. **23:**561, 1966.
Mardh, P., and others: Chlamydia trachomatis infection in patients with acute salpingitis, N. Engl. J. Med. **296:**1377, 1977.
Mardh, P.A., and Westrom, L.: Tubal and cervical cultures in acute salpingitis with special reference to *Mycoplasma hominis* and T-strain mycoplasmas, Br. J. Vener. Dis. **46:**179, 1970.
Mead, P., and others: Incidence of infections associated with the intrauterine contraceptive device in an isolated community, Am. J. Obstet. Gynecol. **125:**79, 1976.
Mishell, D.R., and Moyer, D.E.: Association of pelvic inflammatory disease with the intrauterine device, Clin. Obstet. Gynecol. **12:**179, 1969.
Rees, E., and Annels, E.H.: Gonococcal salpingitis, Br. J. Vener. Dis. **45:**205, 1969.
Rendtorff, R.C., and others: Economic consequences of gonorrhea in women, J. Am. Vener. Dis. Assoc. **14:** 40, 1974.

Stanley, M.M.: Gonococci peritonitis of the upper part of the abdomen in young women, Arch. Intern. Med. **78:**1, 1946.
Studdiford, W.E., and others: The persistence of gonococcal infections in the adnexal, Surg. Gynecol. Obstet. **67:**176, 1938.
Sunden, B.: The results of conservative treatment of salpingitis diagnosed at laparotomy and laparoscopy, Acta Obstet. Gynecol. Scand. **38:**296, 1959.
Sweet, R.L.: Anaerobic infections of the female genital tract, Am. J. Obstet. Gynecol. **122:**891, 1975.
Sweet, R.L.: Diagnosis and treatment of acute salpingitis, J. Reprod. Med. **19:**21, 1977.
Sweet, R.L., and others: Use of laparoscopy to determine the microbiologic etiology of acute salpingitis, Am. J. Obstet. Gynecol. **134:**68, 1979.
Swenson, F.M., and others: Anaerobic infections of the female genital tract, Obstet. Gynecol. **42:**538, 1973.
Targum, S.D., and Wright, N.J.: Association of the intrauterine device and pelvic inflammatory disease, Am. J. Epidemiol. **100:**262, 1974.
Thadepalli, H., and others: Anaerobic infection of the female genital tract: bacteriologic and therapeutic aspects, Am. J. Obstet. Gynecol. **117:**1034, 1973.
Thompson, S.: Personal communication, 1979.
Viberg, L.: Acute inflammatory conditions of the uterine adnexal, Acta Obstet. Gynecol. Scand. **43**(suppl. 4): 5, 1964.
Westrom, L.: Effect of acute pelvic inflammatory disease on fertility, Am. J. Obstet. Gynecol. **121:**707, 1975.
Westrom, L., and others: The risk of PID in women using IUDs as compared to non-users, Lancet **3:**221, 1976.
Wright, N.H., and Laemmle, P.: Acute pelvic inflammatory disease in an indigent population, Am. J. Obstet. Gynecol. **101:**979, 1968.
Wright, R.A.: Pelvic inflammatory disease, Med. Asp. Hum. Sex. July, 1976, pp. 139-140.

CHAPTER 12

Hepatitis type A: a community problem

Sue Iha

Few diseases cause as much chaos in a community as does hepatitis A, the most common type of hepatitis. This diagnosis sends repercussions throughout the neighborhood from home, to work, to church, and possibly to school. The contagious nature of this problem places the primary health care provider in a prime position to assess and plan for afflicted clients and to protect their community from further infection. The clinical course of hepatitis A is uncomplicated, and it rarely proceeds to chronic hepatitis (Sherlock, 1979). Thus the nurse practitioner is invaluable to teach clients and to manage this disease. To accomplish this the provider must have a clear understanding of the disease's pathophysiology, etiology, mode of transmission, and clinical course. The purpose of this chapter is to provide nurse practitioners with the necessary tools to assess and plan for the individual and community, to evaluate the plan of care, and to educate potential and existing communities at risk for hepatitis A.

Hepatitis is an inflammation of the liver, usually caused by a viral agent or by toxic substances. Before the 1940s the definite cause of hepatitis was unknown. Its viral origin was documented in the 1940s and 1950s when a filterable agent was found in the blood and stool of clients with the disease (Dmochowski, 1976). For many years investigators thought only one type of virus caused hepatitis. Later, with the identification of two viruses came the labels "infectious hepatitis" and "serum hepatitis."

Contrary to earlier beliefs, it is evident that more than two viruses are responsible for hepatitis. Thus the titles "infectious hepatitis" and "serum hepatitis" are less accurate, and authorities describe hepatitis as types A, B, and non-A non-B (Table 12-1). Although the antigenic properties of viruses A and B differ, they usually produce similar signs and symptoms in the client. The definite antigenic properties of non-A non-B are unknown.

ETIOLOGY

Synonyms for hepatitis type A include hepatitis A virus (HAV), infectious hepatitis, or short-incubation hepatitis. The virus is present in the liver, bile, stools, and blood during the acute phase and the late prodromal phase of the illness. It is a 27-nm RNA

Table 12-1. Comparison of types of hepatitis

Comparison	Hepatitis A	Hepatitis B	Non-A non-B
Etiology	27-nm RNA virus	42-nm DNA virus	Unknown
Route of transmission	Fecal-oral	Parenteral, venereal	Blood transfusion
Alternate route	Rarely parenteral	Possibly saliva; feces, breast milk, urine, tears, maternofetal	Unknown
Incubation	15-45 days (mean 30)	45-160 days (mean 60-90)	15-160 days (mean 50)
Onset	Abrupt	Frequently insidious	Insidious
Seasonal incidence	Fall, winter	Year-round	Year-round
Age distribution	Children, young adults	Any age	Any age
Clinical course	Short, uncomplicated	Long, often complicated	Variable
Prognosis	Good in absence of prior liver damage	Worse with age and other disease processes	Variable
Potential for chronicity	None documented	10% of cases lead to chronicity	As high as 45%
Carrier state	None documented	0.5% of U.S. population	Yes, prevalance unknown
Bilirubin	Normal to 20 mg/dl	Normal to 20 mg/dl	Normal to 20 mg/dl
SGOT/SGPT	500-4000 IU	500-4000 IU	500-4000 IU
Alkaline phosphatase	Normal or mildly elevated	Normal or mildly elevated	Normal or mildly elevated
Anti-HAV (antibody)	Acute: IgM class Convalescent: IgG class	—	—
HAA (Australia antigen)	—	+, but obsolete test	—
HB_sAg (surface antigen)	—	+	—
Anti-HBs (antibody)	—	IgM: transient IgG: may persist for years	—
HB_eAg (antigen)	—	+ (early in acute disease) + (chronic hepatitis B)	—
Anti-Hb_c (core antibody)	—	+ transiently	
Prophylaxis	0.06 ml/kg of immune serum globulin	0.06 ml/kg of hepatitis B immune serum globulin	Unknown

virus whose various strains belong to one serotype (Deinstag and others, 1980). Researchers had difficulty obtaining the hepatitis A antigen; however, radioimmunoassay techniques have purified the A antigen from feces. This test is primarily used by researchers; since the antigen is detectable in feces only very early in the disease and is usually undetectable in the blood, the test has little clinical value.

Synonyms for hepatitis type B include hepatitis B virus (HBV), serum hepatitis, long-incubation hepatitis, or HB_sAg-positive hepatitis. The hepatitis B virus is a DNA virus. There are three known viral particles related to hepatitis B infection. The first is the large 42-nm Dane particle. This probably is the intact B virus. This particle has an outer coat and an inner core. The others are small, 22-nm spherical or elongated particles. They are thought to represent excess production of the outer surface of the Dane particle.

In the early 1960s researchers developed the first serological test to distinguish hepatitis B from non-B hepatitis. They detected a substance in an Australian aborigine that stimulated an immune response. Thus the first label for this substance was Australia antigen. This antigen results from excess production of the outer surface of the Dane particle. Therefore the Australia antigen was renamed the hepatitis B surface antigen (HB_sAg). The older HAA (Australia antigen) test is obsolete. More sophisticated laboratory methods can quantitate the HB_sAg; thus it provides a specific diagnostic marker of active hepatitis B infection (Gunby, 1979).

Non-A non-B hepatitis may be caused by a number of unidentified viruses. In this situation, clinical signs and symptoms of hepatitis exist, but tests for type A or B are negative. Little is known about this entity, and there are no tests for non-A non-B antigens and antibodies.

EPIDEMIOLOGY

Viral hepatitis ranks fourth among the 30 communicable diseases reported to the Centers for Disease Control (CDC) (Gunby). In 1970 the total number of reported cases of hepatitis A and B in the United States was 62,939. Type A constituted 55,741 cases, or 89%. Non-A non-B hepatitis was not reported at that time. With the introduction of HB_sAg testing in the early 1970s there was more accurate reporting of the disease. Three categories of reportable hepatitis are A, B, and unspecified (for example, non-A non-B, alcoholic, and drug induced). By 1979 a total of 52,983 cases were reported, with 28,237 cases of type A, 14,278 cases of type B, and 10,468 cases of unspecified hepatitis (Center for Disease Control, 1980).

In developed countries reports of type A cases are declining. In 1976 it accounted for 59% of reported cases, while in 1979 it accounted for 53%. This may be due to a number of factors. First, the increasing availability of HB_sAg testing increased the accuracy of diagnosis for type B hepatitis. Before this, providers categorized hepatitis according to the possible route of transmission, incubation period, or clinical symptoms. Second, the number of other types may be increasing because of a higher frequency of parenteral drug abuse. Third, the decline may be due to improved sanitation, since transmission of type A virus is almost entirely by the fecal-oral route.

The hepatitis A virus spreads directly by poor personal hygiene. A contaminated individual may omit hand washing after defecation. Subsequent food handling or intimate physical contact (such as household transmission) may spread the disease. Overcrowded living conditions contribute to the spread of infection. An additional source is childcare programs for preschoolers who are still developing personal hygiene habits. In a study done in Arizona, 40% of all cases of hepatitis type A (or unspecified type) reported in a 10-month period were closely associated with day care centers. All adults who contracted hepatitis had contact with 1- to 2-year-old children who attended the center. The researchers concluded that day care centers appear to be important in the spread of hepatitis type A in the United States. (Hanler and others, 1980).

The question of hepatitis A being sexually transmitted has been posed. In a study done by Corey and Holmes (1980) there was an increase in incidence of antibodies to hepatitis A among homosexual men; there was no increase among heterosexual men. There was correlation with frequent oral-anal sexual contact. Therefore the researchers concluded that if there is oral-anal sexual contact, hepatitis A may be sexually transmitted.

Indirect transmission occurs with the ingestion of contaminated food (shellfish, oysters), water, or milk. This may cause a clustering of cases exposed to a common source. Transmission of type A via the blood occurs rarely. It is not known if the type A virus crosses the placenta. However, no specific fetal abnormalities have been associated with the disease, nor have significant problems for mother or fetus been shown (Siegel, 1973).

In contrast, cases of hepatitis B increased tenfold between 1966 and 1977. There may be as many as 120,000 cases each year (Gunby). The principal modes of transmission include:
1. Direct inoculation by needle of contaminated serum or plasma or transfusion of infected blood or blood products
2. Nonneedle percutaneous transfer of infected serum or plasma, as may occur through minute skin cuts or abrasions
3. Introduction of infected serum or plasma on mucosal surfaces, as may occur through inadvertent introduction of this material into buccal or ocular surfaces
4. Introduction of other infected secretions, such as saliva or semen, into mucosal surfaces through sexual contact
5. Indirect transfer of serum or plasma via vectors or inanimate environmental surfaces (U.S. Department of Health, Education, and Welfare, 1977)

Therefore at risk are blood transfusion recipients, drug abusers, persons with recent tattoos or pierced ears, clients and staff associated with hemodialysis, and homosexual men. For reasons that are unclear, other high-risk groups include clients with Down's syndrome, leukemia, or Hodgkin's disease.

Transmission of non-A non-B hepatitis is usually by transfused blood from asymptomatic donors. Also there is documentation of other routes of transmission similar to type A and B. Non-A non-B accounts for approximately 20% of reported cases of hepatitis.

PHYSIOLOGY AND PATHOPHYSIOLOGY

The functions of the liver are numerous and essential to the body's other organ systems. The functions include storage and filtration of blood, secretion of bile into the gastrointestinal tract, and multiple metabolic functions.

The effects of all viral types of hepatitis on the liver are similar. However, the degree of liver changes varies widely. Changes may be slight, involving individual lobules, the functional units of the liver; or they may be severe, with extensive lobular destruction. Thus varying levels of cell injury, inflammation, and necrosis occur (Robbins and Angell, 1976).

The body responds to acute viral hepatitis with elevated levels of immunoglobulins, particularly IgG and IgM. In acute type A, elevation of IgM levels is more prominent. Additionally, antinuclear antibody, heterophil antibody, and rheumatoid factor may be present. These are nonspecific antibodies that also may increase with other viral or systemic diseases. The data on type A immune complex-mediated tissue damage are limited. However, immunological responses in type B play a major role in the clinical signs and symptoms of the disease.

Hepatitis A antibody (anti-HAV) is present in the body during acute illness. During convalescence anti-HAV titers increase and remain in the body permanently so that a person is protected against reinfection indefinitely. Hepatitis B antibody (Anti-HB_s) persists for years after infection in many cases. It involves a primary response after an acute episode and a higher response subsequently.

Hepatitis A usually does not produce jaundice and is not diagnosed during acute infection. Aach (1978) randomly tested 947 people with no known history of hepatitis. Seventy-five percent of people from the lower socioeconomic groups had a positive hepatitis antibody titer. Twenty percent to 30% of middle-class subjects had a positive titer. In addition, people over 50 were more likely to have the antibody present. In developing countries other investigators find the sequence of exposure, infection, and immunity to be almost universal from childhood on.

ASSESSMENT
Clinical course

The three stages of hepatitis A can be identified clinically and serologically: the prodromal, icteric, and recovery stage. In the prodromal stage symptoms are nonspecific, lasting 1 to 2 weeks; symptoms include general malaise, poor appetite, nausea, vomiting, headache, fatigue, pharyngitis, and coryza. The antigen associated with the hepatitis virus has been detected in stool 5 to 6 days before clinical signs and symptoms appear (Miller, 1980). This is approximately 2 to 3 weeks after initial exposure to the disease. The incubation period is 15 to 45 days, with a mean of 30 days. A temperature between 100° and 102° F may also be present. A frequently reported symptom is abdominal discomfort, which is right upper or generalized upper quadrant pain. As bile stasis occurs the bile is unable to reach the gastrointestinal tract, and stools become light or clay colored. The urine shows increased amounts of bilirubin and takes on a dark orange or brown discoloration. This occurs 1 to 4 days before the onset of jaundice. Pruritus may also be the initial symptom; it is transient and may complicate the initial assessment.

During the icteric stage assessment becomes much easier. Many of the vague prodromal symptoms decrease, and the client usually begins to feel better. The client becomes jaundiced when the serum bilirubin levels are over 2.5 mg/dl. The temperature elevation usually subsides and the client may report mild weight loss. As liver inflammation increases, the liver enlarges, producing complaints of right upper quadrant discomfort. Posterior cervical lymphadenopathy may also be present in about 20% of cases. The hepatitis A virus and antigen usually disappear from the stool by the time jaundice peaks (Miller).

The recovery, or posticteric, stage lasts from a few weeks to several months, averaging 2 to 6 weeks. Signs and symptoms usually subside, except for possible liver enlargement and complaints of fatigue. The client should continue to feel better. During this period hepatic function may still be abnormal, although complete recovery should occur within 3 or 4 months after jaundice begins. Active immunity for hepatitis A exists for an indefinite period of time after the disease is contracted.

Most healthy people recover from hepatitis A without sequelae. However, occasionally the virus attacks differently, or it affects a previously damaged liver. In this situation fulminant or massive hepatic necrosis may occur, though it is most common in type B. The client is usually very ill. The bilirubin value is greater than 20 mg/dl, the liver size decreases, and prothrombin time increases; confusion and coma may ensue. Fortunately, mortality is rare with hepatitis A, occurring in 0.1% to 0.4% of cases. This figure is much higher (5% to 10%) for hepatitis B.

Chronic active hepatitis has not been documented after hepatitis A. It may occur in 10% of type B cases and as high as 45% in non-A non-B hepatitis. It may occur after drug-induced and alcoholic hepatitis as well as Wilson's disease, an inborn error of copper metabolism. The client does not clinically recover; fatigue, anorexia, and liver enlargement continue. In some cases, the client appears well, but laboratory values fail to return to normal within the usual 6 to 12 months. A history of repeated episodes of hepatitis may suggest chronic active hepatitis.

History

A thorough history and a high index of suspicion are the best tools to detect hepatitis A. The practitioner should question the client about the presence and character of abdominal pain; it should be dull rather than sharp and located in upper quadrants. The practitioner should ask about the amount of weight loss, appetite change, or change in the perceived taste or smell of cigarettes or foods. The presence of nausea or vomiting, as well as the color of stools or urine, should be documented. The urine should be orange or brown in hepatitis, not just dark yellow, which signifies urine concentration.

A diet history is extremely important. The client should be questioned about possible new eating establishments during the previous month or the possibility of contaminated foods. Fatty food intolerance needs no special assessment because its association with gallbladder disease has been dispelled (Snodgrass and Abbruzzese, 1977). The incidence of abdominal pain due to hepatitis is not necessarily related to meals. The frequency of alcohol intake with attention toward excess is also a critical assessment factor.

The history of hepatitis or general malaise in friends, family, or close contacts may help determine the source of infection. In addition, the client should be questioned about recent travel in foreign countries, particularly Africa, Asia, South America, or Mexico. Also, the practitioner should ask about any hepatitis contacts during the last month.

The practitioner should search for possible parenteral routes of entry. When appropriate, the client should be questioned about the use of street drugs, heroin, or other substances that the individual could inject.

The client's occupation may provide valuable information for assessment and prevention of hepatitis. Highly suspect individuals are health workers who work with blood products or hemodialysis, or clients hospitalized with hepatitis. In addition, infected food handlers could transmit the disease if they are undiagnosed before jaundice. Occupational exposure to chemicals such as carbon tetrachloride may also cause hepatitis. Inhalation, ingestion, or parenteral administration of many chemical agents can result in liver injury.

Sexual practices may provide a link to disease transmission. The practitioner should ask the client about general sexual activity, specific sexual practices, and possible VD contacts. Finally, the client should be questioned about any medications taken, whether prescribed or over the counter. Idiosyncratic drug reactions may occur with many drugs at any time during therapy. These reactions are not always dose dependent (Table 12-2).

Table 12-2. Examples of primary care drugs that may produce hepatitis-like reactions

Generic name	Brand name
Acetaminophen	Tylenol, Tempra
Aminosalicylic acid	Pamisyl, Parasal
Phenytoin	Dilantin
Erythromycin estolate	Ilosone
Isoniazid	INH
Methyldopa	Aldomet
Phenacetin	Usually in combination with Fiorinal or APC
Sulfonamides	Gantanol, Gantrisin

The practitioner should also question the client about any recent blood transfusions and about a prior history of hepatitis.

Physical examination

Physical assessment may provide a few clues in the diagnosis of hepatitis. During the prodromal phase the examination may be negative except for a low-grade fever and possible right upper quadrant tenderness to deep palpation. The urine may appear brown just before jaundice.

During the icteric phase the skin and scleras appear yellow, posterior cervical adenopathy may be present, and right upper quadrant tenderness is present. Hepatomegaly and occasionally splenomegaly are palpable. The liver edge should be smooth and may be tender, with expansion palpable below the costal margin. In the obese individual the liver may not be palpable, but right upper quadrant tenderness or tenderness over the liver should be present. No rebound tenderness or radiation should exist. Bowel sounds should be present to auscultation. Fever should be absent, weight loss of 5 to 10 pounds may be noticed, and occasionally spider angiomas will appear transiently. Any areas of attempted parenteral injections should be noted. The practitioner should observe for ecchymotic areas, edema, or ascites, which indicates progressive liver disease. The mental status of the client should be noted. At the first signs of altered consciousness or confusion the client should be immediately referred for further evaluation and treatment because this may be the first sign of impending hepatic coma. During the recovery phase liver enlargement may persist, but the remainder of the physical examination should be within normal limits. If perihepatitis associated with gonococcal salpingitis is present, pelvic examination reveals adnexal and cervical motion tenderness.

Laboratory data

HAV is detectable in stool by radioimmunoassay or immune electron microscopy. Most studies reveal that the level of HAV in stool is greatest at or before the time liver enzymes become elevated. Before the onset of jaundice, stool HAV markedly decreases and is usually undetectable even by these sensitive tests (Fig. 12-1). This has implications for preventing transmission of hepatitis A. This test is used primarily by researchers.

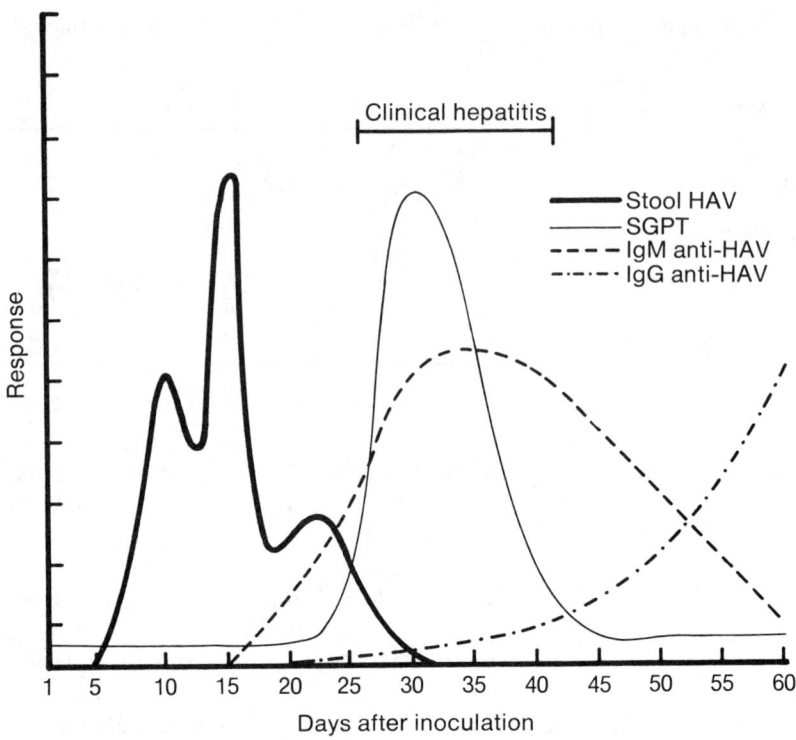

Fig. 12-1. Typical response to infection of hepatitis A virus versus day after inoculation. (Modified from Bradley, D., and Maynard, J.E.: Lab. Manag. **16:**29, Sept. 1978.)

Anti-HAV, the antibody against hepatitis A, is detectable in serum and is specific for the disease. During the acute phase of the illness anti-HAV of the IgM class is detectable and persists for several months. Anti-HAV of the IgG class predominates during convalescence. Presence of a high titer of this antibody is diagnostic for hepatitis A. However, this test may not be available to all laboratories.

$HB_s Ag$ is the hepatitis B surface antigen. It is present in hepatitis B and absent in hepatitis A. This is the only test that is available to most laboratories for distinguishing hepatitis B from non-B. If anti-HAV is unavailable, the diagnosis of hepatitis A is based on absence of HB_sAg, on clinical signs and symptoms, and on high liver enzyme levels. A history of a classical epidemiological setting provides further evidence for hepatitis A. In hepatitis B, serum HB_sAg is usually present before the rise in liver enzymes and is usually undetectable 1 to 2 months after the onset of jaundice. The titer of HB_sAg does not reflect the clinical significance of the disease. Presence of Hb_sAg after 4 months implies the development of chronic hepatitis (Miller).

$HB_e Ag$ is an additional antigen associated with hepatitis B. The presence of $HB_e Ag$ correlates with infectivity and presence of the intact virus. It is present only in HB_sAg-

positive serum. HB_eAg is present early in the course of hepatitis B; if persistent it may be associated with ongoing viral replication and chronic hepatitis. Thus this test may help identify acute or chronic states of hepatitis B; however, this test may not be widely available.

Anti-HB_s is the B virus antibody. Its presence usually indicates past infection, and it confers immunity (Miller).

The *anti-HB_c* antibody is detectable shortly after HB_sAg appears. It can be detected before the appearance of anti-HB_s. There is a period of time during acute hepatitis B when neither the surface antigen nor antibody is detectable. During this time anti-HB_c is present and may be the only means for diagnosis of hepatitis B.

SGOT (serum glutamic-oxaloacetic transaminase) is an intracellular enzyme that catalyzes the transfer of an amino acid group from α-acid to α–keto acid. It is present in various tissues, especially the heart and liver. With liver disease the damaged cells leak the transaminase into the serum. There is a steady increase in SGOT levels during the late prodromal phase of hepatitis; these levels should progressively decrease during the convalescent phase. Levels of the enzyme may increase from 500 to 4,000 units.

SGPT (serum glutamic-pyruvic transaminase) is an intracellular enzyme similar to SGOT and also found in several tissues of the body. A steady increase in SGPT levels is seen in the late prodromal stage also with a decrease in convalescence. The SGPT levels may increase from 500 to 4,000 units. The levels of liver enzymes do not signify the severity of the disease.

Prothrombin time is a test to measure the activity of clotting factors V, VII, X, prothrombin, and fibrinogen, which are sythesized by the liver. In clients with acute hepatitis a prolonged value may signify extensive hepatocellular necrosis and poor prognosis. Normal time is 12 to 15 seconds. This test is difficult to control well in small laboratories and may not be available in some primary care centers.

Bilirubin is a bile pigment produced by the breakdown of heme and subsequent reduction of biliverdin. The liver normally takes up bilirubin and conjugates it to form the water-soluble pigment excreted in bile. Failure of the liver cells to excrete bile or obstruction of the bile ducts can cause increased levels of bilirubin in body fluids. Bilirubin levels are elevated from 5 to 20 mg/dl during the icteric phase of hepatitis. Bilirubinuria, detected by dipstick testing, is present 1 to 4 days before jaundice. Also, urine with increased soluble bilirubin foams when shaken. Otherwise the urine should be normal.

A *white blood count* may be normal or moderately elevated with a relative lymphocytosis. Atypical lymphocytes may be present, as is also the case in mononucleosis. *Alkaline phosphatase* levels may or may not be elevated. Levels are usually higher in obstructive jaundice and rarely greater than 25 Bodansky units in hepatitis. This may be an important diagnostic point. *Total protein* is generally within normal limits, or a slight elevation of the γ fraction is noted.

Initial evaluation should include HB_sAg, a complete blood count with differential, SGOT, SGPT, bilirubin, alkaline phosphatase, and urine for urobilinogen. When available, specific tests for hepatitis A are helpful. Depending on the differential diagnosis, other optional laboratory data might include throat culture, Monospot Slide test, hemoglobin electrophoresis, and cervical gonorrhea culture (Fitz-Hugh–Curtis syndrome).

Differential diagnosis

The assessment of jaundice or right upper quadrant pain is often complicated. The diagnosis of hepatitis A is difficult during the prodromal phase, since specific laboratory tests may be unavailable, and the history is nonspecific. If the symptoms are severe, some physicians prefer hospitalization for more thorough evaluation and testing. In many cases this is infeasible or impractical. Diagnosis during the prodromal phase is by physical examination, negative HB_sAg, elevated bilirubin, rising SGOT and SGPT, and other normal laboratory values. Other common causes of jaundice or right upper quadrant pain are discussed below.

Hemolytic jaundice may be secondary to the breakdown of hemoglobin in the red blood cell. Examples of conditions that produce hemolysis are sickle cell crisis, thalassemia, and glucose-6-phosphate dehydrogenase (G6PD) deficiency. Liver enzyme functions remain normal, while protein-bound bilirubin (unconjugated, or fat-soluble) levels may be elevated. Since the kidneys excrete only water-soluble (conjugated) bilirubin, the urine should not be brown. In addition, the red blood cell count, hemoglobin, or hemotocrit may be depressed. Specific tests such as G6PD or hemoglobin electrophoresis are diagnostic. Splenomegaly may be present. Nausea, vomiting, and weight loss are absent unless hemolysis is extensive.

Jaundice may occur with obstruction of the common bile duct, as with a common duct stone, cholecystitis, or ascending cholangitis. The obstruction prevents the flow of bile from the liver to the intestines. Water-soluble bilirubin then increases in the bloodstream, with subsequent excretion in the urine producing brown urine and clay-colored stools. Right upper quadrant or epigastric pain and jaundice are the prime clinical features of biliary tract disease. Fever, nausea, and vomiting may be present. A sustained fever during icterus with increasing abdominal pain and absence of liver enlargement are helpful clues. SGOT and SGPT levels are not elevated; the bilirubin level is only moderately elevated. Alkaline phosphatase levels may be moderately elevated. The diagnosis may be made only after biopsy or cholangiogram. If biliary tract disease is suspected, physician consultation is required.

Common infectious diseases, particularly mononucleosis, may complicate diagnosis during the prodromal phase. In hepatitis, cervical adenopathy occurs in 10% to 20% of victims, although pharyngitis may occur commonly. In mononucleosis the HB_sAg should be negative, and the Monospot test or Epstein-Barr virus antibody tests may be positive. Hepatosplenomegaly occurs occasionally in mononucleosis. Bilirubin and serum transaminase levels are infrequently elevated. The pharynx may demonstrate secondary infections as documented by a white tonsillar or pharyngeal exudate, although this is not routinely found. Other infectious diseases to consider include cytomegalovirus, herpes simplex, Coxsackie virus, and toxoplasmosis. Specific tests for these should be conducted only after exclusion of other common causes of jaundice and upper quadrant pain.

In alcoholic hepatitis the history of long-term excess alcohol intake is helpful. In addition, the liver may be small and nonpalpable because of extensive, chronic damage. SGOT levels may not be elevated, although alkaline phosphatase levels will be elevated, representing chronic liver inflammation.

Drug-induced hepatitis is most easily determined by past history and negative tests specific for hepatitis A or B. Liver enzyme levels are elevated. In alcoholic hepatitis and drug-induced hepatitis a liver biopsy may be the most helpful test.

Upper quadrant pain and liver tenderness may be present with Fitz-Hugh–Curtis syndrome (perihepatitis), which is associated with salpingitis. There is an increased incidence of this because of the increased incidence of gonorrhea and its sequelae. Liver enzyme levels may be elevated but return to normal rapidly after penicillin therapy. A positive cervical gonorrhea culture and elevated liver enzyme levels in the absence of HB_sAg and anti-HAV are the best diagnostic tools. Pharyngitis, coryza, and cervical adenopathy are absent. Sexually active females with hepatic tenderness or right upper quadrant abdominal pain should have a pelvic examination to exclude salpingitis.

PLAN

With the diagnosis of hepatitis A management should include close observation, supportive care, and client education.

Rest

Activity should be restricted to confinement at home during the prodromal and early icteric phases. In general, most clients do not feel like being active until the middle to late icteric stage. Restriction to bed rest is unnecessary. However, during the prodromal phase restriction to home may also prevent further spread of disease, as in the case of the infected preschooler who attends a child care center. Excessive or strenuous activity should be discouraged. Most clients fatigue easily at this stage. The client usually can resume normal activities when bilirubin or SGOT and SGPT levels begin to decrease. These values do not have to be normal, since this may take months in some clients.

Diet

Since many clients may have anorexia, nausea, or vomiting during the prodromal phase, the practitioner should recommend small frequent feedings throughout the day rather than large meals. Most authorities suggest a high-calorie diet. When fever is present, dehydration may be a problem. A fluid intake of at least 2 quarts per day should be encouraged. Alcohol intake should be discouraged, since this may further damage the liver.

Drugs

The use of all drugs, including birth control pills, should be discouraged during all stages of hepatitis. If the client has viral hepatitis and is taking INH (isoniazid), the practitioner should discontinue the drug and seek consultation about a change of medication and about resumption of antitubercular therapy. If itching is problematic, tub baths with the addition of baking soda should be encouraged.

Prevention of transmission

The most important aspect of prevention for hepatitis A is hand washing after elimination. This includes after urination, since the wiping of the female vulva may inadvertently contaminate the hand as it passes over the rectum in the front-to-back wiping method. Unless the client is incontinent, toilet facilities may be shared with other family members (Favero and others, 1979). Urine and feces may be flushed down the toilet. The practitioner should remember that virus A in stool peaks before changes in liver enzymes are detectable and decreases markedly before the onset of jaundice (Rakala and Mosley, 1977).

Sexual patterns

If the infected client engages in anal or oral-genital intercourse, these practices should be discouraged until 1 week after the onset of jaundice. By this time the HAV content of stool is undetectable. General sexual contact should also be avoided until 1 week after jaundice onset because of inadvertent contamination of hands during sexual activity. Guidelines for sexual activity in HB_sAg-positive clients are different because of the possibility of a carrier state and the mode of transmission.

Isolation

It is unnecessary to force the infected individual to eat alone. The client's dishes and eating utensils may be washed in a dishwasher or in the sink with a detergent after other dishes are washed. Infected clients should not cook for others; household tasks may have to be redistributed. Household items, such as books, magazines, combs, brushes, or clothing, do not need special precautions unless they are visibly contaminated with feces. Contaminated clothing, washcloths, towels, and diapers should be washed separately in hot water with detergent and chlorine bleach. Unless incontinence is present, it is unnecessary to isolate an infected client in one room. Hospitalization may prevent transmission of disease by the incontinent adult or child. If this is infeasible or uneconomical, the caretaker should use disposable rubber gloves when handling excreta. Feces should be bagged twice in plastic, securely sealed, and disposed in trash separately. The hands should be washed afterwards.

Household cleaning

Routine household cleaning is acceptable. In places where visible excreta is present (toilet), the caretaker should clean with a 1:10 chlorine bleach (Clorox) solution while wearing gloves. The hepatitis virus is inactivated by contact with chlorine, formaldehyde, boiling for 1 minute, or ultravoilet irradiation (Deinstag and others).

Prophylaxis

For intimate contacts, such as individuals actually living in the home, immune serum globulin (ISG) should be given. It is unnecessary for office, factory, or school contacts. It is also unnecessary for the elderly, who are almost invariably immune. All ISG contains anti-HAV in varying amounts. If given within 2 weeks of contact, it will prevent clinical signs of hepatitis A in 80% of those receiving ISG (Miller). Unfortunately, hepatitis A is often recognized late in the incubation period. The recommended dose is 0.06 ml/kg (Miller). This dose is higher than some recommended but is necessary because of varying amounts of anti-HAV in different lots of ISG.

Advances have produced hepatitis B immune globulin (HBIG) for prophylaxis. Its uses are still controversial, but many authorities agree that immunization of family members of HB_sAg-positive individuals is unnecessary. In a primary care setting, reasons for giving HBIG include sexual exposure to acute hepatitis B when nonpromiscuity makes subsequent reexposure unlikely, and accidental exposure of health care providers (Mosley, 1979). ISG prophylaxis may be useful with acute hepatitis B, but the data are conflicting (Hoofnagle and others, 1979).

Client education

In addition to the above, the client should know the definition of the disease, its stages, the prognosis, and transmission of the disease. The client should not donate blood. HAV may not be routinely tested by blood banks but HB_sAg normally is. The B virus remains in blood for a variable period after acute infection. Donation of blood may possibly transmit infection to a blood recipient. For the hepatitis A client the virus does not persist after infection, and no chronic carrier state of HAV has been identified. However, clients are still discouraged from giving blood.

Community education

The community can serve either as an important ally or a great source of anxiety. To allay concern, timely and accurate information must be disseminated. The client's community, whether at risk or not, needs education. Written information is helpful and better than word of mouth. The Department of Health and Human Services can provide publication number CDC 78-8271, entitled *Hepatitis,* which may be helpful to the client in answering questions from friends and neighbors. The publication responds to the most frequently asked questions about hepatitis. The local or state health department can be a source of information for the community, providing written material and manpower, if needed. Most health departments supply γ-globulin. In a small community a short article in the local paper may be very effective in transmitting information quickly to more people.

The practitioner should consider the volatile atmosphere surrounding hepatitis and the aggressive feelings associated with fear of spreading the disease: "Johnny gave my Susie hepatitis, and she had to miss 4 weeks of school." It is imperative that the community have accurate information. These feelings are real and cannot be overlooked. The first case frequently is blamed for all subsequent cases. However, if time is taken to explain incubation periods, fault finding can be avoided.

Schools or work settings are important parts of the community. Some schools use a form letter to parents when a child develops hepatitis. Frequently this will cause much concern on the part of the parents, and they may call their health care providers. In order for the practitioner to respond intelligently to this problem, the letter should be read to the practitioner. If still in doubt about exposure and therefore the need for γ-globulin, the practitioner should contact the school to see if exposure did occur. These letters are sent to protect any child who may have been exposed. It is the responsibility of the person managing the client to assess whether exposure could have occurred. It is not unusual for the child who received the note from school to be unacquainted with the infected child. A phone call or succinct note to the school with information about hepatitis and the plan of care for the client can be useful. This can allow the school to plan for students' protection as well as for the client's education while at home.

Many providers voice concern about their own contamination and subsequent transmission of hepatitis. This is an important and valid issue when the provider cares for a client during the prodromal or acute illness stage. The practitioner should remember that

248 *Problems with infectious diseases*

a carrier state for hepatitis type A is not believed to exist. This, however, is not true for type B. This information should be helpful to health providers who may be apprehensive about treating a person with a history of hepatitis. If it can be documented that the client had type A hepatitis, there is little if any need for concern after the client recovers from the disease. The risk of passing the disease to other clients is less problematic because most nurses and physicians do not put their hands in a client's mouth without a glove. The need for thorough hand washing between client visits cannot be emphasized enough for prevention of hepatitis as well as other diseases.

EVALUATION

During the prodromal phase and early icteric phase of hepatitis the client should reduce activity, refrain from drugs and alcohol, and state what preventive behavioral measures he has adopted. If diagnosed early, the client should bring in intimate contacts for prophylaxis.

After initial assessment the client should return in 1 week for observation and reinforcement of teaching. Nausea, vomiting, excessive weight loss, and severe abdominal pain should be absent if the client's condition is stable. At 2 and 4 weeks hepatic function can be tested with a repeat SGOT. Since the range for hepatitis is quite wide (500-4,000 IU), the provider should look for significant declines in SGOT levels from the initial acute value. The client's clinical picture should be an additional indicator for the resumption of activities. Since contagion decreases within the first few days after icterus, the client may return to work or school on a part-time basis. When the client is ready, activity may be increased gradually. Since no carrier state exists in hepatitis A, no antigen-antibody retesting is necessary. Depending on liver enzyme values, the client should return periodically for reevaluation at 2 and 4 months or until values are normal. If SGOT values remain elevated, more frequent observation and consultation are essential. At the end of infection the client should be able to resume normal activities. Jaundice should be absent; SGOT, SGPT, and bilirubin levels should be within normal limits. Hepatosplenomegaly and liver tenderness should disappear.

CASE STUDY
Subjective

The client is a 22-year-old male rice farmer with a 1-week history of fatigue. He complains that he is so tired that it is difficult for him to return to work after lunch. He is also concerned about a loss of appetite. For the last 3 days he has eaten only one sandwich for lunch instead of three. When questioned, he remembered experiencing a vague right upper quadrant abdominal pain only when he would "lie a certain way." He denies use of drugs or alcohol. He has not used any chemicals in his work for over a year. His urine is a little darker, but he is unaware of the color of his stool. He lives with his wife and 1-year-old daughter; both presently have no complaint of illness. He considers himself a relaxed, happy person, but he is concerned about his present illness because he has "never been sick before, except for a cold."

Past history. This is negative. He has had no surgeries, hospitalizations, or serious or chronic illnesses. He takes no medications and has no known allergies. He does not use tobacco.

Review of systems. This is negative except for possibly a few pounds of weight recently lost. There are no positive findings other than those in the history presented.

Family history. This is negative.

Life-style. The client works with his father on the family farm. Even though the hours are long, he enjoys his work because he is doing what he always wanted to do. He is a college graduate with a degree in agriculture. He describes his marriage as happy. His leisure time is spent with his family. He rarely eats away from home and has not done so recently. He is unaware of contact with anyone who has been ill or with known hepatitis.

Objective

General. Ht, 6 ft 1 in; wt, 190 lb; BP, 112/70; T, 99°; P, 74; R, 18. The client appears in no acute distress.

Physical examination. This is within normal limits except for:
1. Sclera: light yellow.
2. Abdomen: mild palpatory tenderness (without rebound) in the right upper quadrant and epigastric areas. There is liver tenderness to "fist" percussion over the right lower ribs. The liver is not palpable. The liver span at the midclavicular line is 8 cm. The spleen is not palpable; there are no masses. Bowel sounds are normal.

Laboratory data. Urine, 1+ bilirubin. Urine appears dark brown and foams when shaken; otherwise urine is within normal limits. WBC 8,400/mm^3, 58 neutrophils, 39 lymphocytes, 2 monocytes, 1 eosinophil. Hct, 45%.

Problems

1. Jaundice: possible hepatitis
2. Alteration in nutrition: decreased appetite and possible weight loss
3. Fatigue

Plan

The history and physical examination are typical of a client with hepatitis A, although no source of contamination can be identified. Thus even though the diagnosis could not be confirmed without further data, precuationary measures for hepatitis A were necessary. The client was instructed that he most likely has hepatitis, a viral infection of the liver. He was told that the most common form of viral hepatitis is not a serious disease and that he should recover fully if he does have this disease. He was told to thoroughly wash his hands after using the bathroom and before meals, since the virus for the common type of hepatitis is initially present in the bowel movements. He was told not to prepare food for others. He was told to rest in bed until his return in 36 hours to inform him of the results of his laboratory tests. He was to telephone the practitioner if his condition worsened or changed in any way.

The following laboratory tests were ordered:
1. SGPT, SGOT, alkaline phosphatase, bilirubin
2. HB$_s$Ag, anti-HAV (these were the only available tests for hepatitis)

Evaluation

The client returned in 36 hours. He reported that his stool was clay colored. His sclera was yellow; otherwise there was no change in subjective or objective findings. Laboratory results were:

SGPT	1,200 IU
SGOT	998 IU
Bilirubin	6 mg/dl
Alkaline phosphatase	9 Bodansky units
HB$_s$Ag	Negative
Anti-HAV	Positive
IgM class	Present
IgG class	Present

Table 12-3. Recommended precautionary measures for hepatitis A

Variables	Precautionary measures
Separate room	No, except with fecal incontinence
Body waste	Wear gloves when handling waste or items contacting intestinal system
	Bag in 2 plastic sacks, seal securely, and discard in trash
Housecleaning	No special techniques; if contaminated with blood or feces, clean with 1:10 chlorine disinfectant (Clorox), wearing gloves
Limitation of visitors	No, except when client is a young child
Gowns and masks	No
Linen	No special precautions unless contaminated with feces; if contaminated, launder separately in hot water, detergent, and chlorine bleach
Dishes	None
Meals	Wash hands before eating
	Client should not prepare food for ingestion by others
Donating blood	Client should not donate blood

The laboratory findings confirmed the diagnosis of hepatitis A. The presence of both IgM and IgG signified acute infection of probably not more than 8 weeks' duration (Miller). The diagnosis was discussed with the client and his wife. Emphasis again was given to the usual short duration and good prognosis of the disease. The fecal-oral route of transmission was explained as well as precautionary measures for hepatitis A (Table 12-3). The client was to continue to rest for 1 week until his next visit. If he is feeling better at his 1 week return he can begin a progressive resumption of work activities, since contagion decreases after the first few days of icterus. Liver enzymes will be reevaluated in 1 month. With the expectation of declining levels, the enzyme tests will be repeated every 2 months thereafter until they are normal. The wife and child received prophylactic ISG.

REFERENCES

Aach, R.D.: Viral hepatitis—A to E, Med. Clin. North Am. **62:**59, 1978.
Ackley, A., and Gockle, D.: Viral hepatitis, Am. Fam. Phys. **21:**156, 1980.
Bradley, D., and Maynard, J.E.: Serodiagnosis of viral hepatitis A by radioimmunoassay, Lab. Manag. **16:**29, 1978.
Center for Disease Control: Morbid. Mortal. Weekly, Reports 1980, Epidemiologic notes and reports, vol. 29, No. 38, Sept. 26, 1980, p. 459.
Corey, L., and Holmes, K.: Sexual transmission of hepatitis A among homosexual men, N. Engl. J. Med. **302:**435, 1980.
Deinstag, J.L., and others: Hepatitis. In Isselbacher, K.J., and others, editors: Harrison's principles of internal acute medicine, ed. 9, New York, 1980, McGraw-Hill, Inc.
Dmochowski, L.: Viral type A and type B hepatitis: morphology, biology, immunology epidemiology—a review, Am. J. Clin. Pathol. **65:**741, 1976.
Favero, M.S., and others: Guidelines for the care of patients hospitalized with viral hepatitis, Ann. Intern. Med. **91:**872, 1979.
Gunby, P.: Clinical trial of vaccine for type B hepatitis to begin next month, J.A.M.A. **241:**979, 1979.
Hanler, S., and others: Hepatitis A in day-care centers, N. Engl. J. Med. **302:**1222, 1980.

Hoofnagle, J.C., and others: Passive-active immunity from hepatitis B immune globulin, Ann. Intern. Med. **91:** 813, 1979.
Ishak, K.: Light microscopic morphology of viral hepatitis, Am. J. Clin. Pathol. **65:**814, 1976.
Mackowiak, P., and others: Oyster-associated hepatitis: lessons from the Louisiana experience, Am. J. Epidemiol. **103:**181, 1976.
Meyers, J.D., and others: Parenterally transmitted hepatitis A associated with platelet transfusions, Ann. Intern. Med. **81:**145, 1974.
Miller, D.J. Seroepidemiology of viral hepatitis: correlation with clinical findings, Postgrad. Med. **68:**137, Sept. 1980.
Mosley, J.W.: Hepatitis B immune globulin: some progress and some problems, Ann. Intern. Med. **91:**914, 1979.
Rakala, J., and Mosley, J.W.: Fecal excretion of hepatitis A virus, J. Infect. Dis. **135:**933, 1977.
Robbins, S.L., and Angell, M.: Basic pathology, ed. 2, Philadelphia, 1976, W.B. Saunders Co.
Sherlock, S.: Clinical aspects of viral hepatitis, J. R. Soc. Med. **71:**430, 1978.
Sherlock, S.: Chronic hepatitis, Postgrad. Med. **65:**81, June 1979.
Siegel, M.: Congenital malformations following chickenpox, measles, mumps and hepatitis, J.A.M.A. **226:** 1521, 1973.
Snodgrass, P.J., and Abbruzzese, A.: Diseases of the gall bladder and bile ducts. In Thorn, G.W., and others, editors: Harrison's principles of internal medicine, ed. 8, 1977, McGraw-Hill, Inc.
U.S. Department of Health, Education, and Welfare: Immune globulins for protection against viral hepatitis, Washington, D.C., 1977, The Department.

CHAPTER 13

Recurrent cystitis in the adult female

Mary M. Crane

Urinary tract infections strike women far more often than men. The problem is widespread; between 10% and 50% of the female population will have at least one urinary tract infection (Santoro and Kaye, 1978; Rubinoff, 1977). Many of these women will have repeated episodes. By comparison, 0.1% or less of young men will experience bacteriuria (Santoro and Kaye). This chapter considers nurse practitioner assessment and management of uncomplicated urinary tract infection in women; initial and recurrent infections are discussed separately. Intervention relates to areas where nurse practitioners may contribute through care and research. New approaches to management and prevention are suggested to reduce the occurrence of this common women's health problem. Although the case presented here focuses on one person, I include approaches appropriate to various other client groups.

A number of factors support the role of the nurse practitioner in caring for clients with uncomplicated urinary tract infections. Guidelines for both the diagnosis and treatment are well established. Clients experiencing recurrences need much support, teaching, and help to make behavior changes necessary to reduce the number of infections. Research demonstrates that nurse practitioners are effective care providers for women with urinary problems. Komaroff and associates (1976) studied nurse practitioner care of respiratory tract and urinary tract infections using protocols. He found that the nurse practitioners were able to provide care for clients in 70% of visits without consultation and that the cost of their care was lower. The following material is based on the experiences and education of nurse practitioners and may prove useful to those who encounter urinary problems in the clinical setting.

EPIDEMIOLOGY

Urinary tract infections are best viewed as multifactorial in cause. Age, sexual activity, pregnancy, history of childhood infections, and the amount of time since the last episode of infection are the best predictors of women at risk for infection. Age plays a significant role. Incidence of infection rises to a peak of 10% to 15% in older women (Santoro and Kaye). Public awareness of "honeymoon cystitis" gives testimony to the increased incidence of infections when women begin to have sexual relations. For women who have had infections during their school years this risk approximates 50% in the first 3 months of marriage (Kunin, 1970). Pregnancy further increases the risk, and the infection rate increases with parity (Kass, 1960). The amount of time since the last infection is another useful predictor. Kraft and Stamey (1977) found the first 6 months after an infection to be the most crucial. They report that infections occur in clusters with long periods of remission. On the other hand, family history and socioeconomic status show no relationship to infection and should not be considered indicators of high-risk individuals.

ANATOMY, PHYSIOLOGY, AND PATHOPHYSIOLOGY
Ascending route of infection

How do high-risk women become infected? The most common route is an ascending path through the short female urethra. Hematogenous and lymphatic routes of entry do not contribute significantly to uncomplicated infections. O'Grady and associates (1970, p. 1210) suggest a sequence of events to explain infection by way of the ascending route. They state:

> In some women, faecal organisms colonize the introitus; in a proportion of those, colonization extends to the urethra; in a proportion of those, urethral organisms enter the bladder during micturition; in a proportion of those, imperfect bladder defense mechanisms allow the admitted organisms to grow.*

If this framework is correct, certain factors along the sequence help determine whether or not infection will occur.

Rees (1978) provides an outline of possible causes of cystitis symptoms in women (Table 13-1). He defines cystitis broadly as "an inflammatory condition of the urinary bladder." The model he uses as the basis for his outline depicts the ascending route of infection (Fig. 13-1). One cause he identifies is introital multiplication of bacteria. Several studies show that women with recurrent urinary tract infections demonstrate a greater frequency of colonization than do normal subjects (Stamey and Sexton, 1975; Fowler and Stamey, 1977). Other fail to find this distinction (Cattell and others, 1974; Elkins and Cox, 1974).

Rees also notes factors that allow pathogens access to the bladder from the introitus, such as short uretha or urethral disorders. In addition to these, coughing, sneezing, or coitus may play a role. The former two occurrences can force urine from the bladder into the urethra, where it may become contaminated. When the pressure is relieved, this infected urine returns to the bladder, predisposing to infection (Riff, 1978). Milking of the urethra, which presumably occurs during sexual intercourse, can also force bacteria into the bladder, with similar results (Santoro and Kaye). Rees's outline further supports the multicausal nature of the problem, which has pertinent implications during establishment of the client's data base.

Symptom complexes as predictors

What client data successfully predict a urinary tract infection? Other conditions, such as vaginal infections and weakened pelvic muscle support, can mimic these infections.

---

*From Cattel, W.R. Cited in O'Grady, F.W., and others: Introital enterobacteria, urinary infection, and the urethral syndrome, Lancet **2**:1208, 1970.

Table 13-1. Urinary tract infection in females

Development of urinary pathogens*	Contributing factors
1. Source of urinary pathogens	Normal bowel flora (usual source) From sex partner Hematogenous via kidney Cross infection in hospital
2. Perianal accumulation of pathogens	Bowel dysfunction Defective toilet hygiene Perianal disorders
3. Progressive colonization of pathogens	Bacterial motility Defective hygiene Sexual activity
4. Introital multiplication of urinary pathogens Any cause of vulvovaginitis	Infection Trauma Chemical Allergy Inadequate vulvar ventilation Postmenopausal atrophy
Other causes of vaginal discharge	Hormonal Chronic cervicitis Intrauterine device

Increased vaginal alkalinity
    Urinary frequency and incontinence
    Other causes of pruritus vulvae
	Leukoplakia
	Pediculosis

5. Factors allowing access of pathogens to bladder	Shortness of urethra (anatomical) Urethral sphincter weakness Coitus Urethrovesical reflux Turbulent urine flow (eddies) Instrumentation or catheterization
6. Defective clearance of pathogens from bladder	Inadequate fluid load Infrequent voiding Incomplete voiding Reduced cellular immunity
7. Other causes of symptoms of cystitis	Almost any urological condition Other pelvic inflammatory disease Spinal dysfunction Sexual and psychosexual problems Psychosomatic problems Anxiety

Modified from Rees, D.L.: Urinary tract infection, Clin. Obstet. Gynaecol. **5**:169, 1978.
*See Fig 13-1.

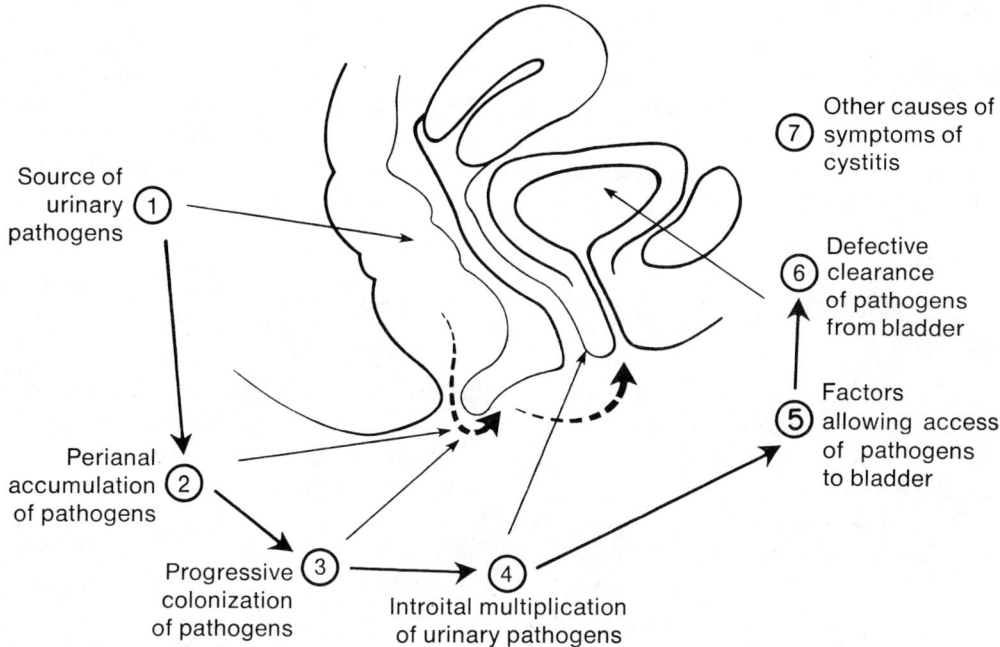

Fig. 13-1. Factors in the etiology of symptoms of cystitis in women, including urinary infection. (From Rees, D.L.: Urinary tract infection, Clin. Obstet. Gynaecol. **5:**169, 1978.)

In the absence of an organic pathological condition, 25% to 50% of women having urinary tract symptoms do not actually have bacteriuria (Stamey, 1972; Kraft and Stamey). Although this is an area ripe for research, some studies provide helpful guidelines. Burger and Wolcott (1978) studied the relationship between symptom complexes and a positive urine culture. Frequency alone did not relate significantly to a positive culture, although dysuria alone did. These symptoms occurred together much more frequently in women with a positive culture. Symptoms of short duration (less than 14 days) and a documented history of a positive culture in the past made the diagnosis of urinary tract infection even more likely. Dysuria and frequency for more than 14 days correlated poorly with positive culture results. Hematuria by itself corresponded highly with a positive culture, but this symptom occurs infrequently. Unreliable symptoms included fever and a history of symptoms in the past.

Komaroff and associates support some of Burger and Wolcott's findings. They found dysuria and frequency more common in women with urinary tract infections than in women with vaginitis. They differentiated internal dysuria (felt inside the body) from vaginal irritation and found the former more frequent in urinary tract infections. Symptoms were more likely to have occurred less than 3 days before women with actual urinary tract infections sought care. They further identified vaginal discharge and irritation as symptoms that should be investigated in patients with urinary tract complaints. The absence of these symptoms with the presence of frequency and dysuria makes the diagnosis of vaginal infection highly unlikely.

ASSESSMENT

A complete and accurate history assumes a major role in the management of urinary tract infections. The physical examination contributes little, and laboratory confirmation (culture and sensitivity) of initial urinalysis is unavailable for 24 to 48 hours. Therefore the burden of proof is on the initial history to establish the presence of a urinary tract infection; however, accurate diagnosis based on subjective data is possible only to a limited extent because of the current level of knowledge in the field.

History

Medication usage. When taking the history, the practitioner should ask about current intake of medications. Knowledge of antibiotics prescribed for other conditions is essential in planning for therapy. When urinary tract infections begin during antibiotic treatment, an unusual organism may be the cause because of changes in bowel flora. Choice of a drug is more difficult, since the causative bacteria may have developed resistance to the antibiotic currently being taken. During antibiotic therapy other drugs, obtained over-the-counter or prescribed, may interfere with absorption and metabolism. Finally, allergies may prevent the safe use of certain drugs.

Past history. In addition to past urinary tract infection, a history of other diseases should be obtained. Research has yet to clearly establish the relationship between certain diseases and urinary tract infections. It is controversial whether the occurrence of urinary tract infections is increased in diabetic women (Burger and Wolcott; Forland and others, 1977). Upper tract involvement (infection above the level of the bladder) appears more common in these clients (Forland and others; Riff). Urinary problems in diabetic clients certainly warrant careful assessment and management. These clients have decreased ability to fight infections; infection may complicate blood glucose control, and diabetic renal impairment may preclude the use of certain antibiotics.

Other diseases show varying relationships to urinary tract infections. Renal disease may increase the susceptibility of the kidney to infection. Organisms located inside renal calculi are inaccessible to antibiotics and are frequent sources of relapse of infection. Black women with sickle cell trait have a higher incidence of bacteriuria during pregnancy than black women without the trait. Some authorities note increased infections in women with hypertension, gout, and chronic hypokalemia, but documentation of these associations is incomplete (Santoro and Kaye).

Questioning for the presence of other diseases in the elderly is particularly important. They may have diminished renal function from past pyelonephritis, arteriosclerosis, or uncontrolled hypertension. These problems alter antibiotic dosage and may cause uneven concentration of the antibiotic throughout the renal parenchyma. Cerebral impairment decreases cortical control of micturition, while relaxation of pelvic structures inhibits complete emptying of the bladder. Aging changes reduce the likelihood of such symptoms as pain and fever. Bone loss may lead to the formation of renal stones. Finally, atrophic changes in the urinary tract may promote infection.

Urinary elimination behaviors may influence the pattern of urinary tract infections. Unfortunately, behavioral research in this area is almost nonexistent. One study, however, showed that voiding patterns significantly influence urinary tract infections. In a student health service Adatto and associates (1979) found that fluid intake and the number of daily voidings differed little between female clients with recurrent urinary tract infections and the normal control group. They did, however, find significant difference between the two groups in voluntary retention of urine. A larger percentage of the client group tended to hold urine more than 1 hour rather than void. Lapides and associates (1968) found that women with recurrent urinary tract infections voided infrequently. The vast majority of these women had abnormally high bladder capacities. He speculated that bladder distention compromises the vesical walls and lowers resistance to bacteria. It may be valuable to ask the client about the number of voidings per day and if she tends to "hold urine" for excessive periods. Another factor to consider is a history of dysuria and suprapubic pain relieved by voiding (Lytton and Epstein, 1977). This symptom complex (Hunner's ulcer) is a nonspecific chronic inflammation of the bladder wall.

Psychological elements may influence urinary tract infections. Rees and Farhoumand (1977) found a higher than normal incidence of psychological symptoms, especially anxiety, in women with recurrent urinary tract infections. Subjects tested higher in free-floating anxiety, obsessionality, and somatization than did the control group. This study, however, included persons with urethral syndrome and frequency-dysuria syndrome. Galland and associates (1977) found that half of the clients related their symptoms to previous emotional stress. Unfortunately, this study did not define "emotional stress" or compare client reports with those of a control group. The practitioner should question the client about urgency or urgency with incontinence as well as the progression of symptoms throughout the day. If symptoms improve throughout the day, psychogenic factors may be the cause.

Sexual history. Client assessment should include aspects of a sexual history. The incidence of urinary tract infections increases with the onset of sexual relations. Adequate foreplay, which is necessary to lubricate the vagina to prevent irritation, may minimize the risk of subsequent urethral bacterial colonization. A rough or traumatic vaginal pentration may also cause irritation and allow bacteria to invade the introital area. Postmenopausal women may experience more urethral trauma during intercourse because of tissue atrophy. Alternate forms of sexual expression, such as oral or anal intercourse, masturbation, and the use of mechanical devices, may also promote transmission of bacteria. The practitioner should ask the client about the frequency of oral, vaginal, and anal intercourse and if there is a recent venereal disease contact.

The type of contraception a client uses may also have an effect on the incidence of urinary tract infection. Although Marsh and associates (1972) found contraceptives to have no influence on colonization of the vaginal introitus, Rees noted a difference in the incidence of symptoms in cystitis among women using various types of birth control. Women taking oral contraceptives were least likely to have symptoms, while users of intrauterine devices expressed urinary symptoms. More work is necessary to clarify this relationship.

Physical examination

The physical examination contributes little to the diagnosis of urinary tract infection; however, it should include temperature, blood pressure, abdominal examination, and palpation for costovertebral angle tenderness. Abnormal findings may suggest upper tract involvement or the presence of other conditions. They do not, however, correlate well with a positive urine culture (Burger and Wolcott). The use of routine pelvic examination is debatable. The symptoms of vaginitis can mimic urinary tract infection, and clients with gonorrhea may experience dysuria. Komaroff and associates suggest that this part of the examination is optional except when vaginal discharge or vaginal-vulvar irritation exists. Others insist that pelvic examination is mandatory. If subjective data can differentiate between vaginal and urinary tract infection, omitting this part of the assessment could reduce the cost of care. In general, routine omission of the pelvic examination is inappropriate if the diagnosis is unclear.

Laboratory data

Bacteriology. *Escherichia coli* is the causative organism for 90% of initial uncomplicated infections (Riff). The presence of *Pseudomonas aeruginosa* or *Proteus* species may suggest structural abnormalities or recent instrumentation. *Klebsiella aerogenes* and *Enterobacter* also indicate that other diseases or defects may be present. A culture that grows multiple organisms is usually contaminated (Riff).

Laboratory data provide the definitive diagnosis of urinary tract infection through quantitative urine culture. Many authorities agree that more than 10^5 organisms per milliliter from an uncentrifuged urine specimen obtained by midstream-voided technique indicate true bladder bacteriuria (Kass, 1965). Colony counts fewer than 10^5 organisms by a clean-voided method are notable when the urine culture identifies gram-positive organisms, fungi, or fastidious organisms. A first specimen yields an 80% probability of bacteriuria. The second specimen increases the accuracy from 90% to 95%. Any organisms recovered from urine by catheterization or bladder aspiration deserve attention.

Although the above appears clear-cut, certain factors may complicate urine culture findings. Urine concentration influences quantitative analysis. Colony counts are higher when the urine remains in the bladder for long periods, as in the first morning specimen. Low to borderline counts in the face of a strongly suspicious symptom pattern may be due to dilution. This may occur when clients begin to force fluids before submitting the specimen for culture. If any doubt exists, a second specimen may prove helpful.

Specimen collection. Careful specimen collection is important for accurate urine culture. Although it is perhaps more reliable, some authorities discourage routine catheterization because of possible infection from catheter insertion. Although this risk is only 1% to 2% in healthy young people, it is higher in the elderly, in persons with obstructive uropathy, and in pregnant women (Kunin and DeGroot, 1975). When a satisfactory voided specimen is unobtainable, an alternative procedure is suprapubic aspiration.

Proper technique in collection of a voided specimen is essential. The practitioner should teach the client to wash hands and to avoid contamination of the specimen container and cover. The client should be instructed to cleanse the perineum thoroughly to prevent vulvar bacteria, epithelial cells, or white blood cells from entering the specimen. Antiseptic soap and benzalkonium chloride (Zephiran) should be avoided because they are irritating and may kill some bacteria if not removed before voiding. The client should pass a small amount of urine into the toilet to clear the urethra before beginning the midstream collection. Women who are menstruating or who have excessive vaginal discharge may need to assume the lithotomy position with the nurse's assistance to ensure a usable specimen. Pregnant, obese, or elderly women may also require assistance because of difficulty reaching the genitalia or because of poor motor control. After obtaining the specimen, the practitioner should plate it on appropriate media within 20 minutes or refrigerate it immediately.

Although ideal, it is often impractical to withhold treatment before positive urine culture results. Client discomfort may preclude waiting. A culture is impractical for some clients; it may be beyond their financial means. In remote areas adequate laboratory facilities may not exist; clients may lack the transportation or travel time to obtain a culture. Insistence on culture may even prevent the individual from seeking care. On the other hand, purchasing expensive antibiotics when no infection exists is wasteful and potentially harmful.

Office screening for bacteriuria. Several low-cost methods are available for office screening for bacteriuria with results in 24 hours. They involve placing a measured amount of urine on agar and counting bacterial colonies. Some methods use different agars to differentiate gram-positive from gram-negative organisms. Many require heat for incubation. Trained laboratory personnel may be necessary to obtain accurate test results. A study done in a university outpatient service showed unreliability when one of these methods was used by nonlaboratory personnel (Martin and McGuckin, 1978). Collacott (1977) found that Microstix dip slides detected 93% of positive culture results with a 9% false positive rate. Kunin showed detection of 90% of positive urines using the same product (Kunin and DeGroot). Other researchers have found less accurate results (Brundtland and Hovig, 1973; Martin and McGuckin). This current lack of consensus on the accuracy of these methods discourages their widespread use. Miriovsky (1979) reviews specific techniques for office analysis of bacteriuria.

Microscopic examination of the urine is helpful initially. The presence of one or two bacteria per high-power field from a midstream, clean catch, Gram-stained, unspun urine specimen correlates closely with culture results of greater than 10^5 bacteria per milliliter (Kunin, 1974). Pyuria may also be present with other conditions, such as trauma, due to calculi or contamination of the specimen with vaginal secretions. Burger and Wolcott did find, however, that a combination of dysuria, frequency, and more than eight white blood cells per high-power field raised the probability of a positive culture to 72%. Color, odor, proteinuria, pH, and specific gravity do not determine the presence of significant bacteriuria. Hematuria alone suggests renal calculi, tumor, or rarely tuberculotic or fungal infection of the urinary tract (Kunin, 1974).

Differential diagnosis

Assessment of dysuria or urinary frequency includes consideration of local disease processes, systemic disease, and psychogenic disturbances. The first conditions to consider are infections of the reproductive system. Komaroff and associates, in studying young women with pelvic complaints, found that the diagnosis of vaginal infection is 6 times more common than that of urinary tract infection. Further, if vaginal discharge or internal irritation was the predominant symptom, vaginitis was almost always the correct diagnosis. Microscopic examination of any vaginal discharge is necessary to identify fungal or trichomonal infections.

Gonorrhea is also suspect because dysuria is a common finding in this disease. Slight dysuria is the only symptom in over half of women with gonorrhea of the lower genital tract (Carrington, 1978). Up to 80% of women with gonorrhea are totally asymptomatic (Green, 1971). Vaginal discharge and cervical tenderness on pelvic examination should lead to a high level of suspicion. The practitioner should keep in mind that the under-25 age group accounts for over half of gonorrhea cases (Green).

The next most common disease process is the urethral syndrome. This is dysuria and frequency with a negative urine culture and the absence of any structural defects. Only 50% to 75% of women with urinary symptoms actually have bacteriuria. In primary health care settings, Kunin (1974) finds the lower figure more common. The urethral syndrome accounts for 20% of symptomatic episodes in women with recurrent infections (Kraft and Stamey). Women with this problem have symptoms similar to true infection, have past history of documented infections, and have future episodes of bacteriuria. Although the cause is elusive, studies find that some of these patients go on to develop bacteriuria. Other clients, however, maintain negative urine cultures (Kunin, 1974; Riff; Stamey). This condition complicates the treatment of urinary tract infections before culture results are available. It frequently mandates obtaining a urine culture, since culture alone differentiates urethral syndrome from true infection. Perhaps future research will assure adequate care at lower cost.

Other, less common urinary tract conditions that produce symptoms similar to urinary tract infections are urethral caruncle and chronic interstitial cystitis. A urethral caruncle may produce profound dysuria. The physical examination reveals a small, cherry red polyp that may or may not protrude from the posterior lip of the external meatus. It is generally extremely tender on palpation. Chronic interstitial cystitis (Hunner's ulcer) is found most often in middle-aged women. A client history is the best tool for establishing its presence. Usual symptoms are dysuria and suprapubic pain relieved by voiding (Lytton and Epstein). Urine cultures for both are negative.

Other disease processes and recent urological treatments may provide the clue to the correct diagnosis. Frequency may be due to congestive heart failure or diabetes rather than to urinary tract disease. Hematuria should lead to suspicion of urinary tract cancer especially if it persists and is painless (Kart and associates, 1978).

When urgency alone or urgency with incontinence is the predominant symptom, psychogenic origin becomes a serious consideration. Frequency can also be due to psychological factors. Frewen (1976) describes this as an autonomic nervous system dysfunction caused by "emotional disharmony." It is most often seen in women aged 45 to 55 but is common in the elderly. Symptoms are usually worse in the morning on waking, with improvement as the day progresses. Most clients can identify events that bring on the difficulty. I find no other source that confirms or refutes the existence of the condition.

PLAN
Medications

When data confirm the diagnosis of urinary tract infection, the provider chooses whether or not to treat with medications. With spontaneous cure rates of 25% to 50%, the decision is complex (Stamey). Kunin (1974) showed that 80% of clients treated with placebos had a sterile urine on posttreatment reculture. Other data show achievement of a 60% to 80% cure rate solely with regular voiding and good hygiene practices (Rees). Thus providers should consider nondrug therapies when cost, drug side effects, or the development of drug resistance is important. Older clients fit these criteria because they have increased risk of side effects, high incidence of urinary tract infections, and often a limited income. However, most authorities still recommend drug therapy because the most commonly used drugs are inexpensive and have few side effects. Drug treatment may also give the client quicker relief of symptoms. Certainly any suspicion of complicated infection such as upper tract involvement, structural defects, calculi, or the presence of chronic disease mandates the use of antibacterial medication.

Sulfisoxazole, 2 to 4 g followed by 1 g four times a day for 10 days, is a standard treatment regimen. Sulfonamides meet all the criteria that should be considered when a drug is chosen. It is inexpensive, achieves high urine concentration in low doses, has few side effects, covers a broad spectrum of bacteria, and is not routinely used in serious infections. Tetracycline also meets these criteria. Pencillin is useful in many cases because it is effective against 80% of *E. coli,* 10% of *Proteus,* 25% of *Klebsiella aerogenes,* and all *Staphylococcus fecalis* (Stamey). I avoid the use of ampicillin. Although it is effective in treating urinary tract infections, it is a frequent drug of choice in more serious infections. The cost of the generic preparation is more economical than the trade name product. Nitrofurantoin is useful in treating urinary tract infections because it provides bacteriostatic levels in urine only. This precludes the development of side effects from the drug's ability to destroy bowel flora. It is, however, fairly expensive and shows frequent intolerance due to nausea. Serious pulmonary reactions have also occurred (Goth, 1981; Rosenow and others, 1968). A combination drug of trimethoprim and sulfamethoxazole (Bactrim) provides greater effectiveness by interfering with two separate steps in bacterial biosynthesis of essential nucleic acids and proteins. The wide use of cephalosporins and aminoglycosides in serious infections prevents their use in uncomplicated urinary tract infections.

Seven to 10 days of treatment is standard for uncomplicated urinary tract infections. Some studies report success with 2- or 3-day therapy; others report success with single-dose therapy (Riff; Bailey and Abbot, 1978). Shorter-term treatment may improve compliance, decrease cost, and reduce side effects.

Some studies also find that lower than usual doses of antibiotics are adequate for urinary tract infections, since a high drug level is achieved in the urine and is more important than the drug's concentration in the blood. Infection of the lower tract usually localizes to the mucosa where a higher antimicrobial level is easily achieved (Riff).

Drug interactions are important considerations. Broad-spectrum antibiotics inhibit intestinal flora and interfere with the synthesis of vitamin K, thus potentiating warfarin. Drug-induced diarrhea due to the destruction of normal bowel flora interferes with further drug absorption. Diarrhea also depletes potassium levels, causing problems with thiazide diuretics and digitalis preparations. Sulfonamides displace drugs, such as tolbutamide and warfarin (Coumadin), from protein-binding sites, which increases their concentration in blood and leads to drug overdosage. Lower doses of the sulfonamides are advisable for the elderly, who have less albumin available for binding. Older persons in general are particularly prone to undesirable drug interactions because of their high drug intake and frequent paradoxical reaction to drugs. Over-the-counter preparations may decrease drug effectiveness. For example, antacids decrease absorption of tetracycline, and a high intake of ascorbic acid may acidify the urine, limiting the antibacterial spectrum of erythromycin.

To use a medication effectively, the client requires more information than the number of pills and times taken per day. The practitioner should instruct the client how to take certain drugs to ensure their effectiveness. Some drugs are more effective when the urine maintains an alkaline pH; others require acidic urine acid pH. A diet high in milk products, fruits, and vegetables alkalinizes the urine. Regulation of urine pH should be appropriate to the drug used. Methenamine, nitrofurantoin, and tetracycline are more effective in an acid urine; erythromycin works better in an alkaline medium (Cimino, 1976). The literature is contradictory regarding optimal pH for the penicillins. Sulfonamides are not dependent on urine pH.

The appropriate accompanying intake of food also varies with different drugs. Clients should take nitrofurantoin with food, they should avoid milk with tetracycline. Ingesting lactobacillus milk, buttermilk, or yogurt with penicillin helps replace intestinal flora and prevent diarrhea. Spacing of doses is also important, since antibiotics are more effective if the client spreads the dose evenly over a 24-hour period. Many clients stop taking drugs when the symptoms subside unless the nurse practitioner teaches them that bacteria may still be present. The practitioner should explain that saving antibiotics and using them later may complicate the diagnosis of other infections. Finally, clients should know symptoms that indicate drug side effects.

Pain relief

Relief of pain may be the client's main concern when coming for treatment. Clients may decrease fluid intake to reduce the frequency of voiding, which may even increase pain. The client should be taught to urinate as a means of ridding the bladder of bacteria. Phenazopyridine (Pyridium) (a bladder anesthetic), 200 mg three times a day for 3 days, and hot tub baths should be used to relieve discomfort. The nurse must prepare the client in advance for the orange discoloration of the urine caused by Pyridium. If discomfort persists past 3 days, reassessment is essential because the bacteria may be resistant to the antibiotic prescribed. Eradication of the infection is the best way to obtain relief. Rest is also important, since it reduces the discomfort of the accompanying malaise.

Behavioral preventive measures

Although few have studied this area well, many authors do not find specific behavioral measures helpful in preventing future infections. The multifactorial cause of urinary tract infections, however, suggests that a highly individual plan might prove helpful. It remains for further study to clarify what measures or combination of measures are effective in prevention.

Elimination patterns. These are particularly relevant to prevention. The practitioner should stress frequent urination, complete bladder emptying, voiding soon after perceiving the urge, and front-to-back wiping after urination and defecation. Complete bladder emptying reduces the number of bacteria in the bladder. Frequent urination discourages bacterial multiplication because *E. coli* doubles every half hour in the bladder (Cimino). One study has shown avoidance of voluntary urine retention and correct wiping to be the most significant factors in behavioral prevention (Galland and others). This study achieved a lower than expected recurrence rate over an 8-month period in subjects who followed a specific preventive regimen. The regimen prescribed eight 8-ounce glasses of fluid per day, urination every 2 hours, urination before and after intercourse, adequate lubrication before vaginal penetration, and correct wiping after elimination.

Sexual activity. If the client is sexually active and the infection is associated with intercourse, sexual counseling is necessary. Voiding before and after intercourse and cleanliness of both partners, especially uncircumcised males, have been suggested as preventive measures (Cattell and others). However, they are not yet supported or refuted by research. If alternate forms of sexual expression are common, hygiene is important. For example, vaginal intercourse should occur before anal intercourse, and the genitals should be cleaned thoroughly afterward. Anal intercourse in the face-to-face position should be avoided. The practitioner should use caution in making these recommendations if changes in sexual practices discourage sexual activity. The provider should include contraception in counseling. Condoms alone provide marginal protection against pregnancy and may explain the pain associated with vaginal penetration. To help them make an informed decision, the client and her partner need accurate information about different types of contraceptives. Another contraceptive may improve the comfort and satisfaction for both.

Diet. A high fluid intake of six to eight 8-ounce glasses of liquids daily should be encouraged. Fluids to avoid in excess are caffeine-containing substances, high-sugar content drinks, and alcohol because they irritate the bladder. Large quantities of cranberry juice are helpful if urine acidification will help the effectiveness of the drug of choice. After treatment, cranberry juice is also useful in prevention because it maintains an acid urine and thus has specific bacteriostatic effects. This bacteriostatic action is due to urinary excretion of hippuric acid, a byproduct of the juice metabolism. The quinic acid in the juice is converted to benzoic acid in the gut. This is then conjugated to hippuric acid in the liver (Kunin, 1974).

Since most aerobic bacteria that colonize the bladder grow best in a neutral or alkaline pH, urine acidification helps prevent infection. Aside from cranberry juice, a diet yielding an acid urine is high in meat, whole grains, eggs, and cheese. This diet limits vegetables and fruits to two servings (except cranberries, prunes, and plums) and milk to 1 pint per day. Carbonated beverages, baked goods containing baking powder or soda, and chocolate should be discouraged (Williams, 1978).

The provider may also recommend ascorbic acid, 500 mg 2 to 4 times daily, to acidify the urine (Kunin, 1974). The provider should be aware that there are difficulties in the use of ascorbic acid for urine acidification. High doses are required to obtain this result. Some studies have implicated high doses of the drug in such problems as increased formation of urinary tract stones, diarrhea, and problems in pregnancy.

Other measures. Several possible preventive measures lack sufficient documentation. Some authors recommend that women at risk for urinary tract infections avoid vaginal hygiene spray, strong soaps, and bubble bath (Jameson, 1976; Cattell and others; Rees). They speculate that these products could cause infection through lowered urethral defense mechanisms due to irritation. I suspect that menstrual hygiene products may also contribute to infection. Tampons might force bacteria into the bladder by milking action during insertion, or the string remaining at the vaginal orifice might help spread bacteria from the anus. Tampons impregnated with deodorant may cause irritation similar to the other feminine hygiene products. However, Kunin (1974) states that menstrual products do not affect bacteriuria. The lack of sufficient study in this area prevents the recommendation of behavior changes unless an infection is clearly associated with the menstrual period. Cotton underwear or underwear and pantyhose with cotton panels may be useful. They permit better air exchange and might decrease introital bacterial growth by reducing the warmth and moisture in the area.

EVALUATION
Expected outcomes

At the end of drug therapy the client's urine should be free of bacteria if the correct medication was prescribed and taken. The client should be free of urinary symptoms in 48 to 72 hours after therapy is initiated. The client should also report the initiation of specific behavioral preventive measures. She should be informed that urinary infections may be recurrent and that care should be sought rapidly if symptoms recur. Assessment for eradication of the infection is part of the return visit. This is done best 48 to 72 hours after completion of antibiotic therapy. A urine culture verifies the absence of bacteria. Where cost and availability are a problem, dip slides or tests for nitrite are acceptable alternatives. Young people enter the health care system infrequently, the evaluation visit provides an opportunity to assess the client's status through developmental tasks and to offer anticipatory guidance for the future.

Recurrent urinary tract infections

Recurrent infections can be tiring and stressful. They take a high-energy toll in both physical illness and psychological stress. Treatment for the infection can be a financial burden to a young family. Much productive time is lost from work and daily activities because of physical illness and frequent visits to health care settings. When a second infection occurs, the provider should consider serious causes of urinary tract infection. The time for extensive testing in the absence of indications is debatable. Early referral may promote instrumentation and surgery. Late referral discounts more serious disease or obstruction, which leads to prolonged infections or damage to the urinary tract. Riff suggests treatment of reinfection as an uncomplicated urinary tract infection unless it appears with great frequency. Asscher (1977) recommends further testing in adult women only if repeated infections occur without linkage to sexual relations. On the other hand, Kunin (1974) advises the continuation of diagnostic evaluation on the second or third infection, especially if there was documented infection in childhood.

Relapse versus reinfection

One question that helps determine need for referral is whether the infection is due to relapse or reinfection (Table 13-2). A relapse is the return of bacteria of the same species, serotype, and antibiotic susceptibility. It usually occurs within 1 week to 1 month after treatment is completed. Reinfection, on the other hand, usually reveals bacteria different in one or all of the above respects and occurs at least 2 to 4 weeks after

Table 13-2. Differentiating types of recurrent infections

Criteria	Relapse	Reinfection
Type of bacteria	Same species, serotype, and antibiotic susceptibility as first infection	Different species, serotype, or antibiotic susceptibility from the first infection
Onset	1 to 4 weeks after treatment for first infection	2 to 4 weeks after treatment for first infection
Involved urinary structure	Often renal involvement when treatment of initial episode was adequate May have underlying structural abnormality	Usually only bladder and urethra without renal involvement
Frequency	20% of recurrences	80% of recurrences
Common causes	Treatment failure: noncompliance, resistance to drug Infected urinary tract stone Remaining microcalculi after stone removal L-form bacteria Renal disease	Different bacteria defined by species, serotype, or antibiotic susceptibility
Disposition	Referral if not due to noncompliance	Consultation preferred

treatment (Riff). If treatment was adequate, relapses are more serious because they usually indicate renal involvement or structural abnormality (Santoro and Kaye; Riff; Turck and others, 1968). Reinfections are usually confined to the lower tract. Fortunately, reinfection accounts for 80% of recurrent infections (Asscher).

Serotyping is a laboratory test used to identify an organism more specifically. It may help differentiate relapse from reinfection. Problems of additional cost and availability make this test impractical in many primary health care settings. Perhaps this test is most useful in patients who, after adequate therapy, show an early return of symptoms or show symptoms of upper tract involvement.

The identification of a relapse places the primary health care provider in an early referral situation. A variety of factors, some known and some speculative, cause relapses. The most common and least serious cause is treatment failure. The client may fail to comply adequately with treatment, or the bacteria may be resistant to the drug used.

After excluding treatment failure, the practitioner should investigate other causes. Urinary tract stones may contain bacteria in their center, which protects them from antibiotic agents. *Proteus* is a common organism in this case (Gleckman, 1979). Some authorities feel that infection may continue after removal of the calculi because of remaining microcalculi.

Another somewhat theoretical cause of relapse is L-form bacteria. L-forms are aberrant bacterial forms with defective cell walls that develop during treatment. These bacteria then revert back to the original organism, causing relapse (Gleckman; Asscher). The hypertonicity of the renal medulla favors persistence of these forms. Penicillin and the cephalosporins also promote their development through interference with the synthesis of the bacterial cell wall. Erythromycin, however, is effective against them, and the increase of fluid intake helps reduce medullary osmolality (Turck and others; Cimino; Asscher).

Renal disease may also cause relapse. Even if the overall renal function seems adequate, patchy disease may cause antibiotics to bypass those nephrons that are diseased (Asscher). Thus bacteria remain there and later emerge. Renal disease may also prevent antibiotics from concentrating sufficiently in the urine to destroy the offending organism.

Upper tract involvement

Early referral is essential when infection involves the urinary tract above the bladder. The provider should seriously consider this possibility when infection becomes recurrent or resistant to treatment or when structural abnormalities exist. Identification of upper tract involvement by history would be ideal; however, this is not possible. Providers associate fever, chills, and flank pain with upper tract infection. Unfortunately, their absence does not exclude the upper tract (Fairley and others, 1971). Rees reported on the significance of backache and loin pain. The incidence of the symptoms was higher in the women with cystitis than in women attending family-planning clinics. However, intravenous pyelograms were normal in most of the study group, and almost 66% remained abacteriuric on repeated testing. The pain disappeared in almost all subjects who practiced regular lumbar spine exercises.

This imprecision causes providers to risk missing an upper tract infection each time they treat without specific tests to identify this. Yet all methods available at this time are invasive, costly, or require referral out of the primary health care setting. Ureteral catheterization provides the most accurate way to tell the difference, but it possesses all three disadvantages. A bladder washout system with serial cultures is also costly and is less accurate.

An antibody-coated bacteria test does provide promise of being reliable, noninvasive, reasonably economical, and possibly available to primary health care settings. The basis for this test is that bacteria that originate in the renal parenchyma become coated with antibodies, while those from the bladder do not. The procedure is as follows: Bacteria from a centrifuged urine specimen are incubated with fluorescin-conjugated antihuman globulin and examined for fluorescence. The antibodies attached to bacteria from the upper tract are reactive with the antihuman globulin and fluoresce, giving a positive test. This test is more reliable when compared with the other two available methods. False negative results occasionally occur when urine is tested too early in the disease process (Segura, 1978; Riff; Hawthorne and others, 1978). If this test becomes economical and available to primary health care settings, providers will no longer overlook upper tract infection and will make more timely referrals.

Further diagnostic procedures

Further diagnostic evaluation uses radiological examination. These tests should be requested by the physician, and at the time of the test the client should be as free from infection as possible. The initial test is plain radiography of the abdomen and pelvis. It may show renal calculi, tumors, cysts, hydronephrosis, or lesions of other systems affecting the urinary tract. The next step is an intravenous pyelogram and excretory urogram. These provide general information on the presence and functional status of the kidney and other parts of the urinary tract. Injection of a contrast medium is required, which may cause allergic reactions in some patients. The examination usually includes a postvoiding film to assess for residual urine. The timing of the passage of the dye through the system assesses the kidney's ability to concentrate and excrete (Kory and Waife, 1971). If the intravenous pyelogram is normal, Kunin (1974) does not recommend further evaluation.

A voiding cystourethrogram may be done if the urologist suspects vesicoureteral reflux or urethral obstruction. Dye is instilled into the bladder, and the lower urinary tract is examined before, during, and after voiding. Since surgery for mild vesicoureteral reflux in adult women is controversial and reflux may occur transiently after infection, the routine use of this test is not advisable (Kunin, 1974; Kory and Waife). If a catheter is used for dye insertion, a small risk of infection secondary to the procedure exists.

Cystoscopy confirms reflux and urethral diverticula or constriction. Combined with retrograde radiography, it further delineates abnormalities in the upper ureters and renal pelvis. Since it is a form of instrumentation, there is a slight risk of infection.

Long-term antibiotic prophylaxis

Unfortunately, most urinary tract infections occur in clusters, with long periods of remission. In adult women, reinfections follow even lengthy remissions. A study by Kraft and Stamey showed a median remission time of 43 weeks. Between remissions, infections occurred in close proximity at a rate of 0.47 per month. Thus the efficacy of any preventive measure is difficult to prove without long-term studies.

Ample data indicate that chemotherapy initiated after eradication of infection markedly reduces the incidence of reinfection (Gleckman). The provider must weigh the benefits against potential adverse effects. Providers frequently use nitrofurantoin and a combination of trimethoprim and sulfamethoxazole (Bactrim) for prevention, since these are least likely to cause resistant organisms.

The cost of prophylaxis may seem high. Kraft and Stamey compared the cost of prophylaxis with the cost of treatment for each infection. They calculated that each patient had two infections before prophylaxis. Treatment included culture and urinalysis before treatment and only culture afterwards. Prophylaxis proved more economical for the group as a whole, although some patients were treated who would not develop infection. The most economical time to begin prophylaxis is after the second infection in 6 months.

Treatment of recurrent infection in the elderly requires careful consideration. Urinary tract infections, with both relapses and reinfections, are common in this age group. However, symptoms usually abate spontaneously without chemotherapy. If obstructive lesions are absent, treatment in this population may do more harm than good. The practitioner should consider the prognosis of the condition versus the dangers of treatment. The elderly frequently experience more adverse effects from the antibiotics because of preexisting conditions, such as decreased renal function. Sulfonamides are safe until only a low level of renal function remains. Tetracycline and nitrofurantoin should be avoided in moderate to severe renal failure. Ampicillin is safe, since fairly high blood levels are tolerable. With this drug, however, the provider must consider the debilitation and potassium loss that might result from destruction of bowel flora and resulting diarrhea. The significance of this for clients taking diuretics or digitalis is profound. The elderly should be carefully monitored no matter what drug is chosen. In addition, the practitioner should consider cost for the elderly, since many of them have limited income.

Surgical intervention

Many providers think that surgical procedures reduce the number of infections that occur in rapid succession. Procedures to widen the urethra and to correct reflux are available but are currently viewed as less useful (Kunin, 1974; Asscher); mild reflux in the adult does not necessarily demand surgical correction. Many of the positive results attributed to surgical intervention may merely be the result of remission of the disease. Just 6 to 10 days of effective antimicrobial treatment results in at least 6 months' remission in 34% of cases (Kraft and Stamey). These surgical procedures are not harmless, any instrumentation carries a risk of infection.

CASE STUDY
Subjective

Myra is a 21-year-old college senior, with a 2-day complaint of "hurting when I go to the bathroom." She describes burning pain "up inside" with voiding, especially at the end of the stream. Myra has had a constant, suprapubic "aching" sensation for the past day, along with urinary frequency (about 4 to 5 times each night). She has not increased her usual 1 quart per day fluid intake. Despite a sensation of urgency, she voids only a few drops of urine. Myra complains of fatigue, sleeping more, and having difficulty concentrating on her studies. She denies fever, chills, flank pain, tenesmus, abnormal vaginal discharge, vaginal bleeding, or perineal or vaginal irritation. Her last menstrual period began 14 days ago. She denies a history of urinary tract infections. She does have a vague recollection of painful urination at age 9 without receiving medical treatment. She also denies any serious illnesses or known allergies. Usual voiding habits reveal that she passes her urine in the morning and again in the late afternoon. After elimination, Myra wipes from front to back. Myra admits to recent increased stress. Exams are approaching. She is sexually active and is taking oral contraceptives. Myra denies any recent venereal disease contact or more than one partner.

Objective

General. Ht, 5 ft 2 in; wt, 110 lb; BP, 116/72; T, 98.6; P, 80; R, 16. The client is a healthy Caucasian female in no acute distress. The physical examination, including pelvic examination, is normal except for the following. There is mild suprapubic palpatory tenderness. Costovertebral angle tenderness is absent. No liver or spleen enlargement or rebound tenderness exists.

Laboratory data. A midstream, clean-catch urine specimen was obtained. The client voided 1 hour before specimen collection. The Gram stain of unspun urine reveals four bacteria and nine white blood cells per high-power field. A drop of centrifuged urine reveals numerous white blood cells and "too-numerous-to-count" motile bacteria. No casts, crystals, trichomonads, red blood cells, or epithelial cells are observed.

Problems

1. Alteration in urinary elimination—probable urinary tract infection
2. Alteration in comfort

Plan

The symptoms of frequency and internal dysuria of recent onset indicate the possibility that Myra has a urinary tract infection. A documented history of a positive culture is necessary to determine the presence of this risk, since the incidence of symptoms without infection is high. She denied vaginal discharge, and irritation and burning were internal, thus making vaginal infection unlikely. Gonorrhea is a possibility in Myra's case. Although the pelvic examination was normal and discharge absent, she gave a history of recent coitus. Additionally, she is in the under-25 age group.

Diagnostic studies included a cervical gonorrhea culture and a urine culture and sensitivity. The urine was a midstream, clean-catch specimen without contamination by the fingers or toilet paper.

Medications. On the basis of the symptoms present and the positive microscopic urinalysis, Myra received sulfasoxazole, 1 g four times a day for 10 days. This drug meets several criteria for usefulness in treating urinary tract infections: It is inexpensive, achieves high urine concentration in low doses, has few side effects, and is not used routinely in serious infections. The nurse practitioner stressed not to discontinue the medication even if Myra felt better, because a full 10-day course is necessary to eradicate the bladder of bacteria.

Comfort. Pyridium, 200 mg three times a day for 3 days, was given to relieve discomfort. If discomfort persisted past 3 days, Myra was instructed to call. She was also prepared for the orange discoloration of urine that accompanies Pyridium intake. The importance of rest to help reduce discomfort and to shorten the course of "feelings of fatigue" was stressed. The practitioner helped identify specific ways to secure rest, including temporary discontinuation of late night studying.

Diet. The practitioner recommended six to eight 8-ounce glasses of fluid a day, and discouraged coffee, tea, and carbonated beverages. Upon the return visit Myra would be instructed on the importance of preventing recurrent infections by acidifying the urine through dietary changes.

Elimination. The provider reinforced frequent bladder emptying to rid the bladder of bacteria. Myra was discouraged from "holding the urine." The importance of wiping from front to back after either defecation or urination was also stressed.

Evaluation

Two weeks' follow-up visit. The results of the urine culture and sensitivity were greater than 10^5 *E. coli* per milliliter of urine. The organism was sensitive to sulfonamides. The gonorrhea culture was negative. The client's symptoms subsided. The nurse practitioner obtained another urine culture, and urinalysis results in the office were within normal limits. The second culture results were negative.

Subsequent visits. Myra married 1 year after graduation. She had two documented infections in the first 6 months of marriage. The infections appeared to be reinfections because the involvement was local and there was 1 month between episodes. All of these infections occurred within 24 hours of sexual intercourse. During the early months of marriage, Myra disregarded instructions on fluid intake, regular undelayed voiding, and voiding after intercourse. Myra was referred to a urologist for evaluation on assessment of the third infection.

The urologist recommended a plain radiogram of the abdomen and pelvis and an intravenous pyelogram. The procedure occurred without complications and showed a normal urinary tract with no residual urine. No further diagnostic testing was recommended at that time.

Because Myra's infections recurred rapidly, specific interventions to prevent further episodes were appropriate. The urologist recommended long-term prophylaxis, one-half tablet of a combination of sulfamethoxazole and trimethoprim (Bactrim) orally after intercourse for 6 months. If infections recurs on the regimen, the urologist would recommend a nightly dose at bedtime.

The importance of health teaching is essential with recurrent urinary tract infection. Myra and her husband were encouraged to use adequate lubrication before vaginal penetration. Voiding before and after coitus to clear the urethra and bladder of bacteria was stressed. The client was instructed to void before taking the prophylactic dose, especially at night, to keep a high concentration of the drug in the urine as long as possible. In reviewing preventive measures, the provider discovered that Myra still passed her urine infrequently and hurriedly because of her busy schedule.

She does, however, wipe correctly after elimination. Myra drinks only 1 quart of fluid daily. To support the pharmacological intervention to stop the cycle of infections, Myra needs to resume her behavioral preventive measures. She had not incorporated these into her daily routine since her marriage. Myra was given specific suggestions for incorporating voiding changes into her daily routine. Myra continued to take her sulfonamide-trimethoprim combination after intercourse for 6 months, and no infection recurred. She also resumed her other preventive measures. At 1-year follow-up, she was still symptom free.

REFERENCES

Adatto, K., and others: Behavioral factors and urinary tract infection, J.A.M.A. **241**:2525, 1979.

American Pharmaceutical Association: Handbook of nonprescription drugs, ed. 5, Washington, D.C., 1977, The Association.

Asscher, A.W.: Diseases of the urinary system: urinary tract infections, Br. Med. J. **1**:1332, 1977.

Bailey, R.R., and Abbot, G.D.: Treatment of urinary tract infection with a single dose of amoxycillin, Nephron, **18**:316, 1977.

Bailey, R.R., and Abbot, G.D.: Treatment of urinary tract infection with a single dose of trimethoprine- sulfamethoxazole, Can. Med. Assoc. J. **118**:551, 1978.

Brundtland, G.H., and Hovig, B.: Screening for bacteriuria in school-girls: an evaluation of a dip-slide culture method and the urinary glucose method, Am. J. Epidemiol. **97**:246, 1973.

Burger, L.M., and Wolcott, B.W.: A clinical algorhythm for urinary tract symptoms, Milit. Med. **143**:476, 1978.

Carrington, E.: Obstetric and gynecologic emergencies. In Schwartz, G.R., and others, editors: Principles and practice of emergency medicine, Philadelphia, 1978, W.B. Saunders Co.

Cattell, W.R.: The management of urinary tract infection in women, Nurs. Mirror **138**:65, 1974.

Cattell, W.R., and others: Periurethral enterobacterial carriage in pathogenesis of recurrent urinary infection, Br. Med. J. **4**:136, 1974.

Cimino, J.E.: Common bacterial urinary tract infections in women, Compr. Ther. **2**:23, 1976.

Collacott, R.A.: "Microstix"—a new diagnostic aid, J. Coll. Gen. Pract. **27**:104, 1977.

Elkins, I.B., and Cox, C.E.: Perineal, vaginal and urethral bacteriology of young women. I. Incidence of gram-negative colonization, J. Urol. **3**:88, 1974.

Erickson, E.H.: Childhood and society, ed. 2, New York, 1963, W.W. Norton & Co., Inc.

Fairley, K.F., and others: Site of infection in acute urinary-tract infection in general practice, Lancet **2**:615, 1971.

Forland, M., and others: Urinary tract infections in patients with diabetes mellitus: studies on antibody coating of bacteria, J.A.M.A. **238**:1924, 1977.

Fowler, J.E., Jr., and Stamey, T.A.: Studies of introital colonization in women with recurrent urinary infections. VII. The role of bacterial adherence, J. Urol. **117**:472, 1977.

Frewen, W.K.: Urgency incontinence, Br. J. Sex. Med. **3**:21, 1976.

Galland, L., and others: Behavioral aspects of recurrent urinary tract infections, J. Coll. Health Assoc. **25**:271, 1977.

Gleckman, R.A.: Recurrent urinary tract infections: therapeutic considerations, Postgrad. Med. **65**:156, 1979.

Goth, A.: Medical pharmacology, ed. 10, St. Louis, 1981, The C.V. Mosby Co.

Green, T.H.: Gynecology: essentials of clinical practice, ed. 2, Boston, 1971, Little, Brown & Co.

Hawthorne, N.J., and others: Accuracy of antibody-coated-bacteria test in recurrent urinary tract infections, Mayo Clin. Proc. **53**:651, 1978.

Holmes, T.H., and Rahe, R.H.: The Social Readjustment Rating Scale, J. Psychosom. Res. **11**:213, 1967.

James, G.P., and others: Urinary nitrite and urinary-tract infection, Am. J. Clin. Pathol. **70**:671, 1978.

Jameson, R.M.: Recurrent urinary tract infections in women, Nurs. Mirror **143**:55, July 22, 1976.

Kart, C.S., and others: Aging and health: biologic and social perspectives, Menlo Park, Calif., 1978, Addison-Wesley Publishing Co., Inc.

Kass, E.H.: Bacteriuria and pyelonephritis of pregnancy, Arch. Intern. Med. **105**:194, 1960.

Kass, E.H., editor: Progress in pyelonephritis, Philadelphia, 1965, F.A. Davis Co.

Komaroff, A.L., and others: Nurse practitioner management of common respiratory and genitourinary infections, using protocols, Nurs. Res. **25**:84, Mar.-Apr. 1976.

Kory, M., and Waife, S.O., editors: Kidney and urinary tract infections, Indianapolis, 1971, Eli Lilly and Co.

Kraft, J.K., and Stamey, T.A.: The natural history of symptomatic recurrent bacteriuria in women, Medicine **56:**55, 1977.

Kunin, C.M.: The natural history of recurrent bacteriuria in schoolgirls, N. Engl. J. Med. **282:**1443, 1970.

Kunin, C.M.: Detection, prevention and management of urinary tract infections, Philadelphia, 1974, Lea & Febiger.

Kunin, C.M.: New developments in the diagnosis and treatment of urinary tract infections. J. Urol. **113:**585, 1975.

Kunin, C.M., and DeGroot, J.E.: Self-screening for significant bacteriuria: evaluations of a dip-strip combination nitrite/culture test, J.A.M.A. **231:**1349, 1975.

Lapides, J., and others: Primary cause and treatment of recurrent urinary tract infection in women: preliminary report, J. Urol. **100:**552, 1968.

Lytton, B., and Epstein, F.: Dysuria, incontinence and enuresis. In Thorn, G.W., and others, editors: Harrison's principles of internal medicine, ed. 8, New York, 1977, McGraw-Hill, Inc.

Marsh, F.P., and others: The relationship between bacterial cultures of the vaginal introitus and urinary infection, Br. J. Urol. **44:**368, 1972.

Martin, M.J., and McGuckin, M.B.: Evaluation of a dipslide in a university outpatient service, J. Urol. **120:**193, 1978.

Miriovsky, M.F.: Office analysis of bacteriuria, Am. Fam. Phys. **19:**121, 1979.

O'Grady, F.W., and others: Introital enterobacteria, urinary infection, and the urethral syndrome, Lancet **2:**1208, 1970.

Pryles, C.V., and Lustik, B.: Laboratory diagnosis of urinary tract infection, Pediatr. Clin. North Am. **18:**233, 1971.

Rees, D.L.: Urinary tract infection, Clin. Obstet. Gynaecol. **5:**169, 1978.

Rees, D.L., and Farhoumand, N.: Psychiatric aspects of recurrent cystitis in women, Br. J. Urol. **49:**651, 1977.

Riff, L.J.M.: Evaluation and management of urinary infection, Med. Clin. North Am. **62:**1183, 1978.

Rosenow, E.C. III, and others: Chronic nitrofurantin pulmonary reaction: report on 5 cases, N. Engl. J. Med. **279:**1258, 1968.

Rubinoff, H.: Urinary tract infections, Prim. Care **4:**617, 1977.

Santoro, J., and Kaye, D.: Recurrent urinary tract infections: pathogenesis and management, Med. Clin. North Am. **62:**1005, 1978.

Segura, J.W.: Guidelines for diagnosing and treating urinary tract infections, Geriatrics **33:**87, 1978.

Stamey, T.A.: Urinary infections, Baltimore, 1972, The Williams & Wilkins Co.

Stamey, T.A., and Sexton, C.C.: The role of vaginal colonization with enterobacteria in recurrent urinary infections, J. Urol. **113:**214, 1975.

Turck, M., and others: Relapse and reinfection in chronic bacteriuria. II. The correlation between site of infection and pattern of recurrence in chronic bacteriuria, N. Engl. J. Med. **278:**422, 1968.

Williams, S.R.: Essentials of nutrition and diet therapy, ed. 2, St. Louis, 1978, The C.V. Mosby Co.

Index

A

Abdominal aortic aneurysm causing low back pain, 17
Abdominal pain, findings and pathological conditions causing, 219-220
Abduction/adduction stress tests to evaluate knee joint instabilities, 43
Abductor muscle
  strengthening exercises for, 64-65
  stretching exercises for, 55-57
Abortion, differential diagnosis of types of, 225
Acetaminophen
  producing hepatitis-like reaction, 241
  for muscle strain, 18-19
Achilles tendon stretching exercise, 53-54
Acidification of urine, 263
Acrisorcin for tinea versicolor, 152
Adductor muscles strengthening exercises, 64-65
Adolescence, 102; *see also* Adolescents
  emotional changes in, problems from, 110
  family tasks during, 105
  physical changes in, problems from, 110
  range of development during, 103
Adolescents; *see also* Adolescence; Minors
  assessment of, 105-107
  autoerotic stimuli and accompanying fantasies in, 110-111
  behavioral characteristics of, 104
  contraceptive counseling for, 111-112
  counseling, about sexuality, 108-110
  family of; *see* Family of adolescent
  interview of, 106-107
  masturbation by, counseling about, 110-111
  nursing care of, legal aspects of, 102
  parents of, guidelines for, 112
  physical examination of, 107
  problems of, managing, 110-113
  questionnaire for, 106
  response to divorce by, 118
  same-sex behavior by, 112
  venereal disease in, counseling about, 112
Adult client
  anemia in, 87-97
  early influences on, that lead to divorce, 115-116
  female, recurrent cystitis in, 252-270
  headaches in, assessing, 68-83
  hematological values in, normal, 90
  male, low back pain in, 3-23
  older, diverticular disease in, 192-208
  response of, to divorce, assessment of, 116-117
Adult runner
  knee pain and injuries in, 26-66
  physical examination of knee in, 32
Afro pick, alopecia associated with, in black client, 158
Akrinol; *see* Acrisorcin

Albinism in black clients, 152-153
Alcoholic hepatitis, 244
Aldomet; *see* Methyldopa
Allergy, cow's milk, in infant, 183-184
Alopecia in black clients, 157-158
American Academy of Pediatrics, Committee on Nutrition, 179, 185
American Medical Association, Subcommittee on Classification of Sports Injuries, 39
American Orthopaedic Society for Sports Medicine, Committee on Research and Education, 43
Aminosalicylic acid producing hepatitis-like reaction, 241
Amoxicillin for salpingitis, 227
Ampicillin
  for cystitis, 261, 267
  for salpingitis, 227
Analgesics
  for headache, 73
  for migraine, 73
  for subdural hematoma, 74
Androgen secretion after menopause, 125-126
Anemia
  in adult client, 87-97
  assessment of client with, 89-93
  iron deficiency, 88
  macrocytic, normochromic, 95-96
  microcytic, hypochromic, 93-95
  paradigm for referral of adults with, 96-97
  pernicious, 89
  plan and evaluation of client with, 93-96
  signs and symptoms of, 89
  simple, assessment factors in, 92
  vitamin B_{12} deficiency, 89
Aneurysm
  aortic, abdominal, causing low back pain, 17
  differential diagnosis of, 75
Angiomas, differential diagnosis of, 75
Ankylosing spondylitis causing low back pain, 16
Annulus fibrosus, 4, 5, 6
Anterior compartment, problems in, assessment and plans for, 30-39
Antibiotics
  for cystitis, 261-262
    long-term prophylaxis with, 267
  for pseudofolliculitis barbae, 157
Anticholinergic drugs for diverticular disease, 203
Anxiety during climacteric, estrogen replacement therapy for, 142
Aortic aneurysm, abdominal, causing low back pain, 17
Apley's test for meniscial injuries, 47
Appendicitis, differential diagnosis of, 224
Apprehension test for patellar instability, 37
Arch supports, 33

Arteritis, temporal, differential diagnosis of, 74
Articular processes, 4, 7
Artificial menopause, 125
Aspirin
  for muscle strain, 18-19
  for salpingitis, 227
  for tendinitis, 42
Autoerotic stimuli and accompanying fantasies in adolescents, 110-111

B

Back
  anatomy and physiology of, 4-8
  ligaments of, 4
  muscles of, 4
  pain in, low; see Low back pain
Bacterial meningitis, differential diagnosis of, 74-75
Bacteriuria, office screening for, 259
Bactrim; see Trimethoprim-sulfamethoxazole
Bed rest for muscle strain, 18
Behavior(s)
  elimination, urinary, and urinary tract infections, 256-257
  same-sex, by adolescents, 112
Behavioral characteristics of adolescent and family, 104
Bellergal for women during climacteric, 143
Biopsy, endometrial, of menopausal women, 134-135
Blacks
  problems of hair in, 157-158
  skin problems common to, 147-158
Bleeding, postmenopausal, 137
Blood cells
  differentiation of, 88
  red, production of, physiology of, 87-89
Blood group and salpingitis, 217
Body fluids, problems with, 85-97
Bottle-feeding, 163-188
  advent of, 163-164
Bowel disease, inflammatory, differential diagnosis of, 225-226
Brain tumor, differential diagnosis of, 74-75
Bran for high-fiber diet, 201-203
Breast self-examination during climacteric, 137
Breast-fed infant, vitamin supplementation for, 184-185
Breast-feeding, 174-179
  benefits of, 175-176
  history of, 163-164
  maternal concerns about, 176-177
  problems in, 177-179
Breast-milk jaundice, 176
Breasts of women during climacteric, 133-134
Burr cells, 91
Bursae of knee, 29
Bursitis, infrapatellar, 35

C

Cancer of prostate gland causing low back pain, 17
Cancer risk with estrogen replacement therapy, 141-142
Carbamazepine for trigeminal neuralgia, 75
Carbohydrate requirements during first year of life, 166
Cardiovascular problems during climacteric, estrogen replacement therapy for, 140-141
Child, response of, to divorce, assessment of, 117-118
Child's perspective of divorce, 116
Chlamydia trachomatis and salpingitis, 214
Chondromalacia patellae, 38-39
Climacteric
  caring for women during, 125-144
  change in menses during, 131
  definition of, 125
  dyspareunia during, 131
  physiology during, 125-126
  psychosocial aspects of, 126-129
  symptoms during, 131-133
  vaginal secretions during, 132
  women during; see Women during climacteric
Climax, information about, for adolescents, 111
Cluster headache, differential diagnosis of, 73-74
Co-counseling of adolescents, 109
Codeine
  for muscle strain, 19
  for salpingitis, 227
Colace; see Dioctyl sodium sulfosuccinate
Colon
  functions and motility of, 196-199
  segmentation activity in, 197
Comfort, alterations in, problems with, 1-83
Committee on Research and Education of American Orthopaedic Society for Sports Medicine, 43
Community education about hepatitis type A, 247-248
Contraception
  counseling about, for adolescents, 111-112
  method of, and salpingitis, 216-217
  in women during climacteric, 138-139
Contraceptives, oral, for women during climacteric, 138-139
Contracts between nurse and adolescent, 108-119
Coping, family, problems with, 99-158
Corticosteroids for temporal arteritis, 74
Counseling
  of adolescents about sexuality, 108-110
  of women during climacteric, 136-139
Cow's milk allergy in infant, 183-184

Cranium, pain-sensitive structures of, 68, 69
Cruciate ligaments, 27
Curves in spine, physiological, 4
Cyanosis in pigmented skin, assessment of, 151
Cyst, ovarian, differential diagnosis of, 224
Cystitis
   in adult female, recurrent, 252-270
      anatomy, physiology, and pathophysiology of, 253-255
      ascending route of infection in, 253
      assessment of client with, 256-260
      bacteriology of, 258
      diagnostic procedures for, 266-267
      diet for client with, 263
      differential diagnosis of, 259-260
      drugs for, 260-262
      elimination patterns and, 262-263
      epidemiology of, 252-253
      etiology of, factors in, 255
      evaluation of client with, 264-268
      history of client with, 256-257
      laboratory data of client with, 258-259
      long-term antibiotic prophylaxis for, 267
      pain relief for client with, 262
      physical examination of client with, 257-258
      plan for client with, 260-264
      reinfection in, 264-266
      relapse of, 264-266
      sexual activity and, 263
      surgical intervention for, 268
      upper tract involvement in, 266
   honeymoon, 252-253

D

Degenerative changes causing low back pain, 13-14
Degenerative disc disease, 14
Depression during climacteric, estrogen replacement therapy for, 142
Dermal melanosis in black client, 153
Dermatosis papulosa nigra, 153, 155
Developmental patterns and nutritional status during first year of life, 174
Developmental tasks during adolescence, 105
Diazepam
   for low back pain, 19
   for muscle spasm, 19
Diet
   for client with cystitis, 263
   for client with hepatitis, 245
   during climacteric, 136
   and diverticular disease, 201-203
   high-fiber, 201-203
Diet history of infant, 172-173
Dietary fiber and diverticular disease, 194-195, 197-198

Dietary patterns and diverticular disease, 194-195
Dilantin; see Phenytoin
Dioctyl sodium sulfosuccinate for diverticular disease, 203
Disc
   degenerative disease of, 14
   herniation of, 14-15
   intervertebral, 4, 5
Disc pressure
   during exercises, 20
   increased, protection of back from, 18
Disease
   bowel, inflammatory, differential diagnosis of, 225-226
   disc, degenerative, 14
   diverticular, in older adult, 192-208
   infectious, problems with, 211-270
   local, causing low back pain, 15-16
   organic, symptoms ascribed to menopause that may signal, 130
   pelvic inflammatory; see Salpingitis, acute
   systemic, causing low back pain, 16
   venereal, counseling adolescents about, 112
   visceral, causing low back pain, 17
Dislocated patella, recurrent, 36-39
Dislocation, patellofemoral, chronic, 36
Diverticula, 192
Diverticular disease in older adult, 192-208
   age, sex, and race and, 195
   assessment of, 199-201
   diet for, 201-203
   dietary patterns and, 194-195
   drugs for, 203
   epidemiology of, 192-196
   evaluation of, 204-205
   geographic distribution of, 193-194
   health education for client with, 204
   historical perspective on, 192-193
   life-style of client with, changes in, 204
   physiology and pathophysiology of, 196-199
   plan for client with, 201-204
   referral for, 205
Diverticulitis, 192-208
   referral of client with, 205
Diverticulosis, 193, 198
   asymptomatic and symptomatic, 200-201
Divorce, 115-124
   adjustment to, evaluation of, 123-124
   adult's response to, assessment of, 116-117
   assessment of client experiencing, 116-118
   assisting child to cope with, 119
   background for, 115-116
   child's perspective on, 116
   child's response to, assessment of, 117-118
   feelings commonly experienced during, 119-121

Divorce—cont'd
  first year after, 121-123
  intervention in early stages of, 118-119
Drawer sign to evaluate knee joint instability, 43
  rotary, 43-44
Drug-induced hepatitis, 244-245
Drugs; see Medications
Dyspareunia during climacteric, 131-132

E

Ectopic pregnancy, differential diagnosis of, 225
Education
  for client with acute salpingitis, 228
  about hepatitis type A, 247-248
  for older adult with diverticular disease, 204
Elimination behaviors, urinary, and urinary tract infections, 256-257
Elimination patterns and cystitis, 262-263
Emancipation of minors, 102
Emotional aspects of skin disorders, 147-148
Emotional symptoms during climacteric, 133
Endocrine process during puberty
  in female, 103-104
  in male, 104
Endometrial biopsy of menopausal women, 134-135
Endometrial cancer and estrogen replacement therapy, 141-142
Endometriosis, differential diagnosis of, 226
Energy requirements during first year of life, 165
Enterobacter and cystitis, 258
Environmental factors in black client with skin problems, 148-149
Ergotamine tartrate for migraine, 73
Eruptions, 150
Erythema in black skin, assessment of, 150
Erythrocyte, 87-89
Erythromycin for cystitis, 262, 265
Erythromycin estolate producing hepatitis-like reaction, 241
Erythropoietin and red blood cell production, 88
Escherichia coli and cystitis, 258, 261
Estrogen replacement therapy for women during climacteric, 139-143
Estrogen secretion after menopause, 126
Examination, physical; see Physical examination
Exercise(s)
  during climacteric, 136-137
  isometric, for client with low back pain, 20
  to relieve muscle strain, 20, 22
  strengthening
    isometric, 58-59
    weight-resistive, 60-65
  stretching, 47-57
Extension, Morton's foot, 34

F

Facets, 4, 7
Family of adolescent
  assessment of, 105-107
  behavioral characteristics of, 104
  developmental tasks of, 105
Family coping, problems with, 99-158
Family tasks during adolescence, 105
Fantasies, autoerotic stimuli and, in adolescents, 110-111
Fat pad, inflammation or swelling of, 35
Fat requirements during first year of life, 166-167
Fat-fold thickness of infants, measurement of, 173-174
Fatigue during first year after divorce, 121-122
Feeding, formula, 179, 183-184
Feeding history during infancy, 172
Feeding schedules for infants, 179
Female
  adult, recurrent cystitis in, 252-270
  endocrine process in, during puberty, 103-104
Femoral-stretch test for nerve root irritation, 15
Fiber
  dietary, and diverticular disease, 194-195, 197-198
  fruit and vegetable, and water-holding capacity, 202
Fitz-Hugh–Curtis syndrome
  with acute salpingitis, 214-215
  with hepatitis type A, 243, 245
Flatfoot, 33-34
Fluids, body, problems with, 85-97
Flushes, hot, 132
Folate deficiency, 88-89
Folic acid deficiency, 88-89
Follicle-stimulating hormone
  level of, in menopausal women, 135
  after menopause, 126
  pubertal changes caused by, 103-104
Foot
  without anatomical variations or previous injuries, running shoes for, guidelines for, 31
  excessive pronation of, 31-35
  Morton's, 31, 33
Foot supports, 31, 33
Formula(s)
  proprietary, 179
    composition, indications, and problems for, 180-182
  soy, 181, 183-184
  special, for infants, 179, 183-184
Formula feeding, 179, 183-184
Formula-fed infants, vitamin supplementation for, 185
Fruit fiber, 202
Fungal infections in black client, 152

Index **279**

G

Gantanol; *see* Sulfonamides
Gantrisin; *see* Sulfonamides
Gastrocnemius stretching exercise, 53-54
Genitourinary system of women during climacteric, 134
Genu valgum, 37
Gland
  pituitary, and pubertal changes, 103, 104
  prostate, cancer of, causing low back pain, 17
Gliding motion of left tibiofemoral joint, 27
Glucose tolerance during climacteric, estrogen replacement therapy for, 141
Gonococcal salpingitis, 214-215; *see also* Salpingitis, acute
Gonorrhea, history of, and salpingitis, 216
Growth standards for infants, 173

H

Hair
  problems involving, in black clients, 157-158
  of women during climacteric, 133
Hair straighteners, alopecia associated with, in black clients, 157-158
Hamstring muscle-tendon unit, 30
Hamstrings
  strengthening exercise of, 63
  stretching exercise of, 49-52
Head circumference of infants, 173
Head pain
  assessment of, 71-76
  history of client with, 72, 76
  origin of, 68, 69
  physical examination of client with, 76, 77
Headache attack diary sheet, 79
Headaches
  in adult client, assessing, 68-83
  differential diagnosis of, 73-75
  migraine; *see* Migraine
  physiology of, 68-71
Health education
  for client with acute salpingitis, 228
  for older adult with diverticular disease, 204
Health-seeking behavior and salpingitis, 217
Heat for muscle strain, 18
Heel lift, medial, 34
Height of women during climacteric, 133
Hematological values in adult, normal, 90
Hematoma, subdural, differential diagnosis of, 74
Hemoglobin, 87
  mean corpuscular, 89
Hemorrhage, subarachnoid, differential diagnosis of, 75
Hemorrhagic ovarian cyst, differential diagnosis of, 224

Hepatitis
  alcoholic, 244
  drug-induced, 244-245
  non-A, non-B, 236, 237
    epidemiology of, 238
  types of, comparison of, 236
Hepatitis type A, 235-250
  assessment of, 239-245
  client education about, 247
  clinical course of, 239-240
  diet for client with, 245
  differential diagnosis of, 244-245
  drugs for client with, 245
  epidemiology of, 237-238
  etiology of, 235-237
  evaluation of client with, 248
  history of client with, 240-241
  infection of, response to, 242
  isolation of client with, 246
  laboratory data on client with, 241-243
  physical examination of client with, 241
  physiology and pathophysiology of, 238-239
  plan for client with, 245-248
  precautionary measures for, 250
  prevention of transmission of, 245-246
  prophylaxis against, 246-247
  rest for client with, 245
  sexual patterns in client with, 246
Hepatitis type B, 236-237
  epidemiology of, 238
  laboratory data in client with, 242-243
  prophylaxis against, 246-247
Hepatitis-like reactions, drugs that produce, 241
Hepatobiliary influence of estrogen replacement therapy, 141
Herniation, disc, 14-15
History
  of client with acute salpingitis, 217-218
  of client with head pain, 72, 76
  of client with low back pain, 8
  of client with skin problems common to blacks, 148
  nutritional, of infants during first year of life, 171-173
  of women during climacteric, 131-133
Honeymoon cystitis, 252-253
Hormone
  follicle-stimulating
    level of, in menopausal women, 135
    after menopause, 126
    pubertal changes caused by, 103-104
  luteinizing
    after menopause, 126
    pubertal changes caused by, 103-104
Hot comb alopecia in black clients, 157

Hot flushes, 132
Hunner's ulcer, 257, 260
Hygiene, personal, during climacteric, 137-138

I

Idiopathic synovitis, 45, 46
Ilosone; see Erythromycin estolate
Infant
    breast-fed, vitamin supplementation for, 184-185
    diet history for, 172-173
    feeding history for, 172
    feeding schedules for, 179
    formula-fed, vitamin supplementation for, 185
    malnourished, 167
    nutrition for, history and trends in, 163-164; see also Nutrition during first year of life
    nutritional assessment of, 171-174
    obesity in, 167, 171
    semisolids for, 185-188
Infected septic abortion, differential diagnosis of, 225
Infections
    fungal, in black client, 152
    urinary tract, 252-270
        differential diagnosis of, 225
Infectious diseases, problems with, 211-270
Infectious hepatitis; see Hepatitis type A
Infertility after acute salpingitis, 230
Inflammation of fat pad, 35
Inflammatory bowel disease, differential diagnosis of, 225-226
Infrapatellar bursitis, 35
"Ingrown hairs" in black clients, 157
INH; see Isoniazid
Injuries
    knee, in adult runner, 26-66
        ligamentous, 42-46
        meniscial, 46-47
        prevention and rehabilitation of, 47-65
    ligamentous; see Sprains
Instability, knee joint, 43-44
Integument of women during climacteric, 133
Intervertebral disc, 4, 5
Interview of adolescent, 106-107
Intolerance, lactose, in infant, 184
Intrauterine device and salpingitis, 216-217
Iron deficiency anemia, 88
Iron requirements for red cell production, 88
Irritability in first year after divorce, 122
Irritable colon syndrome, 199-200
Irritation, nerve root, causing low back pain, 14-15
Isolation of client with hepatitis type A, 246
Isometric exercises for client with low back pain, 20
Isometric strengthening exercises, 58-59
Isoniazid producing hepatitis-like reaction, 241
IUD and salpingitis, 216-217

J

Jaundice
    breast-milk, 176
    with hepatitis type A, 244
    in pigmented skin, assessment of, 151
Joint, tibiofemoral, left, gliding motion of, 27

K

Keloids in black clients, 155, 158
Klebsiella aerogenes and cystitis, 258, 261
Knee
    anatomy of, review of, 27-30
    anterior compartment of, problems in, assessment and plans for, 30-39
    injuries to, prevention and rehabilitation of, 47-65
    ligamentous injuries to, 42-46
    "loose," 45
    medial and lateral compartments of, problems in, assessment and plan for, 39-47
    meniscial injuries of, 46-47
    pain and injuries of, in adult runner, 26-66
    physical examination of, in adult runner, 32
    "runner's," 30
    sprains of
        first-degree, 41, 44
        second-degree, 41, 44-45
        third-degree, 41, 45
    subluxation of, 37
    tendinitis of, 39, 42
    "water on," 45
Knee joint instability, 43-44
Knock knees, 37
Kyphotic curve of thoracic spine, 4

L

Lact-Aid Nursing Trainer, 178
Lactose in infant diet, 166
Lactose intolerance in infant, 184
Lateral compartment of knee, problems in, assessment and plan for, 39-47
Leg length discrepancy, 34-35
Legal aspects of nursing care of adolescents, 102
Length of infant and nutritional status during first year of life, 174
Lesions
    of medial meniscus, 35
    petechial, 150
    skin
        common to blacks, assessment of, 151-158
        description of, 149-150
Life-style and salpingitis, 218
Lift, heel, medial, 34
Ligamentous injuries of knee, 42-46; see also Sprains
Ligaments
    of back, 4

Ligaments—cont'd
  cruciate, 27
Local disease causing low back pain, 15-16
Loneliness during first year after divorce, 122-123
"Loose knees," 45
Lordosis, lumbar, 4, 7
Lordotic curve of cervical spine, 4
Lordotic lumbar curve, 4
Low back pain
  in adult male, 3-23
    approach to causes of, 10-13
    assessment of, 9-17
    drugs for, 19
    essential physical examination for clients with, 9
    history for client with, 8
    local disease causing, 15-16
    nerve root irritation causing, 14-15
    origin of, 7-8
    problems of structural unit causing, 12-14
    systemic disease causing, 16
    tuberculosis causing, 15-16
    x-ray films for, 9, 12
  in menopausal women, 133
Lumbar lordosis, 4, 7
Lumbar spine, 4
  structures of, 7
Luteinizing hormone
  after menopause, 126
  pubertal changes caused by, 103-104

M

Macrocytes, 91
Macrocytic, normochromic anemia, 95-96
Macules, 149
Malassezia furfur, 152
Male
  adult, low back pain in, 3-23
  endocrine process in, during puberty, 104
Malnourished infant, 167
Married women, effect of menopause on, 129
Masturbation
  counseling adolescents about, 110-111
  in women during climacteric, 138
Mature minor, 102
McMurray's test
  for chondromalacia patellae, 38-39
  for meniscial injuries, 47
Mean corpuscular hemoglobin, 89
Mean corpuscular hemoglobin concentration, 89
  formula for computing, 91
Mean compuscular volume, 89
  formula for computing, 91
Media material for counseling of adolescents, 109-110
Medial compartment of knee, problems in, assessment and plan for, 39-47
Medial heel lift, 34
Medial meniscus, lesions of, 35
Medications
  for acute salpingitis, 226-227
  for client with hepatitis, 245
  for cystitis, 260-262
  for diverticular disease, 203
  history of, in black client with skin problems, 148
  for muscle strain, 18-19
  to reduce muscle spasm, 19
  usage of, and cystitis, 256
Melanosis, dermal, in black clients, 153
Membrane, synovial, 27, 30
Meningitis, viral or bacterial, differential diagnosis of, 74-75
Meniscial injuries of knee, 46-47
Meniscus, 27
  medial, lesions of, 35
Menopausal women
  effects of recent role changes on, 128-129
  societal expectations of, 126-128
Menopause, 125
  artificial, 125
  bleeding after, 137
  symptoms ascribed to, that may signal organic disease, 130
Menses, changes in, during climacteric, 131
Menstrual-related migraine, 72
Menstruation and salpingitis, 216
Metamucil; *see* Psyllium
Methenamine for cystitis, 262
Methylcellulose for diverticular disease, 203
Methyldopa producing hepatitis-like reaction, 241
Microcytes, 91
Microcytic, hypochromic anemia, 93-95
Migraine, 68-83
  classic, differential diagnosis of, 73-74
  common, differential diagnosis of, 73
  course of events during, 71
  etiology of, 68-71
  menstrual-related, 72
  physiological factors in, 68-71
  trigger factors in, 69, 70
"Migraine personality," 76
Milk, cow's, allergy to, in infant, 183-184
Mineral requirement during first year of life, 169-170
Minors, emancipation of, 102; *see also* Adolescence; Adolescents
Mittelschmerz, differential diagnosis of, 224
Mongolian spots in black clients, 153
Morton's foot, 31, 33
Morton's foot extension, 34
Motion, gliding, of left tibiofemoral joint, 27

Muscle(s)
  abductor
    strengthening exercises of, 64-65
    stretching exercises of, 55-57
  adductor, strengthening exercises of, 64-65
  of back, 4
  hamstring, 30
  quadriceps, 30
  spasm of, drugs to reduce, 19
Muscle strain
  acute, 17-22
  causing low back pain, 12-13
Musculoskeletal symptoms during climacteric, 133
Mycoplasma and salpingitis, 214

N

Neisseria gonorrhoeae and salpingitis, 213, 214, 217 221, 229, 230, 232
Nerve root irritation causing low back pain, 14-15
Neuralgia, trigeminal, differential diagnosis of, 75
Nitrofurantoin for cystitis, 261, 262, 267
Nodules, 150
Non-A, non-B hepatitis, 236, 237
Nongonococcal salpingitis, 214-215; see also Salpingitis, acute
Nonpigmented and pigmented skin, differences between, 150-151
Novocaine; see Procaine
Nucleus pulposus, 4, 5, 6
Nursing care of adolescents, legal aspects of, 102
Nutrition during first year of life
  assessment and guidance of, 163-188
  evaluation of, 188
  history and trends in, 163-164
  laboratory data on, 174
Nutritional alterations, problems with, 161-208
Nutritional assessment of infant, 171-174
Nutritional history of infant during first year of life, 171-173
Nutritional requirements during first year of life, 164-171

O

Obesity, infant, 167, 171
Occupational factors in black clients with skin problems, 148-149
Office screening for bacteriuria, 259
Oral contraceptives for women during climacteric, 138-139
Organic disease, symptoms ascribed to menopause that may signal, 130
Orgasm, information about, for adolescents, 111
Osteomyelitis causing low back pain, 15
Osteoporosis during climacteric, estrogen replacement therapy for, 140

Ovarian cyst, differential diagnosis of, 224
Ovarian torsion, differential diagnosis of, 224-225
Overnutrition during first year of life, 167, 171

P

Pain
  abdominal, findings and pathological conditions causing, 219-220
  back, low; see Low back pain
  of cystitis, relief of, 262
  head; see Head pain
  knee, in adult runner, 26-66
  pelvic
    differential diagnosis of, 223
    laboratory data in and pathologic conditions causing, 221
  peripatellar, 30-35
  of salpingitis, relief of, 227
Pain-sensitive structures of cranium, 68, 69
Pallor in pigmented skin, assessment of, 150
Pamisyl; see Aminosalicylic acid
Papules, 149-150
Papulosquamous eruptions, 150
Paradigm for referral of adults with anemia, 96-97
Parasal; see Aminosalicylic acid
Parents
  of adolescents, guidelines for, 112; see also Family of adolescent
  single, 122-124; see also Divorce
Patella, 30
  dislocated, recurrent, 36-39
Patella alta, 37, 39
Patellar tendinitis, 35-36
Patellofemoral dislocation, 36
Pelvic inflammatory disease; see Salpingitis, acute
Pelvic pain
  differential diagnosis of, 223
  laboratory data in and pathological conditions causing, 221
Penicillin
  for cystitis, 261, 262, 265
  for salpingitis, 227
Peripatellar pain, 30-35
Pernicious anemia, 89
Personal hygiene during climacteric, 137-138
Personality, "migraine," 76
Pes planus, 33-34
Phenacetin producing hepatitis-like reactions, 241
Phenophen for salpingitis, 227
Phenytoin producing hepatitis-like reaction, 241
Physical examination
  of adolescent, 107
  of client
    with acute salpingitis, 218-220
    with cystitis, 257-258

Physical examination—cont'd
  of client—cont'd
    with diverticulosis, 200-201
    with head pain, 76, 77
    with hepatitis type A, 241
    with low back pain, 9
    with skin problems common to blacks, 149
  of infants for nutritional status, 173-174
  of knee in adult runner, 32
  of woman during climacteric, 133-134
Pigmentary disorders in black clients, 152-155
Pigmentation, skin, social significance of, 148
Pigmented and nonpigmented skin, differences between, 150-151
Petechial lesion, 150
Pituitary gland and pubertal changes, 103, 104
Posterior capsule of knee, 30
Postmenopausal bleeding, 137
Posttraumatic headache, differential diagnosis of, 73
Pregnancy, ectopic, differential diagnosis of, 225
Pressure, disc
  during exercises, 20
  increased, protection of back from, 18
Pro-Banthine; see Propantheline bromide
Probenecid for salpingitis, 227
Procaine penicillin G for salpingitis, 227
Progesterone secretion after menopause, 126
Pronation of foot, excessive, 31-35
Propantheline bromide for diverticular disease, 203
Proprietary formulas, 179
  composition, indications, and problems for, 180-182
Prostate gland, cancer of, causing low back pain, 17
Protein requirements during first year of life, 165-166
Proteus sp. and cystitis, 258, 261, 265
Pseudofolliculitis barbae in black clients, 156, 157
Pseudomonas aeruginosa and cystitis, 258
Psoralen for vitiligo, 153
Psychosocial problems and infant nutrition, 171
Psychosocial support for client with salpingitis, 228
Psyllium for diverticular disease, 203
Puberty, 102
  anatomical, physiological, and behavioral changes during, 102-104
  endocrine process during
    in female, 103-104
    in male, 104
  sexuality during, 101-113
Purpura, 150
Pustular eruptions, 150

Q

Quadriceps muscle, 30
  strengthening exercise of, 58-59
    extensor action, 60-61

Quadriceps muscle—cont'd
  strengthening exercise of—cont'd
    flexor action, 62
  stretching exercise of, 48
Questionnaire for adolescents, 106

R

Race and salpingitis, 217
Recurrent cystitis in adult female, 252-270
Recurrent dislocated patella, 36-39
Recurrent urinary tract infections, 264; *see also* Cystitis in adult female, recurrent
Red blood cell production, physiology of, 87-89
Referral of adults with anemia, paradigm for, 96-97
Relaxation training instructions, 80-81
Rest
  for client with hepatitis, 245
  for muscle strain, 18
Reticulocyte counts to measure bone marrow activity, 91
Reticulocytes, 87
Retirement, planning for, by women during climacteric, 139
Reverse leg-raising test to test nerve root irritation, 15
Role changes, effects of, on menopausal women, 128-129
Rotary drawer sign to evaluate knee joint instability, 43-44
Runner, adult
  knee pain and injuries in, 26-66
  physical examination of knee of, 32
"Runner's knee," 30
Running, 26
Running shoes for feet without anatomical variations or previous injuries, guidelines for, 31
Ruptured ovarian cyst, differential diagnosis of, 224

S

Sacrum, 4
Safety measures for women during climacteric, 139
Salpingitis, acute, 213-232
  activity for client with, 227
  assessment of client with, 215-226
  differential diagnosis of, 222-226
  epidemiology of, 213-215
  etiology of, 213-214
  evaluation of client with, 228-230
  gonococcal, 214-215
  health education for client with, 228
  history of client with, 217-218
  infertility after, 230
  laboratory data of client with, 221-222
  medication for, 226-227
  nongonococcal, 214-215

Salpingitis, acute—cont'd
   pain relief for client with, 227
   pathogenesis of, 214-215
   physical examination of client with, 218-220
   plan for client with, 226-228
   psychosocial support for client with, 228
   recurrent, 230
   referral of client with, guidelines for, 229-230
   risk factors for, 216-217
   sexual activity for client with, 228
   signs and symptoms of, 222, 224
Same-sex behavior by adolescents, 112
Scars in black clients, 158
Schober's test, 16
School-aged child, response to divorce by, 117-118
Seasonal factors in black clients with skin problems, 148-149
Secretions, vaginal, during climacteric, 132
Selenium sulfide suspension for tinea versicolor, 152
Selsun; *see* Selenium sulfide suspension
Semisolids, introduction of, to infant, 185-188
Septic abortion, infected, differential diagnosis of, 225
Sexual activity
   for client with salpingitis, 228
   and cystitis, 263
Sexual counseling of women during climacteric, 138
Sexual history
   of client with cystitis, 257
   of client with salpingitis, 218
Sexual partners, number of, and salpingitis, 217
Sexual patterns of client with hepatitis type A, 246
Sexuality
   counseling of adolescents about, 108-110
   during puberty, 101-113
Shoes, running, for feet without anatomical variations or previous injuries, guidelines for, 31
Sickle cell ulcer, 158
Sickle cells, 91
Single parents, 122-124; *see also* Divorce
Single women, effect of menopause on, 129
Sinus headache, differential diagnosis of, 73
Skin
   anatomy and physiology of, 147
   disorders of, emotional aspects of, 147-148
   pigmentation of, social significance of, 148
   pigmented and nonpigmented, differences between, 150-151
   problems of, common to blacks, 147-158
      assessment of client with, 147-151
      history of client with, 148-149
      laboratory data of client with, 151
      physical examination of client with, 149
      planning and evaluation of selected lesions of, 151-158

Skin lesions
   common to blacks, assessment of, 151-158
   description of, 149-150
Smears, vaginal, of menopausal women, 135
Smoking by women during climacteric, 139
Social Readjustment Rating Scale, 19-20, 21
Societal expectations of menopausal women, 126-128
Somatic symptoms during climacteric, 133
Soy formula, 181, 183-184
Spasm, muscle, drugs to reduce, 19
Specimen collection, urine, 258-259
Spherocytes, 91
Spine
   lumbar, 4
      structures of, 7
   physiological curves of, 4
Spondylitis, ankylosing, causing low back pain, 16
Spondylolisthesis causing low back pain, 13
Sprains
   classification of, 39, 41
   of knee
      first-degree, 41, 44
      second-degree, 41, 44-45
      third-degree, 41, 45
Staphylococcus fecalis and cystitis, 261
Sterilization of bottles for infant feeding, 179
Straight leg–raising tests to test nerve root irritation, 15
Strains
   classification of, 39, 40
   muscle
      acute, management of, 17-22
      causing low back pain, 12-13
Strengthening exercises, 58-65
   isometric, 58-59
   weight-resistive, 60-65
Stretching exercises, 47-57
Stress management to relieve muscle strain, 19-20
Stress tests, abduction/adduction, to evaluate knee joint instabilities, 43
Subarachnoid hemorrhage, differential diagnosis of, 75
Subcommittee on Classification of Sports Injuries of American Medical Association, 39
Subdural hematoma, differential diagnosis of, 74
Subluxation of knee, 37
Sulfisoxazole for cystitis, 261
Sulfonamides
   for cystitis, 261-262, 267
   producing hepatitis-like reaction, 241
Surgical intervention for recurrent cystitis in adult female, 268
Swelling of fat pad, 35

Syndrome
  Fitz-Hugh–Curtis
    with acute salpingitis, 214-215
    with hepatitis type A, 243, 245
  irritable colon, 199-200
Synovial membrane, 27, 30
Synovitis, idiopathic, 45, 46
Systemic disease causing low back pain, 16

T

Target cells, 91
Tears of meniscus, 46-47
Teens; see Adolescents
Tegretol; see Carbamazepine
Temporal arteritis, differential diagnosis of, 74
Tempra; see Acetaminophen
Tendinitis
  of knee, 39, 42
  patellar, 35-36
Tendon, Achilles, stretching exercises for, 53-54
Tension headache, differential diagnosis of, 73
Test(s)
  Apley's, for meniscial injuries, 47
  apprehension, for patellar instability, 37
  McMurray's
    for chondromalacia patellae, 38-39
    for meniscial injuries, 47
  of nerve root irritation, 15
  Schober's, 16
  stress, abduction/adduction, to evaluate knee joint instabilities, 43
Testosterone, pubertal changes caused by, 104
Tetracycline
  for cystitis, 261, 262, 267
  for salpingitis, 227
Threatened abortion, differential diagnosis of, 225
Tibiofemoral joint, left, gliding motion of, 27
Tinea versicolor in black client, 152, 154
Torsion, ovarian, differential diagnosis of, 224-225
Traction alopecia in black clients, 157
Training, relaxation, instructions in, 80-81
Transactional analysis for counseling of adolescents, 109
Triceps fat-fold thickness of infants, 174
Trigeminal neuralgia, differential diagnosis of, 75
Trigger factors in migraine, 69, 70
Trimethoprim-sulfamethoxazole for cystitis, 261, 267
Tuberculosis causing low back pain, 15-16
Tumor, brain, differential diagnosis of, 74-75
Tylenol; see Acetaminophen

U

Ulcer
  Hunner's, 257, 260
  sickle cell, 158

Ulcerations, 150
Undernutrition during first year of life, 167
Urinary elimination behaviors and urinary tract infections, 256-257
Urinary symptoms during climacteric, 132
Urinary tract infections, 252-270; see also Cystitis in adult female, recurrent
  ascending route of infection in, 253
  assessment of client with, 256-260
  differential diagnosis of, 225
  epidemiology of, 252-253
  in females, summary of, 254
  history of client with, 256-257
  recurrent, 264
Urine
  acidification of, 263
  specimen of, collection of, 258-259
Urticarial eruptions, 150

V

Vaginal changes during climacteric, 134
Vaginal secretions during climacteric, 132
Vaginal smears of menopausal women, 135
Valium; see Diazepam
Values clarification in counseling of adolescents, 109
Vasomotor symptoms during climacteric, 132
  estrogen replacement therapy for, 140
Vastus medialis muscle-tendon unit, stress on, 35
VD national hot line, 228
Vegetable fiber, 202
Venereal disease, counseling adolescents about, 112
Vertebrae, 4
Vertebral column, lateral view of, 5
Vesicular eruptions, 150
Viral meningitis, differential diagnosis of, 74-75
Virus
  hepatitis A; see Hepatitis type A
  hepatitis B, 236-237
Visceral disease causing low back pain, 17
Vitamin B_{12}, deficiency anemia, 89
Vitamin requirements during first year of life, 168-169
Vitamin supplementation
  for breast-fed infant, 184-185
  for formula-fed infant, 185
Vitiligo in black clients, 153

W

"Water on the knee," 45
Water requirements during first year of life, 164-165
Weight
  of infants and nutritional status during first year of life, 174
  of women during climacteric, 133
Weight-resistive strengthening exercise, 58-59

Wingspread Conference on Early Adolescent Sexuality and Health Care, 101
Women
  during climacteric
    assessment of, 130-135
    caring for, 125-144
    counseling of, 136-139
    estrogen replacement therapy for, 139-143
    evaluation of, 143-144
    laboratory data of, 134-135
    physical examination of, 133-134

Women—cont'd
  married, effect of menopause on, 129
  menopausal; *see* Menopausal women
  single, effect of menopause on, 129
  working, effect of menopause on, 128-129
Working women, effect of menopause on, 128-129

X

X-ray films for low back pain, 9, 12